Reproduction on the Reservation

CRITICAL INDIGENEITIES

J. Kēhaulani Kauanui and Jean M. O'Brien, series editors

Series Advisory Board

Chris Anderson, University of Alberta
Irene Watson, University of South Australia
Emilio del Valle Escalante, University of North Carolina at Chapel Hill
Kim TallBear, University of Alberta

Critical Indigeneities publishes pathbreaking scholarly books that center Indigeneity as a category of critical analysis, understand Indigenous sovereignty as ongoing and historically grounded, and attend to diverse forms of Indigenous cultural and political agency and expression. The series builds on the conceptual rigor, methodological innovation, and deep relevance that characterize the best work in the growing field of critical Indigenous studies.

Reproduction on the Reservation

Pregnancy, Childbirth, and Colonialism in the Long Twentieth Century

Brianna Theobald

The University of North Carolina Press CHAPEL HILL

The University of North Carolina Press has been a member of the
Green Press Initiative since 2003.

Library of Congress Cataloging-in-Publication Data
Names: Theobald, Brianna, author.
Title: Reproduction on the reservation : pregnancy, childbirth, and colonialism
    in the long twentieth century / Brianna Theobald.
Other titles: Critical indigeneities.
Description: Chapel Hill : University of North Carolina Press, [2019] | Series:
    Critical indigeneities | Includes bibliographical references and index.
Identifiers: LCCN 2019004398 | ISBN 9781469653150 (cloth : alk. paper) |
    ISBN 9781469653167 (pbk : alk. paper) | ISBN 9781469653174 (ebook)
Subjects: LCSH: Indian women—North America. | Maternal health services—
    North America. | Reproductive rights—North America. | Indians of
    North America—Health and hygiene.
Classification: LCC RG962.5.I6 T44 2019 | DDC 362.198200973—dc23 LC record
    available at https://lccn.loc.gov/2019004398

Cover illustration: *Of a Path Known to the Old Ones*, mixed media. 2017. By Ben
Pease—Apsàalooke (Crow)/Tsitsistas (Northern Cheyenne) Creative.

A previous version of chapter 3 was published as "Nurse, Mother,
Midwife: Susie Walking Bear Yellowtail and the Struggle for Crow Women's
Reproductive Autonomy," *Montana: The Magazine of Western History* 66, no. 3
(2016): 17–35.

This book is dedicated to those in the struggle for reproductive justice — past, present, and future.

Contents

Illustrations and Map

Acknowledgments

They say it takes a village to raise a child, and given the subject of this book, the metaphor seems particularly apt. I am so grateful for the village that has supported this project. My first thanks go to Valerie Jackson. I met Valerie in Arizona, and she quickly became this book's biggest supporter. She has generously shared her memories and materials, including much of her own powerful writing. She has also become a dear friend. Aho. Other Yellowtail women have made equally valuable contributions. My heartfelt thanks to Connie Jackson, Jackie Yellowtail, Lesley Kabotie, and Anita Morin. These women opened their homes to me, ensured that I was well fed, invited me to countless functions and family events, and patiently answered my fumbling questions. I am especially grateful to Connie for allowing me access to the rich documents she has accumulated regarding her own and her mother's history. Aho. Indeed, the entire Yellowtail family cheerfully tolerated my presence over the past few years and warmly welcomed me upon each return.

Several others helped make my trips to the Crow Reservation both enjoyable and productive. Thank you to Mardell Hogan, historian and former archivist at the tribal college, for a lovely dinner in Billings on an early trip to Montana. Mary Elizabeth Wallace and Janine Pease graciously agreed to share their knowledge and experiences in interviews. Their contributions, as well as those of a handful of Crow women who opted to have their interviews remain anonymous, have made this a much richer book. Janine has supported this project in other ways as well, and I am especially grateful to her for welcoming my participation in the Crow Language Summer Institute in June 2016. When it comes to Tim McCleary, words are inadequate. His gracious feedback and his generosity in sharing sources and insights have immeasurably strengthened this book, and his friendship has enriched the experience of writing it. Aho. My sincere thanks to Ben Pease for allowing his striking painting *Of a Path Known to the Old Ones* to grace this book's cover. I am a huge fan of Ben's work, and this is a real honor. At Little Bighorn College Library and Archives, thanks are due to Tim Bernardis and Jon Ille.

I owe thanks to individuals throughout Montana and Indian Country. Marina Brown Weatherly was exceedingly generous with me as I began this project, opening her beautiful home and sharing materials as well as her knowledge of her friend Susie Yellowtail's life. Marina's ongoing work in telling Susie's story has been a consistent source of inspiration. I met Father Peter Powell, who currently resides in Chicago, at a birthday party on the Crow Reservation, and I am grateful for his kindness and his willingness to share his memories regarding many of the people and events covered in this book. The talented Cinnamon Spear introduced me to women on the Northern Cheyenne Reservation, and I am especially grateful to her mother, Gladys Limberhand, who spent an afternoon sharing stories with me. Thanks as well to the Northern Cheyenne women who must remain anonymous but made valuable contributions to my understanding of the history of reproductive health care on and off the reservation. Although it would be impossible for me to thank each Native woman who contributed to this project, I would be remiss not to mention the illuminating and energizing conversations I had with Nicolle Gonzales, Ursula Knoki-Wilson, and June Strickland.

This research took me to archives across the country. Thanks to the following institutions that provided the funding to make this research possible: the American Historical Association, Arizona State University, Charles Redd Center, Coalition for Western Women's History, Smith College, University of Illinois at Urbana-Champaign, Western Association of Women's Historians, and the Western History Association. Thank you to the many archivists who facilitated my research, especially Eric Bitner at the National Archives and Records Association (NARA) in Colorado, Mary Frances Ronan at NARA in Washington, D.C., Joyce Martin at Labriola American Indian Center, Amy Hague at Smith College, Anna Trammell at University of Illinois at Urbana-Champaign University Archives, Joan Miller at Big Horn County Historical Society, John Ille at the Little Bighorn College Archives, and Natalie Navar at the Center for Oral and Public History at California State University, Fullerton. Thanks as well to the staff at the Montana Historical Society, Mansfield Library at the University of Montana–Missoula, the Minnesota Historical Society, the Buffalo Bill Center of the West, and the Newberry Library.

I have many people to thank at Arizona State University (ASU), where I had the good fortune to have Susan Gray as my adviser. If only all graduate students could have such a devoted and rigorous mentor. Thank you, Susan. I will strive to pay it forward. I have benefited from Ann Hibner Koblitz's immense knowledge of the history of medicine, and I am equally grateful for her commitment to feminist historical scholarship. Katherine Osburn arrived at ASU shortly after I did, and she immediately became a valued mentor.

Thank you, KO, for your ongoing support. Thanks also to Tsianina Lomawaima and Karen Leong. These women are phenomenal people and fantastic scholars, and I count myself fortunate that each took an interest in my work. Myla Vicenti Carpio offered early guidance, and her own work on sterilization abuse and reproductive justice provided a critical foundation for my research. Donald Fixico, Catherine O'Donnell, Christopher Jones, and Matt Delmont each offered welcome advice and guidance along the way.

My Americanist cohort was simply the best: thanks to Cali Pitchel Schmidt, Paul Kuenker, Monika Bilka, and Lauren Berka. Thanks to Ben Beresford, Melissa Beresford, James Dupey, Tanya Dupey, Dave Dupey, Keri Dupey, Cody Ferguson, and John Goodwin for (probably too many) happy hours. Shout-out to Aletheia, who brought so much joy to all our gatherings. I owe Aaron Bae a tremendous debt for his generosity in sharing sources. I owe Pete Van Cleave a year's worth of pumpkin porters for reading several "shitty first drafts" and for never tiring of my seemingly endless requests for advice. I hope he knows the requests won't end anytime soon.

This book took shape at the University of Illinois at Urbana-Champaign (UIUC), where a Chancellor's Postdoctoral Fellowship in American Indian Studies allowed me the gift of time and space in which to work. I am grateful to those who helped make my two years in central Illinois so productive and rewarding. Thanks to Robert Warrior for creating an environment that allowed postdoctoral fellows to focus almost exclusively on their research. Thanks to Adrian Burgos, who took over as interim director after Robert's departure. Matt Gilbert was—and remains!—an exceptional mentor and has become a good friend. Thanks, Matt. I lucked out in sharing the third floor with Jenny Davis, who was generous with time and resources and is a role model in so many ways. I was also fortunate to have arrived at UIUC a year before Fred Hoxie's retirement. Fred's research on Crow history has been indispensable, and I am grateful for his support of this project. Thanks to my fellow fellows Silvia Soto and Kora Maldonado. They, along with Raquel Escobar, helped keep me sane. John McKinn and Dulce Talavera skillfully handled all manner of logistics; for that and for so many other things, I am grateful.

I completed this book at the University of Rochester (UR). Thanks to Dean Gloria Culver for granting me a course release in the fall of 2017 and for providing subvention support that aided in this book's publication. Matt Lenoe, chair of the History Department, went above and beyond in facilitating my transition to UR, and I am so grateful for his support. Stewart Weaver was similarly fantastic in his capacity as interim chair. Thanks to him as well as to Laura Smoller, who took over as chair in this book's final stages. Laura has been a gracious mentor from the moment I entered the department, and I cannot thank her enough for her camaraderie. I feel fortunate to have joined UR's History Department, and although I cannot thank each of my colleagues by name, I do want to single out Molly Ball, Thomas Fleischman, and Pablo Sierra, who are fabulous colleagues and have become fast friends. Thanks as well to Joan Rubin for her support and her work as director of the Humanities Center. My sincere thanks to Jacqui Rizzo and Kristi Packusch, as well as to the department's talented team of student workers, for all they do to keep the department running smoothly and to make my life easier. At a critical moment in the revision process, I taught a seminar on the history of reproduction, and I benefited tremendously from the intellectual contributions of these students. Thanks to Lily Deng, Jessica Hunsicker, Lisa Kim, Hedy Ludwig, Piffanie Rosario, and Katie Turi. Through her painstaking research exploring Native women's collective responses to sterilization abuses in the 1970s and 1980s, Lisa introduced me to a couple of primary sources that I—after studying the issue for several years—had not previously encountered. My sincere thanks, Lisa. Outside the History Department, Kate Mariner organized a weeklong writing refuge for junior faculty at just the right moment for me. Thanks, Kate!

Thanks to the many people whose input has directly improved this book. Cathleen Cahill and Jacki Rand read an early and much different version of the manuscript, and their astute feedback informed the new directions it took over the last several years. Lesley Kabotie, Margaret Jacobs, Jane Simonsen, and an anonymous reader provided constructive feedback on a version of chapter 3, which was previously published as "Nurse, Mother, Midwife: Susie Walking Bear Yellowtail and the Struggle for Crow Women's Reproductive Autonomy" in *Montana: The Magazine of Western History* 66, no. 3 (2016): 17–35. Thank you to *Montana* magazine for granting me permission to reprint portions of this article. My sincere thanks to Susan Gray, Fred Hoxie, Ann Koblitz, Colleen O'Neill, and Katherine Osburn for making time to read chapter drafts, as well as to the scholars who participated in not one but two workshops during my tenure at UIUC. At UR, Tom Devaney and the students in his graduate methods seminar offered insightful feedback on the introduction and two chapters. Tim McCleary's feedback on drafts, already noted above, has been invaluable.

I knew within moments of talking to Mark Simpson-Vos that I wanted to publish with the University of North Carolina Press, and I am grateful to the entire team at the press for making my experience as a first-time author as painless as possible. Thanks especially to Mark for his faith in this project and his clear and patient guidance at each step in the process. Lucas Church assisted in the very early stages, and Jessica Newman has been an absolute joy to work with since I first met her at the Berks in 2017. My sincere thanks to series editors Jean O'Brien and J. Kēhaulani Kauanui, scholars whom I have long admired. Thank you to the two scholars who reviewed the manuscript for the press. The anonymous reader offered encouragement as well as several critical insights, and Rose Stremlau provided generous and constructive feedback on three separate occasions. For so many reasons, I count myself extremely lucky to have come to know Rose throughout this process. Finally, I appreciate Liz Schueler's work in copyediting the manuscript.

The contributions of other colleagues and friends have sometimes been less direct but no less necessary. Thanks first and foremost to the Western History Association crew. Elaine Nelson and Kent Blansett have supported my work in so many ways that I will never be able to repay. I am always grateful for my feminist cohort: Lindsey Passenger Wieck, Alessandra Link, and Rebecca Wingo. Thanks as well to Michael Childers and Leisl Carr Childers. Outside academia, Jill Pitsch and Cari Rothluebber have been the very best friends I could have asked for since well before this book was even an idea. I love you both. Crystine Miller and Canon Luerkens hosted me on a research trip to Helena, Rob Hartwell and Heather Guith put me up on multiple visits to Washington, D.C., and Dave and Judy Kuenker were always willing to put me up when I was in the Denver area. Thank you all.

I've been unusually fortunate when it comes to family. My parents always encouraged me to "just do your best," and I know that they will love me just the same if this book is a total flop. Thanks to my mother, Jan Simmons, for patiently responding to my many grammatical queries. Thanks to my father, Paul Theobald, for instilling my love of history. I am so lucky to have Renee and Alayna as sisters. I am the oldest, but more often than not, I am the one looking up to them. They also make life more fun. I am grateful that Maureen, Nathan, and Carly are family; thank you all for consistently modeling righteous politics. Thanks to each of my siblings for choosing great partners: Lora, Eric, Derek, and Derek (yes, you read that right) complete the family. Shout-out to Jordan and Meelah. Emmett Carroll remains the world's best nephew. Your aunties love you like crazy.

Partnering with Rio Hartwell brought so many good people into my life. Lexie Thompson graciously welcomed me into the family before we had even met. I can always count on Tom Hartwell and Melissa Caraway to provide good food, good wine and cocktails, and good conversation. Words fail me when it comes to thanking Rachel, Dexter, Anne, Marsalis, Kai, and whoever happens to be living at the Adriano-Stowell residence when this book is published. You all are a constant inspiration, and you have enriched and expanded my conception of "family." Shout-out to Karan, who, thankfully, finds my neuroses endearing.

Remarkably, Rio did not once complain about reading draft after draft of each chapter. This book would be a shadow of itself were it not for his brilliance and keen editorial eye. He may very well be the best human being on the planet, and I could not have chosen a better partner in life's adventures. Thank you for loving, supporting, putting up with, and inspiring me.

Onward.

Reproduction on the Reservation

Introduction

In our birth stories we carry the stories of our people.

—METÍS ELDER MARIA CAMPBELL (2012)

Women from more than thirty Native American Nations gathered in Rapid City, South Dakota, in 1978 for the first conference of the Women of All Red Nations (WARN). No novices to political struggle, many of these women had been active in the American Indian Movement (AIM) over the previous decade, and a few had attended the United Nations Convention on Indigenous Rights in Geneva, Switzerland, in 1977 or the International Women's Year Conference in Mexico City in 1975.[1] Katsi Cook, a young Mohawk mother who was visiting relatives in South Dakota at the time, had dropped out of Dartmouth College a few years earlier to devote herself full time to activism.[2] The "grandmothers, mothers, aunties, nieces, [and] sisters" who came together in Rapid City believed that a separate organization was necessary to tackle issues of particular importance to women and children. In defending Native families, cultures, and communities, these women endeavored to fulfill "their duty as native women."[3] Over the next several months, WARN women organized locally in their communities and established national and international networks with Native and other women. The following summer, more than 1,200 Native people, mostly women, met in Seattle, Washington, for a second meeting.[4] The label "reproductive justice" would not be coined for another decade and a half, but in these annual meetings and in their grassroots organizing, WARN women articulated an early vision of Native reproductive justice.[5]

Above all, WARN protested the sterilization abuses that had gained widespread publicity in activist circles by the end of the decade. Scholars estimate that beginning in 1970, physicians sterilized between 25 and 42 percent of Native women of childbearing age over a six-year period.[6] Some of these procedures occurred in government-operated hospitals, while others occurred in facilities contracted by the federal government to provide health services to American Indians. WARN leaders alleged that in many cases physicians performed these procedures coercively and with genocidal intentions. They further argued that such abuses could not be separated from other reproductive challenges facing Native women, including the lack of

1

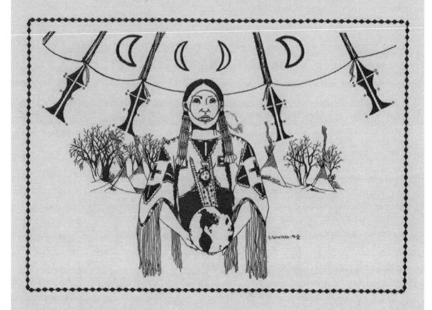

WOMEN OF ALL RED NATIONS

W.A.R.N. REPORT II

This drawing of a Plains Indian woman holding the world in her hands and an infant in a cradleboard graced the cover of the Women of All Red Nations' annual report in 1979, as well as some of the organization's promotional materials. Library Hill Foundation Records, 20th Century Organizational Files, Southern California Library (Los Angeles, California).

access to culturally appropriate sexual and reproductive health education; the environmental degradation of reservation land, which threatened maternal and infant welfare; and the removal of Native children to white foster and adoptive homes.[7] WARN and other Native women transformed the ongoing struggle for Native sovereignty and self-determination by insisting that women's reproductive health and autonomy be recognized as fundamental to these efforts.[8]

WARN's early activism thus offers a poignant starting point for this book, to date the first book-length history of reproduction that places Native American women at the center of the analysis.[9] This book owes much to the historical questions, and often answers, that I discovered upon my introduction to WARN women's writing nearly a decade ago. After this introduction, however, WARN does not reappear in these pages until the book's final chapter. The story recounted here begins a century before the organization's founding and explores the intersecting histories of colonialism and biological reproduction in which these women and their contemporaries were embedded. My contention is that we can better understand WARN's mission, significance, and legacy by stepping outside the militant moment of the group's birth and exploring the deeper roots of these 1970s developments.

These intersecting histories require definition and elaboration. WARN and other activists in the Red Power movement readily employed the label "colonialism" to describe the federal government's historical and ongoing relationship with Native peoples. Today, scholars are more likely to specify "settler colonialism." In settler-colonial societies like the United States, Canada, and Australia, among others, the principal objective of governments and settler-citizens is the acquisition of land for permanent occupation and dominion. This contrasts with so-called classic or extractive colonial contexts in which colonial objectives center on the exploitation of labor and the extraction of resources. The imperatives of what the anthropologist Patrick Wolfe refers to as "territoriality" — "settler colonialism's specific, irreducible element" — underpin much of the story that follows.[10] As WARN was acutely aware, Native women's bodies had long been on the front lines of white Americans' often-brutal quest for Native land. Furthermore, the presence of settlers and settler institutions unquestionably shaped Native women's reproductive experiences in the twentieth century. Yet, as several scholars have demonstrated, settler colonialism and extractive colonialism are not dichotomous models. Nor did the various Euro-American actors in the pages that follow always act in ways that settler colonial theory might predict. In this book's title, I have chosen the more general "colonialism" to underscore the flexibility of colonial power. In doing so, I take my cue from WARN's own political analysis and from group members' pursuit of anticolonial coalitions with Indigenous peoples throughout the globe.

Biological reproduction is defined here as the labor of conceiving, carrying, and delivering a child, as well as early infant care. These forms of reproductive labor are often closely linked to the productive labor women have historically performed in Native communities, and women's prominence in the realm of biological reproduction is matched by their valued role in the reproduction of social relationships and cultural lifeways. In foregrounding biological reproduction, my intention is not to privilege biology above the many other and often more significant means by which Native peoples understand family and kinship. Rather, it is to take seriously Maria Campbell's observation in this introduction's epigraph that attitudes, practices, and rituals surrounding birthing—and by extension, menstruation, pregnancy, and other reproductive experiences—contain and reflect important histories. Here, too, WARN provided a framework that persists in twenty-first-century reproductive justice organizing and that has informed my approach to this book: reproductive matters cannot be separated from broader political struggles or from the economic, social, and cultural contexts that shaped women's lives. At times, I use the phrase "reproductive health" to refer—as the World Health Organization currently defines it—to women's "reproductive processes, functions, and systems," but readers should know that this terminology dates only to the 1970s.[11]

Reproduction on the Reservation demonstrates the extent to which colonial politics have been—and remain—reproductive politics.[12] This history could begin well before the late nineteenth century, as Native women's reproductive bodies proved symbolically and materially central to European objectives from the first days of conquest. Seventeenth-century European playwrights and authors circulated fantasies about staking claims in the lands they viewed as the "New World" through sexual conquest—a form of domination that emasculates Native men, terrorizes Native women, and appropriates the latter's reproductive capacity in the service of creating new European subjects. The historian Kathleen Brown observes that the male characters in the English comedy *Eastward Ho!*, first performed in 1605, fantasized about acts of sexual conquest that produced English rather than Anglo-Indian children.[13] While the arrival of these "English-faced children" was tantalizingly convenient and at least somewhat tongue-in-cheek, the outcome is consistent with English expectations of patrilineal descent. The often-told and frequently distorted story of the Virginia Algonquian woman whom most twenty-first-century Americans know as Pocahontas can be read as a further example of the appropriation of a Native woman's reproductive labor for colonial ends. Although Pocahontas's own life ended tragically when she died in England at the age of nineteen or twenty, the birth of a son a few years earlier—fathered by Pocahontas's English husband John Rolfe—meant that subsequent generations of English colonists and eventually American citizens could remember Pocahontas as "The Mother of Us All."[14] This genealogical fiction proved irresistible for a population invested in establishing claims to the territory that is currently the United States.[15]

Well into the eighteenth century, Europeans employed images of fertile Indigenous women to represent the continent they had committed to explore, conquer, and settle. The Native studies scholar Rayna Green has documented the ubiquity of the "Indian Queen," a "Mother-Goddess" figure who was voluptuous and maternal but also "powerful" and "dangerous"—the embodiment, Green argues, of "the opulence and peril of the New World."[16] The meanings colonizers attached to Native women's reproductive bodies derived from their own needs and desires, and often this meant viewing Indigenous reproduction as a marker of difference. Travel writers, artists, and other observers caricatured Native women's breasts and hips, and they characterized Native childbirth as "animal-like."[17] To the degree that English colonists and their American descendants depended on a clear line between their own "civilized" society and the "savagery" they ascribed to Native peoples, biological reproduction provided one means of delineating these boundaries.

In the nineteenth century, growing numbers of American citizens looked westward, spurred by the alluring and self-serving doctrine of Manifest Destiny. American settlement of the West required the disappearance or displacement of the Native peoples who resided in the region, a feat the U.S. Army pursued in a series of battles and massacres collectively remembered by many non-Natives as "the Indian wars." In a number of documented instances, U.S. soldiers and militiamen, some of whom understood their task to be the total extermination of their Native opponents, eagerly killed women alongside men. If the latter presented an immediate wartime threat, the former—by virtue of their reproductive capacity—embodied a more fundamental peril. The explanation attributed to the commanding general of the U.S. Cavalry as to why cavalrymen killed so many Cheyenne and Arapaho women and children at Sand Creek in the early 1860s—"nits make lice"—encapsulates this view.[18] In the aftermath of the massacre, allegations circulated regarding the genital mutilation of female victims at the hands of U.S. forces.[19] Reminiscent of earlier fantasies of sexual conquest, soldiers, miners, and settlers also sexually assaulted Native women, producing trauma, fear, and social instability and sometimes pregnancy and disease.[20]

In the last decades of the nineteenth century, the historical moment in which the story recounted here begins, the federal government's approach to U.S.-Indian relations shifted gradually and unevenly from violent conquest to cultural assimilation, another form of violence. By this time, the federal government had embraced the reservation system, envisioned by policy makers as an "alternative to extinction."[21] Confined to shrinking tribal lands, Native peoples navigated familiar life processes, including birthing and childrearing, in unfamiliar and disorienting circumstances and sometimes in new physical environments. Not all Native women lived on reservations in the late nineteenth century, but many did, and federal Indian policy was almost entirely oriented toward western reservations.[22] The title *Reproduction on the Reservation* derives from my initial interest in this early period, as biological reproduction and reproductive politics took new forms on emerging reservations in the West.

Three themes emerge in the years surrounding the turn of the twentieth century—recounted in chapters 1 and 2—that remain salient throughout the century and thus throughout this book. First, even absent any explicitly reproduction-related policies, Native women's reproductive experiences have been profoundly shaped by colonial policies and processes that produced the material realities of reservation life. In the early reservation years and thereafter, these realities included but were not limited to economic underdevelopment, poverty, malnutrition, and cultural repression. These developments contributed to a notable deterioration in maternal as well as infant health, although the latter has consistently received more attention from policy makers, health professionals, and other non-Native individuals and organizations.

Second, the reservation system facilitated heightened scrutiny, sometimes even surveillance, of Native women's reproductive bodies and lives, and this documentation was employed for a wide range of purposes. Employees ranging from agency farmers to lowly clerks to boarding school teachers and ultimately to field relocation officers in urban centers throughout the West and Midwest had something to say about individual women's reproductive lives as well as about the reproduction-related policies and practices of the Bureau of Indian Affairs (BIA).[23] Finally, as government employees intervened more directly in Native pregnancy and childbirth beginning in the early twentieth century, justifications for these intrusions derived from a politics of blame. BIA officials and employees diverted responsibility for population and land loss, poor maternal and infant health outcomes, and, following World War II, overpopulated and underresourced reservations to the bodies and behaviors of childbearing women and the women who cared for them.

The first decades of the twentieth century witnessed the start of a multidecade federal effort to persuade women to reject the reproductive practices of their mothers and grandmothers; replace midwives with government physicians, nurses, and field matrons as authorities on reproductive knowledge; and give birth in the government hospitals being built on some reservations in these years. Many government officials, missionaries, and social reformers came to view biological reproduction as a marker of assimilation and a valuable tool in advancing the federal government's assimilation agenda. Pregnancy and childbirth were deeply rooted in Native social, cultural, and spiritual life, and birth—like other reproductive-related events such as menarche—functioned as a key site of female power and the affirmation of clan and familial relationships. The federal government's attempt to transform birthing was thus closely connected to contemporaneous efforts to restructure Native families and households, initiatives that have been ably addressed in recent scholarship.[24] In carrying out all such initiatives, reservation employees relied on a combination of moral suasion and the coercive power of the state.[25]

As this book will emphasize, federal efforts to intervene in Native biological reproduction were implemented unevenly, in fits and starts, and often in a nonlinear or contradictory fashion. In the first decades of the twentieth century, for example, government bureaucrats, health workers, boarding school teachers, and many missionaries touted the superiority of trained government physicians and hospitals, even as many reservations lacked the medical manpower and infrastructure to provide the obstetric care they advocated. Nevertheless, as Native women came to rely increasingly on the BIA and later the Indian Health Service (IHS) for their reproductive health needs over the course of the century, a development that occurred at different rates in different locations, these federal agencies assumed a more prominent role in shaping the parameters of women's options regarding birth control, prenatal care, and obstetric services. These developments affirm the sociologist Barbara Gurr's recent observation that for Native women, the provision of "imperialist medicine" has been articulated through a "double-discourse of control and neglect."[26]

Although Gurr only briefly addresses the sterilization rates that WARN and other groups protested in the 1970s, this episode exemplifies the dual forces of control and neglect that she identified. In these years, as in the prewar period, some women with the means to do so procured reproductive health services from private physicians off the reservation, and some certainly received guidance from female kin. But most women living on reservations—and many living in cities—found their options for reproductive care limited to the government services and practitioners on their reservation, regardless of their satisfaction with this care. When IHS was unable to provide necessary gynecological and obstetric services on or near a reservation, the federal agency contracted with medical institutions off the reservation, an arrangement that required some women to travel two or more hours to deliver a baby. As became clear during the investigations prompted by 1970s activism, the Department of Health, Education, and Welfare failed to provide adequate oversight for the care Native peoples received in contract hospitals.[27] Activists further argued that inconsistent access to temporary birth control measures and obstacles in procuring abortions—the result of federal policies as well as unwritten practices—encouraged women to "choose" more permanent measures like tubal ligations.[28] Katsi Cook spoke out at WARN's first meetings against women's "absolute dependence" on these medical systems, which she argued left Native women vulnerable to abuse.[29] Ironically, the controversy and publicity surrounding sterilization procedures in the 1970s limited some women's reproductive options still further, as IHS increasingly steered clear of services that could be deemed controversial.[30]

My analysis of the reproductive abuses of the 1970s builds on scholarship in Native studies, Native history, and women's history while emphasizing the need for a more expansive chronology. To date, most scholarship on the coercive sterilization of Native women presents the sterilizations that occurred in the late 1960s and 1970s as largely anomalous. Scholars have deftly illuminated the racialized fears about global overpopulation and the domestic welfare state that gained ascendance in the post–World War II period. These scholars demonstrate how such fears contributed to the disproportionate sterilization not only of Native women but of women of color more broadly.[31] With limited exceptions, however, historians have taken for granted or explicitly argued that Native women remained outside of early twentieth-century eugenic campaigns, as eugenicists' emphasis on heredity seems contrary to the prevailing assimilation agenda in Indian affairs. One historian, for example, has argued that eugenicists "did not seek out Indian women as candidates for eugenic control."[32] *Reproduction on the Reservation* complicates this argument, demonstrating that colonial power dynamics, racialized and class assumptions, and a growing pessimism regarding assimilation created conditions that made Native women and sometimes men vulnerable to the eugenic proclivities of superintendents, physicians, and social workers. This book documents the involuntary sterilization of Native women on one reservation in the 1930s; these operations generally were not officially classified as "eugenic" because they did not follow the state's legal procedures but were motivated at least in part by eugenic logic and explained using eugenic language. The book further points to evidence suggestive of broader patterns throughout some corners of Indian Country. These findings should spur further exploration of how eugenics functioned on reservations, a crucial topic for historians of American eugenics as well as for Native and western historians.

Analyzing the politics and circumstances surrounding permanent sterilization in the early twentieth century and in the 1960s and 1970s reveals several patterns. Patrick Wolfe has argued, and many Native studies scholars and historians have demonstrated, that settler societies like the United States are predicated on a "logic of elimination," an ongoing impetus to orchestrate the disappearance of Native peoples through assimilation, removal, or annihilation.[33] Within this context, these two historical moments should surely be read as particularly blatant instances of this eliminatory logic being expressed through assaults on Native women's bodies and reproductive capacities. On the ground, the potential for abuse stemmed less from specific written policies and more from the lack thereof, resulting in individuals — physicians, social workers, and bureaucrats — wielding tremendous discretionary power. It is also not coincidental that the two historical moments in question were periods of Native population growth, as well as of cultural and political resurgence on reservations and, in the latter period, in urban centers. Finally, as demonstrated more fully below, growing awareness of unethical hospital practices spurred activist agendas spearheaded by women and sometimes men who recognized the multilayered threat coercive sterilization posed to Native women, families, and communities.

WHEN MARIA CAMPBELL OBSERVED that in their birth stories Native women "carry the stories of our people," she referred in part to the kind of colonial intrusions and abuses briefly outlined above.[34] She and others who gathered in Toronto in 2012 to share their vision for an Indigenous birth center spoke about how colonization had disrupted cultural processes in ways that are particularly visible in the realms of birthing and women's health. But these were not the only stories the women who met in Toronto told, nor were they the only stories that evoked rich histories. Campbell and others told stories about kinship, cultural knowledge, women's role in families and communities, and women's power—power that manifests and is symbolized through pregnancy, childbirth, and mothering. Such stories resonate on the U.S. side of the border. As a Nez Perce woman explained in the 1980s, "Woman is strong when she is pregnant, woman is strong on her moon. She is creator at time of pregnancy."[35] Native women's stories carry the knowledge that federal policies and practices sought to eradicate. These stories and their survival are equally critical for a history of Native reproduction.

Reproduction on the Reservation traces the reproductive histories of generations of Native women over the long twentieth century. In this book, policy and politics obtain meaning and import as they intersect with women's lives. I heartily reject the reverse formulation that Native women's lives and reproductive experiences obtain meaning and import through their voluntary or involuntary engagement with colonial policies and processes. When Native women remain at the margins of histories of reproduction and histories of health care, entering the story at the moment in which physicians performed unethical procedures on them, one unintended consequence is that in the eyes of nonspecialist readers these events become the defining feature of Native women's reproductive experiences, if not their lives more generally. The most frequent response I received over the past several years upon telling nonspecialist colleagues that I study the history of Native reproduction is some version of "You mean sterilization?" This history is simultaneously submerged and defining. This book aims to strike a delicate but necessary balance: while exposing additional layers to the history of coercive sterilization in Native America, it nonetheless frames the discussion so as not to overshadow the full range and complexity of women's reproductive lives.

By focusing attention on what women said and did, *Reproduction on the Reservation* advances two additional arguments that foreground Native women's agency. First, this book demonstrates that women navigated pregnancy and birthing throughout the twentieth century in myriad ways that disrupt any tidy dichotomy between "traditional" and "modern" reproduction—or between the "old" and "new" birthing methods that government documents and many anthropological studies contrasted so starkly. Women's needs and desires evolved alongside their circumstances. So-called traditional childbirth—typically described as birth outside a hospital with the assistance of an empirically rather than medically trained Native midwife—

was far from static; midwives adapted and expanded their practices over time. Peyote serves as an illustrative example. In the first decades of the twentieth century, midwives in some communities began incorporating peyote into their repertoire, a practice some twenty-first-century midwives continue to this day.[36] Peyote use in some Indigenous birthing spaces thus coincided with the federal government's introduction of medicalized birthing on reservations, including hospital childbirth.[37] Although Euro-American observers have often viewed these developments as entirely distinct, characterizing peyote as a "traditional" practice and the hospital as its opposite, women experimented with both reproductive options. For some women, this meant bringing peyote, like other elements of Indigenous birthing cultures, into the hospital. We must be wary of accepting too easily the federal government's vision of reservation hospitals and their function.

Some Native women strove to incorporate field matrons, nurses, physicians, and even hospitals into their reproductive lives on Native terms. These efforts did not necessarily signal a loss of faith in midwives or an inevitable decline in the midwife's status, although her role did change over time. When births occurred outside the hospital, female kin, including midwives, continued to attend births also attended by a field matron or physician, and often wielded significant control over the process. Women who might have acted as midwives in other circumstances also accompanied women to the hospital, where their efforts to serve as patient advocates and authorities on birthing were met with varying degrees of success in different contexts. Furthermore, because most Native midwives carried reproductive knowledge that extended far beyond obstetrics, women who chose or felt pressured to give birth in a hospital continued to consult midwives before and during pregnancies and after their deliveries, as childbirth was one stage in what Native communities recognized as a much broader reproductive process.

Eschewing the traditional/modern binary creates space for richer stories than previous narratives have allowed. It makes room, for example, for the reproductive trajectory of Susie Yellowtail (Crow), who delivered her first child in a private hospital in Sheridan, Wyoming, her second child in the government hospital at Crow Agency, and her third child at home with the assistance of an experienced Crow midwife.[38] It also makes room for Rose Maney's (Ho-Chunk) story. Maney gave birth to her first child on the Winnebago Reservation in the late 1930s, a few years after Susie Yellowtail delivered her third child at home. Maney then moved to Chicago and gave birth to two children but returned to the reservation during her fourth pregnancy because she "wanted my baby to be born in Winnebago hospital." The

Ho-Chunk mother apparently delivered her three subsequent children in Chicago after the family returned to the city.[39] As these examples suggest, individual women's childbirth experiences did not always follow prescribed patterns. They moved in and out of hospitals according to a host of factors, and they did not necessarily view all such institutions as interchangeable.

This argument merits a note of caution. In making it, I draw on the work of historians including Phil Deloria, Colleen O'Neill, and Mary Jane Logan McCallum, who have emphasized the constraining effect of a traditional/ modern binary.[40] In this context, as McCallum argues, "traditional" has been used "to discipline, manage, simplify, and reduce Aboriginal people's broad experiences of the world." But it is equally true, as McCallum also notes, that "tradition" "has been a useful political strategy of resistance" for Native peoples.[41] This certainly applies to the women who have been working since the 1970s to decolonize Indigenous reproduction, an effort that has included—indeed, necessitated—an exploration of tribal as well as pan-Indigenous traditions and teachings. I in no way intend to undermine this effort, which I wholeheartedly support. Rather, my intention is to underscore a point that practicing Native midwives have themselves made: "tradition" has never been static or monolithic but rather is a historical process that is continually negotiated.[42] Throughout the twentieth century, and continuing to the present, Native women have displayed fortitude and creativity in navigating the federal government's often contradictory demands on their bodies and behaviors and in meeting their perceived parturition and childbirth needs in evolving historical contexts.

My second argument regarding Native women's agency can be viewed as an extension of the first. *Reproduction on the Reservation* demonstrates that the roots of WARN women's activism are not only in Native struggles for sovereignty and self-determination in post–World War II decades but in Native women's reproductive-related activism on—and sometimes off—reservations throughout the century. Much of this activism was carried out by women who did not identify with militancy. After spending decades working to improve the health and well-being of Native women and children, Susie Yellowtail, the Crow nurse whose personal and professional history is recounted in chapter 3, insisted that "the Indian is not militant."[43] Some women, including Yellowtail, may not have viewed themselves as activists. Jackie Yellowtail, Susie's granddaughter, recalls that the family did not view Susie in such terms. Jackie lived with her grandparents for much of her childhood, and years later she explained that she and her siblings understood their grandmother's work on behalf of Crows and other Native peoples as "natural." In the Yellowtail household, one was simply expected "to advocate for our community, for each other . . . our people."[44] Susie Yellowtail and countless other women performed "politically purposeful work" by advocating for and supporting pregnant and childbearing women, including themselves, in tribal councils, local clubs, federal committees, and professional organizations, as well as in diverse birthing spaces.[45]

Extraordinary in so many ways, Susie Yellowtail's story nonetheless reveals critical themes about Native women's reproduction-related activism in the twentieth century. It underscores, for example, how midwifery has served as a political act of resistance for women. Some Crow women responded to sterilization abuses in the 1930s much as some Native women would respond to the abuses of the 1970s: by turning once again to midwives whom they trusted or by taking up midwifery themselves. Yellowtail and other women also pursued reformist agendas. They worked to secure the best possible care for Native women, and by the mid-twentieth century many had concluded that much of this care would necessarily occur in hospitals. They advocated for women's health and the health and well-being of their communities by pressuring federal agencies to uphold Native "treaty rights." They marshaled this language to demand that Native women receive services comparable to what a white woman with private insurance might receive off the reservation, but they also demanded that government health workers provide culturally appropriate care. Following Yellowtail's story also leads to a network of Native nurses and other health professionals who assumed roles as watchdogs and patient advocates in colonial medical institutions. In the 1970s and 1980s, these women struggled for Native women's reproductive autonomy alongside WARN—with sometimes differing tactics but often overlapping goals.

The Path Forward

Reproduction on the Reservation integrates an analysis of federal reproduction-related policies and practices targeting Native women with a local history of childbearing, motherhood, and activism in a single location—the Crow Reservation in southern Montana. The study of reproduction inevitably raises questions of scale: individual decisions are connected, as the historian Lynn M. Thomas explains, "to debates and interventions that flow from community, colonial, and international regimes."[46] In this case, my interest in reproductive policies and politics came first; my recognition of the need to ground this history in an extended case study derived from the research process. "Policy" pertaining to intimate matters such as reproduction was often informal and sometimes unwritten, and in other cases practices on the ground diverged notably from the directives emanating from Washington, D.C. The implementation—or lack thereof—of reproduction-related policies was shaped by local conditions, the availability of resources, the whims of individual employees, and perhaps most significantly Native response and engagement.

This dual approach is reflected in the book's structure: the study alternates between chapters that zoom in to provide ethnohistorical analyses of the Crow Reservation and chapters that zoom out to address trends throughout Indian Country. The book's interwoven chapters represent my attempt to reflect what the historian Devon Mihesuah refers to as "the commonality of difference." Mihesuah argues that "Indian women share the common context of gender and the 'common core' of struggle against colonialism," yet she cautions that the "intricacies of Indian women's lives must be specific to time and place."[47] More recently, Kent Blansett has warned of the homogenizing effect that settler colonial theory can impose on historical narratives, flattening out or erasing localized Indigenous experiences. Blansett calls on Native and western historians to remain attentive to "unique points of difference, departure, diversity, and sophistication."[48] My argument is not that the Crow case and Crow women's experiences are representative of all reservations and all Native women. Rather, I contend that, crucial common trends notwithstanding, there is no "representative" case; thus, the contingencies, particularities, and possibilities that a Crow case study reveals matter.

The book's alternating chapters represent different methodological approaches. In researching the chapters that focus on Crow, my priority was depth. These chapters rely on diverse and wide-ranging sources. I consulted virtually every source I could access pertaining to the reservation or Crow people, as I never knew where biological reproduction would pop up in the historical record or what would emerge as important context. Conversely, in researching the chapters that zoom out from the Crow Reservation, my priority was breadth. These chapters rely primarily on bureaucratic records, oral history collections, sociological and anthropological studies, and activist literature for several locations and tribal nations. Here, my analysis centered on identifying chronologies, patterns, and themes, as well as divergences and exceptions. When a person, issue, or event achieved particular prominence in one of these source sets, as when WARN sponsored

Native midwifery training and women's health programming in the Twin Cities in Minnesota in the late 1970s, I followed these leads.

Why the Crow Reservation? The simplest answer is that I followed the sources. My preliminary survey of BIA records revealed that federal records for the reservation were particularly robust and relatively complete. In addition, Crow has often been selected as a site for government studies and surveys, resulting in statistical data on topics ranging from hospital attendance at midcentury to family planning usage in the 1970s.[49] Crow-produced sources are similarly voluminous. Beginning in the early 1930s, when Pretty Shield, a respected elder, collaborated with the amateur ethnographer Frank B. Linderman to tell a version of her life story for publication, Crow women have produced several memoirs and as-told-tos in which they—often mediated by the participation of a scholar or editor—discuss gender, family, childbearing, and motherhood.[50] These perspectives are supplemented by the writing, speeches, and stories held in the tribal archives at Little Bighorn College Library, as well as by Crow individuals' participation in oral history projects, with interviews currently stored in archives from Montana to South Dakota to Illinois.

A fortuitous connection with Valerie Jackson, a Crow woman living in Arizona, paved the way for my richest source material, the oral history interviews that I conducted with Native women over the past several years. Jackson facilitated my introduction to her mother and sisters on my first trip to the reservation, and she later introduced me to women from the neighboring Northern Cheyenne Reservation.[51] In turn, these women introduced me to expanding circles of female kin. Working through families is an Indigenous methodology—Jackson referred to it as "the Crow way"—and it is one that has particular value for a history of reproduction, as my inquiries involved stories and knowledge that have historically been and, in many cases, continue to be transmitted through female networks.[52]

Reproduction on the Reservation proceeds chronologically. Chapter 1 sets the stage for the book's Crow-focused chapters, providing readers with an overview of Crow history to the late nineteenth century and establishing the parameters of a Crow birthing culture that thrived through the turn of the century, as did birthing cultures in most Indigenous societies. This chapter documents growing federal intervention in Crow reproductive practices in the years surrounding the turn of the century, as the regulation of reproduction dovetailed with the growing management—or attempted management—of Native life in the early reservation era. Chapter 2 traces the introduction of medicalized pregnancy and childbirth on reservations, including but by no means limited to Crow, in the first decades of the twentieth century. The context and justification for medicalization was the BIA's progressive campaign to combat infant mortality, a reality that shaped the reproductive experiences of successive generations of Native women. Returning to the Crow Reservation, chapter 3 explores the competing (and gendered) pressures regarding assimilation, self-determination, and elimination during John Collier's tenure as commissioner of Indian affairs and considers what this meant for Crow women's reproductive autonomy.

When, in the years after World War II, policy makers rejected Collier's agenda and devised policies and programs intended to assimilate Native peoples once and for all, these midcentury developments affected Native pregnancy and childbirth in various and not always predictable ways. Although this is primarily a reservation-centered study, chapter 4 necessarily ventures away from reservations, following the thousands of Native women of childbearing age who migrated to cities after the war. Some migrated through the federal government's relocation program, while others did so on their own or a family member's initiative. Policy makers and government employees expected that through employer health insurance and/or the use of public hospitals and low-income clinics, biological reproduction in the city would facilitate assimilation. In reality, women's reproductive decisions often strengthened rather than diminished ties to the reservation and to reservation-based kin. As demonstrated more fully in chapter 5, hospital childbirth itself was not new to many of the women who migrated to cities in these years. By the 1950s, most reservation women delivered in hospitals, yet the terminationist priorities of postwar policy makers threatened the government-operated reservation hospitals in which so many women received reproductive services. Crow women responded to this very real threat by organizing in defense of maternal and infant welfare. In tracing this story, this chapter reveals the centrality of health- and reproductive-related activism to Native resistance to termination.

The disproportionate sterilization rates in many Native communities in the 1970s conjure the terminationist ethos that had waned by many other measures. Beginning with IHS's introduction of family planning services in 1965, chapter 6 explores the sometimes-contradictory web of federal policies surrounding the reproductive technologies of artificial contraception, abortion, and permanent sterilization. WARN and other activists understood women's reproductive autonomy as fundamental to contemporary struggles for Native sovereignty and self-determination, and the chapter documents women's diverse attempts to regain "control of reproduction" in these tumultuous years.[53] The self-determination era ostensibly continues in the twenty-first century, yet Native women's ability to determine where, when, and what kind of sexual health, prenatal, and obstetric services they receive remains limited. In some cases, their options are more circumscribed than they were in the 1970s. These realities—as well as the reproductive justice agendas that Native women are waging in response to them—are addressed in the epilogue.

CHAPTER ONE

Childbearing and Childrearing

A year or two before her husband, Goes Ahead, scouted for General George Armstrong Custer in the fateful Battle of the Little Bighorn, a young Crow woman named Pretty Shield gave birth to her first child. When Pretty Shield went into labor, her mother and Left-hand, a "wise-one"—healer and midwife—directed her to a lodge constructed for birthing. Once in the lodge, Left-hand placed four live coals on the ground in each cardinal direction and dropped grass on each coal. She then instructed Pretty Shield to "walk as though you are busy." As Pretty Shield recalled the experience decades later, the delivery proceeded quickly from that point: "I had stepped over the second coal when I saw that I should have to *run* if I reached my bed-robe in time. I *jumped* the third coal, and the *fourth*, knelt down on my robe, took hold of the two stakes; and my first child, Pine-fire, was there with us." Left-hand wrapped a strip of tanned buffalo skin around Pretty Shield's waist to help expel the afterbirth, cleaned and dressed Pine-fire, and left the infant in the care of her mother and grandmother.[1] The story of Pretty Shield's first delivery reveals key features of a Crow birthing culture: she labored in a female-only space, and knowledgeable—in Left-hand's case powerful—older women played a critical role in her experience.

In the decades after Pine-fire's birth, Pretty Shield and other Crows experienced major changes to their way of life, as formerly dispersed people relocated to a new and reduced reservation and government employees and missionaries sought to transform the Crow people's world. Despite hardship and demoralization, Crows persisted and in fact proved remarkably adaptive. Barney Old Coyote Jr., a Crow educator and spokesman, later argued that "flexibility" was Crow society's "greatest strength."[2] In the realm of biological reproduction, a Crow birthing culture endured the disruptions of early reservation life, albeit not without adaptation to colonial circumstances.

This chapter explores Crow reproduction from the 1880s through the early 1900s, the years after Pine-fire's birth and the first decades after Crows' relocation to the flatland along the Little Bighorn River. Relying on oral histories, contemporary ethnographic sources, and recollections recorded in the early twentieth century, the chapter establishes the parameters of a Crow birthing culture as it existed in the years surrounding the turn of the century. The above account of Pretty Shield's delivery provides only a glimpse of a longer reproductive process extending at least from pregnancy, if not before, through early infant care. As in many Indigenous societies, Crow reproduction was not only a biological process but a social, cultural, and spiritual one. Gender roles, clan and kin relationships, and a distinctly nonnuclear conception of child care that I call "flexible childrearing" were expressed and buttressed through reproductive practices.[3] The chapter further considers government employees' attitudes toward and interventions in Indigenous pregnancy and childbirth in the early reservation years. Through the turn of the century, Native reproduction was a source of fascination for many Euro-Americans, including Office of Indian Affairs (OIA) employees.[4] Although the reproductive process remained almost entirely outside government purview, reservation employees scrutinized and theorized women's reproductive practices. Ultimately, Native reproduction, much like Native family life more broadly, came to occupy a significant symbolic and material position in the federal government's assimilationist agenda.

Crow Life after "Nothing Happened"

Before the nineteenth century, Crows had minimal contact with Euro-Americans. According to the tribal historian Joseph Medicine Crow, the ancestors of modern-day Crows originally migrated from northeastern North America, crossing the Mississippi River during the 1500s. The bands that would eventually become the Crow Nation separated from the Hidatsa sometime in the seventeenth century and traveled farther west to present-day northern Wyoming and southern Montana, where they created a new homeland.[5] After acquiring horses in the early eighteenth century, Crows developed a lifestyle of mobility in a land equipped with water, vegetation, and game. As Arapooish, a Crow chief, explained in the nineteenth century, "The Crow country is a good country. The Great Spirit has put it exactly in the right place."[6] Crows lived and traveled first in two and then in three groups: the River Crow resided in the plains between the Yellowstone and Missouri Rivers, the Mountain Crow dwelled in the mountain ranges to the south, and the Kicked in The Bellies splintered off from the Mountain Crows.[7]

Life changed dramatically for Native peoples in the West in the nineteenth century. Like other Plains Indians, Crows established closer relationships with Euro-American fur traders early in the century. The growth of the fur trade in the region intensified military conflict between Crows and their Native neighbors, including the Blackfeet, Cheyenne, and Lakota, as these groups increasingly competed for environmental resources, Euro-American goods, and commercial opportunities. Crows also established a more formal relationship with the federal government during this period. In 1825, leaders signed the tribe's first treaty with the United States, a pledge of friendship to which the former has remained faithful.[8] At midcentury, the U.S. government transferred the OIA from the Department of War to the Department of the Interior, a transition that did not mean the end of military violence but that signaled the federal government's shift toward the reservation era. In 1851, Crow and other Plains Indian leaders signed the first Fort Laramie Treaty, in which the U.S. government recognized 33 million acres in present-day Montana and Wyoming as Crow land. In a second Fort Laramie Treaty of 1868, the U.S. government recognized only 8 million acres as Crow land, and other Plains Nations faced similar reductions. Despite repeated betrayals, Crow leaders maintained a military alliance with the United States, and Crow warriors fought alongside the U.S. military in a series of battles against the Lakota, their primary rivals in the region, in the 1860s and 1870s.[9]

In the early 1880s, U.S. officials reduced Crow land still further and moved the tribe's agency headquarters to its current location along the Little Bighorn River. The once-dispersed people moved to their newly bounded reservation in 1884, settling in decentralized groups according to band and kin networks. The government eventually subdivided the reservation around these settlements, creating five bureaucratic districts. (A sixth would be added in the first decade of the twentieth century.)[10] Additional land reductions followed. In 1890, 1899, and 1904, government representatives persuaded Crow leaders to agree to land cessions. These cessions followed the passage of the General Allotment Act of 1887, the centerpiece of policy makers' objective to privatize Indian land. Policy makers and social reformers hoped that allotment would transform the way Native Americans related to land and to one another. To the delight of encroaching Euro-American settlers, it also facilitated the transfer of vast swaths of land from Native to non-Native hands. The Crow Nation lost more than three-quarters of its homeland during the allotment era, which continued until the early 1930s.[11]

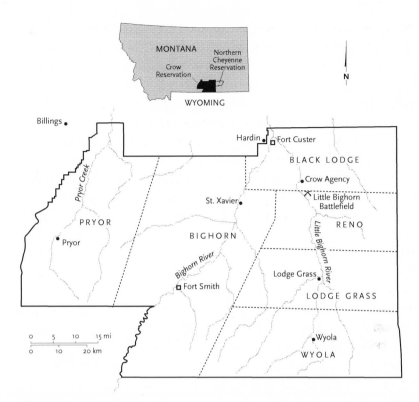

The Crow Reservation.

Although policy makers envisioned the reservation system as an "alternative to extinction," for many groups the first decades of reservation life were characterized by suffering and death.[12] Crows struggled to survive within new geographic constraints at the same moment that the buffalo almost completely disappeared from the region, depriving them and their Native neighbors of sustenance and their livelihoods.[13] Increasingly reliant on inadequate government rations, some families endured extreme hunger.[14] Malnutrition, combined with a forced sedentary lifestyle, created the conditions for the rapid spread of diseases. At Crow as elsewhere, these circumstances resulted in an alarming demographic decline. The historian Frederick Hoxie has concluded that nearly one-third of the Crow population died in the 1890s, and youth were disproportionately affected. The demise of the younger generation had demographic consequences into the next century.[15]

Pretty Shield was a young mother during these dislocations. Like many of her peers and many Crow elders, she found life on the reservation disorienting and demoralizing. Decades later, she refused to talk about this period, insisting "there is nothing to tell, because we did nothing."[16] Pretty Shield responded not only to her people's newly restricted mobility and the morbidity and mortality she witnessed but also to the new set of expectations that government employees and missionaries imposed on her people. In the decades after the Civil War, policy makers, social reformers, and government bureaucrats embarked on a multifaceted campaign to assimilate Native peoples. Many optimistically believed that Indians could be transformed into American citizens quickly, perhaps within a single generation. Crows had mostly managed to evade these ad hoc assimilation efforts before the 1880s, but the government's presence and reach increased after the move to the Little Bighorn.[17]

Along with land reform, the education of Native children was a cornerstone of the government's assimilationist agenda. Social reformers and policy makers reasoned that at boarding schools, separated from their families, Native youth could be trained to reject their cultural beliefs and practices and adopt English, Christianity, and Western ways.[18] The government had operated a boarding school for Crow children in the 1870s, which Pretty Shield briefly attended, but the school rarely attracted more than a dozen Crow students at any given time.[19] In subsequent decades, the Indian Service resorted to more coercive measures to enforce attendance at the new government school at Crow Agency, methods that employees simultaneously implemented on other reservations. Superintendents dispatched tribal policemen to act as truant officers, and they withheld rations from families that proved uncooperative. In some cases, authorities resorted to bribery and outright deceit.[20]

Native children later described the lengths to which their families went to resist these coercive methods. Tall Woman, a Navajo woman also known as Rose Mitchell, recalled the fear that accompanied policemen's efforts to fill the reservation boarding school that was constructed in the 1880s: "I guess some children were snatched up and hauled over there because the policemen came across them while they were out herding, hauling water, or doing other things for the family. So we started to hide ourselves in different places whenever we saw strangers coming to where we were living."[21] Tom Tobacco, who first went to school in the late 1890s at the age of six or seven, had similar memories of Crow policemen, who traveled the reservation on horseback to "round [children] up just like rounding horses up."[22] The paternal grandmother of Robert Yellowtail, one of Tobacco's contemporaries, took her

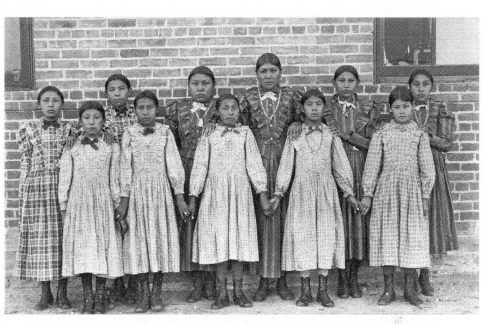

Government employees on the Crow Reservation were under significant pressure to fill the boarding school at Crow Agency in the late nineteenth century. These young women attended the school in the late 1890s and received academic, vocational, and assimilationist training at the government-run institution. Catalog number 955-926, Legacy Photograph Collection, Montana Historical Society (Helena, Montana).

grandson into the hills each day to avoid capture by policemen, just as she would later do with Robert's younger siblings. Eventually, a member of the tribal police force discovered the duo and delivered Robert to Crow Agency.[23]

Robert Yellowtail, like many Native children, later journeyed still farther from his family when he left Montana to attend a government boarding school in Riverside, California. Some of his peers attended Carlisle Indian School in Pennsylvania, and his younger brother Thomas later attended Bacone Indian School in Oklahoma. At government or denominational boarding schools, students learned English and other elements of a Western education and also received a steady dose of gendered vocational training. For Robert Yellowtail and his peers, boarding school often meant years separated from their land, families, and culture. For the older generations who remained at home, it meant an extended disruption in their ability to pass down cultural knowledge and beliefs. Particularly in the early years of off-reservation Native education, families experienced both grief and fear when their child was sent to boarding school, as they did not know when their loved one would return, or if he or she would come home alive.[24]

Whether on or off the reservation, the curriculum at Indian schools included Christianity, as policy makers and social reformers viewed conversion to Christianity and rejection of Native spiritual systems as a critical step in the assimilation process. A few missionaries had lived among the Crow before the move to the new agency, but they rapidly descended on the reservation beginning in the mid-1880s—first the Unitarians, then the Catholics and Congregationalists, and finally, shortly after the turn of the century, the Baptists. At Crow as in other locations, missionaries were agents of domestic imperialism. They intended to colonize the hearts and minds of their Indigenous flock, while generally acting as advocates and enforcers of other aspects of the government's assimilation campaign. But Crows sometimes used missionaries' objectives to their advantage. In the early 1900s, Crow leaders persuaded the Baptists to establish a day school in Lodge Grass, allowing Crow children to be educated closer to home, at least when they were young.[25] Joseph Medicine Crow suggests that his kin approached the missionaries' agenda selectively, taking advantage of the material benefits of church membership and incorporating Christian precepts and rituals into what Medicine Crow viewed as "their traditional religion."[26]

Native peoples also faced new expectations regarding gender roles and familial relationships in the final decades of the nineteenth century. Social reformers and many government bureaucrats took for granted that the nuclear family unit—consisting of husband, wife, and biological children—was the most moral and civilized domestic arrangement. Thus, imposing the nuclear family unit on Native families with very different systems of familial reckoning became a primary objective of late nineteenth-century federal Indian policy. The nuclear family, organized around a male head of household, also implied particular gender roles. The Indian Service expected Native men to provide for their families—not through hunting or raiding but rather through farming an individually owned plot of land. The Indian Service envisioned a simultaneously expanded and diminished role for women within the household: they would occupy a more prominent position in relation to extended female kin but a subordinate position in relation to their husbands.[27] Generally satisfied with Crow gender, familial, and social arrangements, Crow women had reason to resist the Indian Service's efforts.

Gender, Family, and Kinship

In the nineteenth century, gender relationships in Crow society, as in many North American Indigenous cultures, are better described as complementary than hierarchical.[28] Until the federal government prohibited such activities in the 1880s, Crows celebrated men's achievements as warriors and hunters, and they continued to value men's qualities of bravery and leadership after settling on the reservation. Likewise, Crows valued women's work preparing and distributing food and producing tepees, clothing, and most household items. This value was reflected in control of resources: women owned a household's food, home, and all domestic equipment. Women's labor in the realm of reproduction—as life givers, mothers, and midwives—garnered them status and a role in public and ceremonial life.[29] One Crow man later described gender complementarity in Crow society without using this language. He explained that Crows had never been matriarchal in terms of political affairs, where men assumed a more public role, but that something of a "matriarchy" had always existed in the realm of familial and social relations.[30]

Crows distinguished between one's sex and his or her gender role; biology did not determine destiny. As Frederick Hoxie has argued, "The successful fulfillment of one's social obligations was far more significant to the Crow community than an individual's anatomical makeup."[31] Although rare, women could and did fight as warriors before the government prohibited intertribal warfare.[32] The community included a handful of men who dressed and lived as women, and all evidence suggests that these individuals were well respected by fellow community members, who pushed back against government employees' efforts to force such men to conform to Euro-American gender standards.[33]

Men, women, and children related to one another through clans and kinship networks, and Crows recognized more than ten exogamous clans in the nineteenth century.[34] The Crow clan system was—and remains—matrilineal, which meant that children joined their mother's clan at birth. Perhaps more than most matrilineal societies, however, Crows also recognized close ties with the father's clan and kin, and such relationships carried a number of social obligations. The father's clan, for example, assumed responsibility for bestowing blessings for a healthy and accomplished life.[35] Because Crows placed significance on the extended rather than the nuclear familial unit, marital unions were fluid. A husband or wife could dissolve an unhappy union with relative ease because Crows cherished individual autonomy and because the dissolution did not cause serious social disruption.[36]

In raising children, Crows practiced—and in many cases continue to practice—flexible childrearing. As Robert Yellowtail's daughter later explained, "When a child is born, the parents are not the ones really responsible for their upbringing. It's the aunts and the uncles and the grandparents."[37] Flexible childrearing was not bound by nuclear structures and instead incorporated communal child-rearing practices and a variety of temporary and long-term adoption procedures. Yellowtail's younger sister Agnes Deernose observed that "Crows like to share children"; "they don't think of adoption as a giving a child up."[38] Female kin occupied a prominent role in childrearing. As the historian Theda Perdue has observed for Cherokees, another matrilineal society, "mother" signified a social rather than exclusively biological relationship, and children had many mothers.[39] Robert Yellowtail and his siblings, for example, used the same word to refer to Elizabeth (Lizzie) Yellowtail, their biological mother, as they did to refer to Mary Takes the Gun, Lizzie's sister.[40] Robert Yellowtail also lived with Mary Takes the Gun off and on throughout his early years. In turn, Takes the Gun's two boys lived with the Yellowtails in their youth.[41]

As on many reservations, grandmothers often assumed responsibility for daily child care. In many cases, grandmothers lived in the same house as their children and grandchildren. Well into the twentieth century, it remained a common practice for grandparents to adopt the first child of their own children after the grandchild had been weaned. Thomas Leforge, a white man who spent much of his life among the Crows, emphasized the practical benefits of this custom: "This old-time practice was good for the young parents, it was good for the elderly foster-parents, it was good for the tribe, as it left physically capable young couples free from the worries of providing for their children and thus enabled them to go on producing others."[42] Crows had a word to describe a child who for one reason or another was raised primarily by his or her grandparents: *káalisbaapite*, or "grandmother's grandchild."[43] The tribal historian Joseph Medicine Crow later explained that his mother Amy—Lizzie Yellowtail's oldest daughter and Robert's younger sister—had been adopted by her maternal grandparents. The grandparents lived "just across the railroad tracks" from Lizzie and her husband, Hawk with the Yellowtail, so Amy saw her biological parents frequently.[44]

Flexible childrearing mitigated the potentially disruptive effects of hardship and loss, a feature that became increasingly important in the context

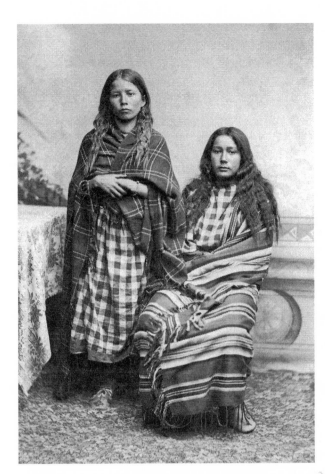

Orlando Scott Goff photographed sisters Mary Shane (Takes the Gun) and Lizzie Shane (Yellowtail) in 1888. Lizzie likely gave birth to her first child, Robert Yellowtail, a year or so after this photograph was taken. Catalog number 955–777, Legacy Photograph Collection, Montana Historical Society (Helena, Montana).

of colonization. If a child's biological mother and/or father died or became seriously ill, that child generally had no shortage of parents and grandparents with whom to live. In an era of unusually high infant and child mortality, the sharing of children also helped alleviate parents' heartbreak. Take, for example, one adoption that occurred just after the turn of the twentieth century. Faced with the tragic albeit unfortunately relatively common experience of losing a child—in this case, a daughter—who succumbed to diarrhea, a Crow mother was overwhelmed with grief. The family spent a week out in the hills, where they performed a burial, fasted, and mourned. Shortly thereafter, the woman visited a family who had a three-year-old daughter. She took so much joy in seeing the little girl that the girl's biological parents said, "You better take her with you. You can keep her and she can stay there." The woman gained a daughter, and the young girl gained another mother and father, as well as another set of extended kin. Once the girl reached school age, she moved back and forth between the two homes, as well as the home of her adopted father's sister.[45]

Adoption not only mitigated loss; in some cases, Crows believed it could prevent it. If an infant or child was ill or sickly and remained so for an extended period of time, his or her parents might announce a *baakáatawaxiia*, a "throwaway" ceremony. Although the term translates awkwardly into English, the ceremony was an effort to improve the infant's welfare. The parents left the child in a prearranged location, and a clan relative or friend picked the child up and took him or her home, where the ill child was given a new name and new clothing and effectively treated as a newborn. If the child survived, the adoption might be brief, but in most cases, it was permanent.[46] This practice did not signify neglect or abandonment. Rather, it was rooted in Crows' understanding of the *iláaxe*, which the anthropologist Timothy McCleary explains is "often translated as a person's will-power, drive, or soul."[47] Crows believed the *iláaxe* to be capricious and wont to stray from the physical body, particularly during one's infancy or early childhood, and the *iláaxe's* departure resulted in illness. New parents attempted to avoid this outcome by having a respected elder, often within the extended family, select a name for the child in the days following birth, as Crows believed that names tethered the *iláaxe* to the body. If the child became ill, family members suspected the *iláaxe* had disliked the name. Often, a family member selected a new name for the child, and if that failed to improve his or her condition, the parents arranged an adoption.[48]

The above practices all reflect Crows' conviction that one's wealth was measured in relatives, a belief that was reflected in every step of the reproductive process. The bonds between a child and his or her kin began even before birth, in the ways that relatives cared for a mother during her pregnancy. Crows often placed significance on the presence of female kin at an infant's birth. For example, when Alma Hogan Snell related the story of her birth decades later, she emphasized her maternal grandmother's presence: "She was with me when I was born."[49] In the days immediately following birth, relatives and clan members performed rituals to solidify the newborn's position within the Crow social world. It was often a grandmother, for example, who cut an infant's umbilical cord and pierced the child's ears. A paternal relative, either an aunt or grandmother, typically produced a cradleboard for the infant's support and safety.[50] The birth of a child, even more than a marital union, created bonds between the child's patrilineal and matrilineal kin, who were now, in the ethnographer Fred W. Voget's words, "bound together" in service of the child's well-being.[51]

Pregnancy and Childbirth in the Early Reservation Years

Throughout the nineteenth century and into the twentieth, Crows viewed reproduction as a sex-segregated process. This was common, although not universal, in Native societies.[52] Crow women navigated pregnancy and childbirth through female generational networks, but their gendered education had begun much earlier. As young girls, they came to understand the meanings attached to and the responsibilities associated with Crow womanhood through subtle instruction but especially by observing the women around them. Lillian Bullshows Hogan, born in Pryor shortly after the turn of the century, learned to be a "good woman" from watching her biological mother's industriousness within their home.[53] Other female kin were equally valued teachers. Agnes Deernose later recalled that she "learned more from my mother's sister than my own mother."[54] Alma Hogan Snell spent her childhood days accompanying Pretty Shield, her maternal grandmother, as the elder woman went about her daily tasks, telling stories and offering advice for proper living.[55] Through observing women like Pretty Shield and Deernose's aunt Mary Takes the Gun, Crow girls witnessed the faith community members placed in these women as healers and midwives.

Menarche marked a Crow girl's transition to womanhood. When a young woman first menstruated, she typically consulted an older woman in the family, often her grandmother, who provided instruction as to sanitary care and appropriate behavior. After distancing themselves from the larger group, the teacher informed her pupil of the need to stay away from men during menstruation, as her blood weakened them.[56] In some Native cultures, this belief manifested in women's residence in separate tents or lodges for a few days each month.[57] Crow women did not sojourn in separate dwellings during menstruation in the late nineteenth century, although they may have done so previously.[58] Many missionaries and government agents opposed this and similar practices, and external pressures forced women in many societies to circumscribe or stop honoring this custom.[59] Non-Native observers often misunderstood prescriptions for women's behavior during menstruation, interpreting taboos for menstruating women as evidence that tribal members viewed them as unclean. More recent scholarship pushes back against these Euro-centric assumptions and instead contends that menstruating women in many Native societies held "great power," requiring all of a woman's energy and focus, and that this power could be dangerous to men.[60] Unlike other Native groups, Crows apparently did not commemorate menarche with a ceremony, but a woman often married shortly after her first menstruation, and extended families marked these unions with public gift giving.[61]

Crow women maintained a significant degree of sexual and reproductive autonomy, which included their ability to terminate undesired pregnancies. Midwives' and herbalists' extensive knowledge of women's health often included abortifacients, and women in Plains societies used medicinal herbs, such as calamus, tansy, juniper, and horsetail, for this purpose.[62] Crow women also likely used bearroot. In the early twenty-first century, Alma Hogan Snell, by this time a highly regarded herbalist in her own right, recalled that her grandmother Pretty Shield and other midwives always had a piece of bearroot on hand. Among other gynecological functions, Snell explained, bearroot "constricts the womb" and thus could be used to facilitate deliveries. Snell, whose religious beliefs led her to oppose the termination of pregnancies, warned that the root should not be given to a woman before the onset of labor "for fear of abortion" — a warning that underscores Crow women's knowledge of this potential and possibly previously practiced use.[63] Women who specialized in gynecological and obstetric matters had recourse to other techniques as well. According to Crow cosmology, the stars supplied the people with critical knowledge. The Seven Sacred Brothers, also known as the Big Dipper, had introduced massage techniques and methods for kneading the stomach to terminate pregnancies as well as to treat "belly ache" and colic.[64] As a Crow elder later explained, a woman who wanted to end a pregnancy visited an older woman known to be skilled at this practice, and, as when requesting the assistance of a healer in any context, she bestowed gifts on the older woman as payment for the service.[65]

Crow sources point to several circumstances in which a woman might decide to end a pregnancy. Emphasizing Crows' mobility, their habit of "traveling from place to place" in the late nineteenth century, women later explained that a woman utilized postcoital birth control methods when a pregnancy or child would be burdensome — for example, when a particularly brutal winter had left the tribe with inadequate resources, or if the mother was not in good health. One woman, whose grandmother had been a skilled midwife and had performed abortions, explained that it was important for a woman to be confident that she would give birth to a strong, healthy infant who had a fair chance of survival.[66] Some Crows later recalled that unmarried women sometimes opted to end pregnancies.[67] Regardless of motivation, Crow sources make clear that this was a woman's decision and that she had the autonomy to make it. Although cloaked in cultural arrogance and moralism, a physician stationed at Crow Agency in the 1880s likewise emphasized the pregnant woman's prerogative and authority in these matters.[68]

Women also turned to kin to guide them through pregnancies. Crow women encouraged expecting mothers to rise early, stay active, and drink plenty of water, injunctions that were common in many Native societies. They also offered instructions that were more tribally specific but that in all cases were intended to facilitate the labor process and/or ensure a healthy child. Kin instructed Crow women, for example, to sleep with their feet facing a doorway throughout their pregnancy because they believed this act would bring about an unobstructed delivery. Elders also urged parturient women to avoid looking at anything deformed, "for fear," a male elder later explained, that "it may come out in the child."[69] At some point during the pregnancy, the expecting parents asked a clan aunt or uncle to pray and request blessings for the child.[70]

As had been the case for Pretty Shield's first delivery, family members often arranged for a midwife to be in attendance ahead of time, whom they paid generously with a horse, blankets, foodstuff, or money.[71] If a member of the woman's extended family had midwifery experience, the woman would turn to her for birthing assistance. For example, Pretty Shield, who in the decades after the birth of her first child earned a reputation as a skilled midwife in her own right, attended her daughters' deliveries.[72] Although it is not clear who assisted Lizzie Yellowtail in the births of her oldest children, her sister Mary Takes the Gun served as Yellowtail's midwife in the early 1900s.[73] A woman's mother and/or grandmother typically attended her deliveries, regardless of whether either of them acted as midwife. If a pregnant woman's mother did not live nearby—if, for example, she lived in another district—it was common for the woman to go stay with her mother in anticipation of delivery and remain in her mother's home for a few weeks postpartum.[74]

The nature of birthing locations evolved between Pretty Shield's first delivery in the 1870s and those of her daughters in the 1910s and 1920s, but much of what occurred within these spaces remained relatively consistent. Pretty Shield reported having delivered in a "lodge," and other Crows recalled that in "the old days" babies had been born in tepees.[75] In the 1880s and thereafter, however, births increasingly took place in tents. Within the tent, birthing attendants encouraged the laboring woman to move around, much as Left-hand had done for Pretty Shield. When the infant's arrival was imminent, attendants directed the woman to deliver in a kneeling position, working with rather than against gravity and often grasping two sticks that had been planted into the ground for her support.[76] Most midwives had techniques to facilitate the birthing process, beginning with the prohibition of men from the birthing area; they warned that a man's presence made delivery more difficult for the woman.[77] They also concocted juices or teas from roots, herbs, or other plants and employed sage as incense.[78]

When one midwife's techniques or powers proved inadequate for any given birth, someone sent for another with different, or stronger, medicine. As late as the early 1920s, Pretty Shield called on another midwife to assist in the birth of her daughter Helen Goes Ahead's last child. The midwife sent one of Goes Ahead's sons to the river with a bowl and instructed him to return with a fish. The young boy heroically set himself to the task, despite the fact that these events occurred in the middle of a Montana winter. After breaking through the ice, he returned with a fish and some water. The woman swirled her finger in the water, took out the fish, and directed the laboring woman to drink the remaining liquid. "As soon as she drank that water," Goes Ahead's daughter Alma later reported, "my mother had me. I was born." Yet the midwife's work was not done. She sent the boy back to the river to return the fish, and when he reported that the fish swam swiftly upon release, the old woman declared with confidence that "the baby will live."[79] Given the circumstances of her own birth, Alma Snell always felt a strong connection with water.[80]

Some late nineteenth-century Euro-American observers recognized the skill of Native midwives.[81] Walter Hoffman, a German ethnologist who visited the Crow Reservation in the late 1880s, reported favorable maternal health outcomes. He observed that puerperal fever—a significant risk in nineteenth-century childbirth that is now understood to be caused by uterine infection—was "rare" on the reservation.[82] Hoffman further noted that it was unusual for women to die during or following childbirth. Relatively low maternal mortality, combined with women's faith in the importance of their role as life givers, contributed to women's generally positive attitudes toward childbirth, another trend that caught the ethnologist's attention. Hoffman's observations contrast with the fear and danger that the historian Judith Walzer Leavitt has argued many middle- and upper-class Euro-American women endured "under the shadow of maternity" in the nineteenth century.[83]

Childbirth was not without danger, however, and Native midwives were not without limitations. At Crow, most parties agreed that the most challenging task typically occurred after a child's birth with the removal of the placenta.[84] A. B. Holder, the physician at Crow Agency in the late 1880s, reported that women relied on external compression of the uterus, usually through the application of a "binder" around a new mother's waist, to assist the delivery of the placenta.[85] A few decades later, an older woman living in the Pryor district could recall five women who died during or immediately after childbirth, and she attributed three of the five to the attendants' inability to expel the afterbirth.[86] Breech births—a condition that twenty-first-century physicians believe occurs in about 3 percent of maternity cases—may also have posed risks to the infant and mother, but it should be noted that some Native midwives were well known for their ability to manually alter the position of babies who were "turned around."[87] The Pryor woman attributed the other two maternal deaths in her recollection to disease and malnutrition, two conditions that defined early reservation life for many Native women.

Crow Reproduction and Colonial Scrutiny

Native midwives attended virtually all reservation births at the turn of the twentieth century. In the preceding decades, the federal government had begun assigning physicians to many reservations, but high turnover left Native patients with limited government health services for extended periods of time. The training and ability of government physicians varied widely, but in the 1880s, the commissioner of Indian affairs took strides to standardize qualifications for the position. As the historian Robert Trennert explains, under Commissioner Hiram Price, the OIA began "requiring that a physician prove graduation from a recognized medical school, be actively engaged in the practice of medicine, and possess a high moral character."[88] Nevertheless, Native peoples remained suspicious of government physicians, and relatively few Crows visited the physician for care in the late nineteenth century.[89] As a result, A. B. Holder, the physician at Crow Agency, reported that life for a reservation physician was "dull to a serious degree." Holder further observed that Crow and other Native women rarely called on physicians for obstetric services, which he attributed to their expectation that childbirth was a sex-segregated event and to their understanding of parturition as a "physiological process" that did not require "skilled assistance."[90] The physician was accurate regarding the former point and overly simplistic with regard to the latter. As suggested above, it is more likely that Crow women believed their female attendants were equipped with critical birthing-related skills.

Reflecting the fascination of many Euro-Americans with Indigenous biological reproduction, Holder dedicated himself to gathering information about Crow and other Native women's bodies and sexual and reproductive practices. The physician explained his motivations for such investigations through the discourse of evolutionary theory, which held that human societies gradually progress from stages of savagery to barbarism to civilization, and he understood his work as a kind of salvage anthropology: "As the years go by, the Indians, as a race, lose their distinctness; as savages, their characteristics. The time for investigation is passing."[91] Holder solicited information from fellow physicians, government agents, and school superintendents throughout Indian Country regarding menstruation, childbearing practices, the prevalence of venereal disease, and women's level of "chastity." It is not always clear how Holder or his peers arrived at their data; many relied heavily on female matrons, and some pronouncements, such as those regarding women's virtue, read as little more than one individual's subjective assessment. At any rate, the receptiveness of Holder's colleagues to his many inquiries underscores the scrutiny Native women endured during these years.[92]

Under the banner of "scientific methods," Holder reached conclusions shaped in large part by Euro-American "knowledge" regarding "primitive" or "savage" women, including long-standing tropes about Indigenous promiscuity. For example, the physician attributed what he termed "precocious menstruation," by which he meant menstruating at an earlier age than white women, to early sexual activity and "the entire absence of modesty in Indian thought and conversation."[93] Holder then shared the results of his investigations with medical colleagues in multiple articles in the *American Journal of Obstetrics and Diseases of Women and Children*, providing a body of additional colonial "knowledge" on which successive generations of physicians and scholars could draw.[94] Holder joined a vibrant field of scholarly inquiry. A decade earlier, the American obstetrician and gynecologist George Engelmann had begun publishing scholarly articles on Indigenous biological reproduction, and in 1882 Engelmann published *Labor among Primitive Peoples*, an ambitious attempt to document, as the book's subtitle explained, *the Natural and Instinctive Customs of All Races, Civilized and Savage, Past and Present.*[95]

Like Engelmann before him, Holder dedicated particular energy to the long-standing myth of painless Indigenous childbirth. This line of thinking, which was pervasive throughout the eighteenth and nineteenth centuries and extended into the twentieth, held that women in so-called primitive societies, closer to nature, gave birth with relative ease, and thus pain in childbirth was an indication of a woman's—or a tribe's or a race's—level of civilization.[96] Indeed, Engelmann argued that a people's degree of contact with civilization could be measured by the average length of labor; hence, a Modoc woman might expect to labor for an hour or less, while Kootenai women generally labored a bit longer. Engelmann remained confident that Native women seldom labored more than two hours.[97] The notion of painless Indigenous childbirth had some skeptics by this period—the ethnologist Walter Hoffman among them—and Holder himself acknowledged the occasional occurrence of long, challenging deliveries.[98] Nevertheless, Holder boldly declared that "it is universally admitted that labor is easier, quicker, and safer with savage than with civilized women, and my experience confirms this."[99]

Assumptions regarding pain and childbirth served as an umbrella for divergent if not necessarily contradictory understandings of the evolutionary process. Holder reported that Native women typically labored in a kneeling or squatting position or situated themselves on all fours, practices he acknowledged had the advantage of utilizing gravity. Lest one suspect, however, that the relative ease of Indigenous childbirth could be explained by laboring postures, Holder proclaimed that "half-breeds" experienced more difficult deliveries than "full-bloods," a phenomenon he attributed to the "infusion of white blood."[100] Engelmann was at times equally dismissive of the significance of laboring postures, and he placed comparable emphasis on the negative consequences of interracial sexual and marital relationships: "The Umpqua mother," he argued, "will be easily delivered of an offspring from an Umpqua father, but the head and body of a half-breed child is apt to be too large to pass through her pelvis."[101] At first glance, Holder's emphasis on biology—blood—as a marker of difference seems to coexist uneasily with the cultural assimilation campaign of which he was at least temporarily an agent. Yet missionaries and government agents had long linked blood and culture, implicitly or explicitly associating white ancestry with progress toward civilization. Furthermore, the amount of "Indian blood" was a crucial factor in the implementation of some of the government's most important assimilationist policies, such as land allotment.[102] Other government physicians placed less emphasis on blood but nonetheless described a similar process, interpreting the difficult deliveries they observed as a sign of progress toward civilization.[103]

None of this theorizing affected Crow women's reproductive experiences in any meaningful way in these years, nor did such theories align with women's own perceptions. In the twentieth century, older women would concur that childbirth had become more difficult for Crow women. They explained women's increased suffering in childbirth by pointing to altered birthing practices, changes in women's attitudes, and a decline in women's health.[104] In addition to interracial mixing, Engelmann attributed Native women's "rapid and easy" deliveries to the active lives they led, and some twentieth-century Crow women seem to have agreed that decreased activity on the reservation hindered women's preparedness for birthing.[105] Yet neither Holder nor most of his colleagues alluded to the material and demographic conditions on their respective reservations, which placed new pressures on women's bodies and shaped many women's experience of pregnancy and childbirth.[106] The chronic malnutrition that resulted from Crows' increasing reliance on inadequate government rations for sustenance took a particular toll on women of childbearing age. Alma Snell attributed her mother's difficulty in her own birth to poor nutrition and further noted that her mother had been "pretty well undernourished" throughout all of her pregnancies.[107] Malnourishment further increased women's susceptibility to diseases like tuberculosis, which plagued many reservations at the turn of the century. Women of childbearing age were disproportionately vulnerable, and American physicians warned that pregnancy and childbirth were dangerous for tubercular women. When Snell was two years old, her mother succumbed to the disease.[108]

The high morbidity and mortality on the reservation encouraged high fertility, as families feared that they would not have offspring who survived to adulthood, and leaders worried about the tribe's survival. Frederick Hoxie has argued that "only the maintenance of extraordinarily high birth rates prevented the tribe from dropping into oblivion."[109] The demographic decline of youth in the late nineteenth century also meant that there were fewer women of childbearing age to carry this increased reproductive burden. More frequent pregnancies undoubtedly took a physical toll on Crow and other Native women, with cycles of pregnancy and lactation exacerbating the malnourishment many mothers endured at the turn of the century.[110] At Crow as on many reservations in the years surrounding the turn of the twentieth century, birth rates increased in the same years that women's health decreased by many measures.

Familial and Reproductive Politics in the Early Twentieth Century

Samuel G. Reynolds arrived on the Crow Reservation just over a decade after A. B. Holder had left it. Commissioner of Indian Affairs William Jones had recently appointed Reynolds, a banker from Billings, as the new agent at Crow Agency. Reynolds's 1902 appointment reflected a shift in Indian affairs toward local (white) control and in service of local interests.[111] The banker turned agent had little patience for gradual approaches to assimilation. He believed that the time had come for Indian self-sufficiency, even if this outcome had to be accomplished forcibly. Reynolds immediately reduced government rations; after four years on the reservation, he eliminated them completely. Viewing "camp life" as a relic of the past, not to mention a potential breeding ground for political dissent, he prohibited the congregation of Crows in camps.[112] The new agent took a similarly authoritarian approach to gender, sexuality, and family life on the reservation. Although Reynolds's administration was not a complete departure from that of his predecessors, his tenure as agent accelerated many of the pressures facing the Crow Nation and in doing so illuminated connections between diverse federal objectives, including those related to reproduction and family life.

Above all, Reynolds's administration reflected a shift in Indian affairs toward more predatory land policies. During his seven years as superintendent, Reynolds advocated for the rapid completion of tribal allotment, oversaw the Crows' 1904 land cession, and eased the process by which white ranchers and farmers could lease reservation land. These trends could be seen throughout much of Indian Country under Commissioners William Jones and Francis Leupp, resulting in the transfer of hundreds of thousands of acres from Indian to white control.[113] The allotment of Crow land had begun in 1885, two years before Congress passed the General Allotment Act, but the process had proceeded in fits and starts, with progress limited by inadequate resources and Crow resistance.[114] A 1903 Supreme Court decision, combined with the eagerness of encroaching white settlers—the border town of Hardin would be founded in 1907—produced unprecedented land pressures for Crows under Reynolds. In *Lone Wolf v. Hitchcock*, the court ruled that Congress could, in the words of the historian Charles Crane Bradley Jr., "do as it pleased with the reservation" with or without tribal consent, a fact that Commissioner Jones as well as Agent Reynolds regularly emphasized to Crow leaders.[115]

In the eyes of many policy makers, government employees, and social reformers, questions of land were closely related to questions of morality. They expected that policies pertaining to the former would further concomitant objectives regarding cultural and moral "uplift." As the historian Rose Stremlau has demonstrated, social reformers and many policy makers viewed allotment as a means of forcibly reforming Native families. Allotment policies centered on the nuclear family and the "civilized" gender roles that familial model implied.[116] Allotting agents issued allotments to men as heads-of-household, an arrangement that allotment proponents hoped would instill a sense of responsibility in Native men as providers of their families. The arrangement further facilitated a patriarchal and biological line of inheritance that was legible to the colonial bureaucracy. As the allotting agent at Crow realized in the late 1880s and his successors confirmed in subsequent decades, this system was virtually impossible to implement on the Crow Reservation, due to the ease and frequency with which men and women dissolved marital unions and the fluctuating makeup of any given household.[117]

These bureaucratic imperatives served as the backdrop for Reynolds's aggressive approach to what he viewed as the reservation's "grave" moral situation, by which he meant Crows' continued refusal to abide by Euro-American expectations regarding gender and familial arrangements.[118] Reynolds's efforts to shore up the nuclear family included continuing his predecessors' practice of disciplining those who disregarded marriage vows. The superintendent relied on agency farmers—men the OIA had hired to teach Indian men to farm their allotments—to enforce this requirement. He urged farmers to keep "strict watch" on all unions or instances of cohabitation in their district and to send any couples who lived together without a marriage license to the agency immediately, where "proper punishment will be meted out to them." The agent further authorized farmers and tribal policemen to order men or women who had left their partners to return home or face "severe punishment."[119] Reynolds left the specific punishment for these particular infractions unstated; common punitive methods in these years included the denial of resources for individuals and their families and the temporary incarceration of individuals, especially men, who proved uncooperative.

Superintendent Reynolds also intensified his predecessors' "rightful homes" policy, which required that all children live with their biological parents. Missionaries on the reservation helped enforce this policy by rejecting the day school applications of children who lived with their grandparents. These children were thus more likely to have to attend school at some distance from their homes.[120] Two years after arriving at Crow Agency, Reynolds apparently believed that he and his staff had made real progress in eliminating Crow adoption practices. His annual report claimed that "the adoption of children of one family by another is an evil we have completely stamped out during the past year."[121] In retrospect, Reynolds's boast appears comical, as Crow sources offer no indication of change in this regard. In fact, the adoption described above, in which the woman who had recently lost a daughter became so enamored with another young girl that the girl's biological parents encouraged the grieving woman to take their daughter home with her, occurred in 1906 or 1907—a few short years after the agent's declaration of victory, despite Reynolds's continued employment on the reservation.[122] His claim nonetheless underscores his investment in restructuring Crow families.

Allotment—and early twentieth-century land policies more generally—furthered government employees' moral agendas in other ways as well. In the 1860s, many American physicians launched a national campaign to criminalize abortion. The feminist scholar Rosalind Petchesky emphasizes that this was "overwhelmingly a *moral* crusade," rather than a medical initiative, and other scholars have demonstrated that physicians' appeals reflected contemporary gendered and racial politics.[123] The antiabortion campaign was ultimately successful; in Montana Territory, the practice was criminalized in the 1870s.[124] Over the next few decades, government employees, including but not limited to Holder, issued reports lamenting the practice of abortion at Crow and on other reservations. Such reports drew on and perpetuated tropes of Indigenous sexual promiscuity, implicitly or explicitly justified colonial presence and intervention, and diverted blame from colonial policies and processes to women's bodies and behaviors.[125] As in Euro-American assessments of Native biological reproduction more generally, the authors of these reports seldom mention material conditions, which undoubtedly affected women's reproductive decisions.[126] For his part, Agent Reynolds blamed the tribe's precarious land situation not on policies in which he himself was implicated but on Crow women's ability to terminate pregnancies.

In the summer of 1905, Reynolds engaged in a regular correspondence with Commissioner Francis Leupp regarding the progress of allotment on the reservation. One letter stands out and at first glance appears incongruous: "In reply to 'Land,' dated June 30," the agent began, "I beg the honor to say that the *frequent cases of abortion* practiced among these Indians during my time as agent has been a matter that I have given much thought and energy towards stopping."[127] Reynolds reported that through regular appeals to Crow men in council meetings and private conversations, he had presented reproductive and land politics as linked. Aware of Crow men's very real anxieties regarding the tribal land base, Reynolds argued that if Crow women terminated their pregnancies, there would be fewer Crows to receive allotments, resulting in less land for the tribe as well as for any given family.

Walter Q. G. Tucker, the government physician, had a role to play in this effort as well. Tucker had arrived at Crow Agency in 1903 after working for three years on the Rosebud Reservation in South Dakota. Much to his frustration and in contrast to his experience at Rosebud, Tucker quickly learned that Crow women had little interest in his obstetric services, although he reported that, in general, reservation residents were "rapidly learning the value of medical treatment."[128] The obstetric situation thus had not changed significantly since A. B. Holder's tenure in the late 1880s. In contrast to Holder, Tucker conducted no formal investigations while on the Crow Reservation, but Reynolds ensured that the physician dedicated a portion of his time to surveilling women's bodies and especially pregnancies. In his 1905 letter to the commissioner, Reynolds explained that Tucker had spent the "last several months" engaged in detective work. Relying on information provided by "policemen, Indian judges, Indian employees, and his personal friends throughout the tribe," Tucker set himself the task of discovering all pregnancies on the reservation and then visiting the pregnant woman—as well as, Reynolds emphasized, her husband—to make a case for "the importance of raising babies."[129] Although Reynolds does not mention the possibility of punishment, the illegality of abortion in Montana and his eagerness to impose punishments for other infractions make it likely that his and Tucker's many discussions with Crow men and women also included the threat of punitive measures.[130]

Reynolds's missive to his boss in Washington, D.C., is revealing in at least two ways. First, the agent's decision to call on Native men to "use their influence to eliminate this practice" did not occur in a vacuum. Native feminist scholars have demonstrated the extent to which turn-of-the-century federal Indian policy hinged on the destabilization of gender norms on reservations and specifically the imposition of patriarchal relationships.[131] The agent's letter first demonstrates the extent to which government employees viewed land ownership and land politics as the concern of men, even though government documents underscore Crow women's active interest in allotment and other land issues. It then reveals Reynolds's conviction that land provided the pretext for men's increased influence in reproductive matters. While it is not clear what, if any, steps Crow men took in response to the agent's appeals, this would not have been the first time that colonial pressures had spurred Native men to adopt new positions regarding the termination of pregnancy. Decades earlier, the all-male Cherokee Council passed a law that criminalized abortion, imposing a penalty of "fifty lashes" for any woman found guilty of the practice. As the historian Theda Perdue has emphasized, the council's action marks Cherokee men's intrusion into what had to that point been "woman's prerogative."[132] Some Native women have been critical of Native men's interference in this and related reproductive matters during the nineteenth and early twentieth centuries, but others emphasize that all such actions should be understood within the often-desperate context of the times.[133]

Second, years before Crow childbirth came under government purview in any meaningful way, government employees scrutinized Crow women's pregnancies, and colonial processes affected their reproductive experiences. Evidence suggests that women carried more pregnancies to term in the early 1900s than they had in the late 1880s and early 1890s.[134] Regardless of whether Reynolds himself had any influence, Crow men and women were well aware that high fertility was critical for the group's survival. A woman born in the early 1900s later reported that around the time of her birth, elders had encouraged women not to terminate pregnancies both for the good of the tribe and for their family's own security in a period of high infant and child mortality.[135] It is also possible that the gradual spread of Christianity on the reservation altered community members' attitudes toward the termination of pregnancies, but there is no evidence of this in Crow sources until decades later.

Three years after Reynolds's exchange with Leupp, allotment had been completed, and white settlers' seemingly insatiable demand for Crow land continued apace. In February 1908, the OIA sent a representative to pressure Crow leaders to sell all "surplus" land. Although the stresses of recent years had created divisions among tribal leaders, the men who met with the OIA negotiator were united in their opposition to the cession of additional land. Big Medicine, a tribal policeman, framed the issue as follows: "Among my people, many of the women are in a pregnant condition and expect to have healthy children, and we need our land to share and share alike in the making of allotments."[136] Women's role as life givers, their close association with "reproduction, nurturance, growth, and population increase," had long been celebrated in Crow society and was a source of women's status and influence.[137] As Crow men and women looked ahead to the new century, women's reproductive labor appeared as the bulwark that would protect against further colonial encroachments.

AS TRIBAL NATIONS STRUGGLED to adjust to reservation life in the late nineteenth and early twentieth centuries, clan and kinship systems and a vibrant flexible childrearing system functioned as a stabilizing force in Crow society. In the midst of economic and political upheavals, relative cultural and social stability allowed women some continuity in their approach to pregnancy and childbirth. While specific to local contexts, the Native birthing cultures that prevailed at the turn of the century shared many common features, including an understanding of biological reproduction as a social process. Women's historians have warned of the dangers of romanticizing "social childbirth," a caution that is perhaps especially warranted when considering Native reproduction in the early reservation years, as these years were characterized by hardship and loss for many women and their families.[138] Romanticization also runs the risk of implying that birthing cultures were static and that women opposed adaptations, both false assumptions. Nevertheless, all evidence suggests that Crow and many other Native women had faith in their birthing attendants and in female healers more generally in these years.

Although direct government intervention in Native reproduction remained minimal through the turn of the century, the early reservation years altered the circumstances in which Native women experienced biological reproduction. Most immediately, confinement to shrinking boundaries and disruption of subsistence patterns produced severe morbidity and mortality, sparking demoralization and anxiety about the tribe's future. Materially and demographically, the early reservation years placed new pressures on women, whose bodies and behaviors came under increased scrutiny. Government employees, like other Euro-American observers, incorporated reproductive practices into a familiar evolutionary discourse of "savagery" versus "civilization." As Native women and families faced mounting assimilationist pressures, some non-Native observers believed that reproductive norms served as one means of assessing the "progress" of individuals and groups. In the late nineteenth and early twentieth centuries, the ostensibly private domains of home life, childbearing, and childrearing emerged as a touchstone in federal Indian policy.

In the fall of 1908, Lizzie Yellowtail gave birth to her fifth and final child. As her daughter Agnes later recounted, the Yellowtail family was camped at Crow Agency for the annual agricultural fair, so the recently constructed government hospital was "right across the way." Despite this potentially fortuitous proximity, Lizzie did not consider entering the one-room institution for childbirth, nor is there evidence that other women did so in the hospital's first years. Instead, Yellowtail gave birth under circumstances not unlike those of her first delivery two decades earlier.[139] Five years later, Lizzie's oldest daughter, Amy, gave birth to her first child. Amy delivered at home, and her son later emphasized that "there were no doctors or nurses around with their instruments"; a trusted and knowledgeable midwife assisted his mother.[140] In the following years, however, physicians and hospitals would attain increased prominence in the reproductive experiences of some women at Crow and on other reservations. The federal policies and local practices that facilitated this development are the subject of the next chapter.

CHAPTER TWO

To Instill the Hospital Habit

W. W. Scott replaced Samuel G. Reynolds as superintendent of the Crow Reservation in 1909.[1] After four years at Crow Agency, Scott traveled more than 1,000 miles southeast to take up the post of superintendent at the Cheyenne and Arapaho Agency in Oklahoma. His tenure in Oklahoma coincided with a pronatal campaign called Save the Babies, a multipronged Office of Indian Affairs (OIA) effort to combat infant mortality on reservations. The superintendent's correspondence and annual reports illuminate the campaign's three basic components: home visits conducted by field employees; annual baby shows, where medical staff evaluated infants; and the promotion of hospital childbirth. By mid-decade, Scott noted with satisfaction that Cheyenne and Arapaho women had come to understand that their housekeeping and mothering skills were under "constant inspection."[2] These same women proved less compliant when it came to Scott's effort to persuade them to eschew midwives. Much to the superintendent's frustration, virtually all women resisted pressures to give birth in the hospital throughout the decade.[3]

OIA employees carried out some version of these initiatives on reservations throughout the West beginning in 1912 and often extending beyond the official conclusion of Save the Babies in 1918. The pronatal campaign was part of a national—indeed, international—movement for infant and maternal health during the Progressive Era. This movement took on a distinctive cast in colonial settings, as European and American powers displayed a growing investment in the management of colonial populations.[4] As the historian Lynn M. Thomas has argued, early twentieth-century pronatalism exemplified the dual moral and material objectives of colonial rule.[5] In the United States, growing awareness of high Native infant mortality prompted something of an existential crisis for the OIA. "We cannot solve the Indian problem without Indians," one commissioner of Indian affairs declared on more than one occasion.[6] The Save the Babies campaign—the OIA's proposed solution to the problem of Indian infant mortality—dovetailed with and furthered the federal government's ongoing assimilationist agenda. Although one of the campaign's defining characteristics was its uneven and sometimes sparse implementation, in this chapter I present Save the Babies as a cornerstone of early twentieth-century federal Indian policy.[7] In addition to saving infant life, OIA officials and many reservation employees envisioned a transformation in Native childrearing, birthing, and familial arrangements, all of which required a transformation in the attitudes and practices of Native women.[8]

Cheyenne, Arapaho, and other Native women's reproductive experiences in the first decades of the century were shaped to varying degrees by both infant morbidity and mortality and the OIA's sluggish response to this suffering. For Native women and families, infant mortality, which on some reservations had climbed rapidly and in other locations had begun a slow decline, was a personal tragedy. At a moment when the American Indian population was near its nadir, high infant mortality, combined with other health crises on reservations, also represented a collective tragedy that was often intensely felt at the tribal level.[9] For the mothers targeted by OIA pronatalism, Save the Babies was a double-edged campaign that at its best brought some degree of assistance in improving the health of their families but that also brought heightened scrutiny and false promises. The campaign's initiative likely improved the health of some Native women, but as the sociologist Barbara Gurr has argued, Save the Babies relegated women's health "to a secondary status in relation to potential or real children."[10]

Most importantly for this study, the OIA's pronatal campaign served as the context for the office's concerted promotion of medicalized pregnancy and childbirth, the latter ideally in a hospital setting.[11] Although this component of the Save the Babies campaign has received the least scholarly attention, it had the longest-lasting and farthest-reaching consequences. Indian Service officials increasingly presented hospital childbirth as a panacea for reservation infant mortality and other indicators of poor health—one that dovetailed with assimilationist objectives regarding the eradication of Native health ways and the diminished influence of elders and extended kin networks. Yet as with so much of federal Indian policy during the Progressive Era, the vision presented in OIA and social reform records outpaced the Indian Service's bureaucratic and institutional capacities, which meant that Native women received messages of medicalized reproduction and hospital childbirth before they experienced notable changes in birthing. Most women continued to deliver their children under circumstances that were familiar to them, even as some began to selectively incorporate aspects of the federal government's expanding health services. Nevertheless, the beginning of what would become a notable change was under way. The chapter concludes by considering the experiences of the minority of Native women who accepted hospital obstetric services as soon as government employees began promoting them. As maternity patients, women revealed the limitations of these federal institutions, but they also disrupted the OIA's vision of how a hospital should look, how it should sound, and how it should function.

Progressive Pronatalism in Indian Country

By the turn of the twentieth century, the poor health conditions that had plagued some reservations for decades had become difficult for both the OIA and its critics to ignore. Surveys and statistics, favored technologies of progressive Americans within and outside the Indian Service, demonstrated that reservations suffered rates of illness and disease that surpassed those of their white neighbors. These studies further demonstrated that despite the establishment of a rudimentary medical infrastructure, conditions were not improving; if anything, they were deteriorating.[12] Although OIA employees typically attributed poor health outcomes to tribal "customs" and the alleged primitivism of "medicine men" rather than colonization and federal policies, they nonetheless recognized that the prevailing health situation hindered their assimilation agenda at a moment when many policy makers and bureaucrats hoped to accelerate the assimilation of Native peoples.[13] In response to these dire findings, the OIA launched health campaigns targeting tuberculosis, trachoma, and infant mortality.

The historian Diane T. Putney has demonstrated that progressivism, although frequently associated with urban settings, permeated the Indian Service and gave federal Indian policy new "respectability" in the early twentieth century.[14] Nowhere is this more evident than in the OIA's health campaigns, which reflected the era's faith in the transformative power of education and the authority of experts and ostensibly objective science. OIA health campaigns further reflected federal and state governments' increasingly explicit investment in the well-being of the nation's citizens — or in the case of Native Americans, "wards" and "future citizens" — an investment that manifested in an expansion of public policy.[15] Because tuberculosis and trachoma disproportionately affected Native peoples in the early twentieth century, these campaigns arguably foregrounded Indians' conceptual and physical distance from the mainstream. The campaign to combat infant mortality, in contrast, linked Indian Country to a broader progressive movement for infant health.

In the United States, a flurry of activity signaled an unprecedented level of attention to infant welfare. The White House sponsored the Conference on the Care of Dependent Children in 1909, the American Association for the Study and Prevention of Infant Mortality held its first meeting in 1910, and the U.S. Children's Bureau was founded in 1912, immediately launching a series of studies that investigated infant mortality.[16] These developments were driven in part by the demands of middle- and upper-class women who were determined to make their private sorrows a matter of public policy, and in part by the development of reasonably reliable methods of measuring infant mortality, which public health officials recognized as a sensitive indicator of community health. Infant mortality rates (IMRs) seemed to provide objective data on the problem that could then be solved through scientific means, and the global use of this measure facilitated comparisons that further galvanized sectors of the American public. Early Children's Bureau investigations determined, for example, that the United States lagged behind most other industrialized nations — ranking eleventh of twenty — in infant mortality and lagged still further in maternal mortality.[17]

Domestic comparisons were equally illuminating. In contrast to Europe, where public health officials typically measured mortality rates by socioeconomic position, Americans tended to view infant mortality (and so much else) through a racial prism. As a result, mortality rates functioned to buttress and reify racial stereotypes. Near the turn of the century, for example, the statistician Frederick Ludwig Hoffman documented the disproportionate IMRs in southern black communities; Hoffman attributed this disparity to "race traits."[18] By and large, however, public health officials and humanitarian organizations ignored black infant mortality. Instead, they associated the problem with the urban immigrant poor and attributed it to some combination of ignorance, backwardness, and poverty.[19]

Public health officials and social reformers discovered and began to publicize rural infant mortality in the late 1910s, but the Indian Service's open discussion of infant mortality on reservations preceded this development by a few years.[20] OIA inspectors and reservation field staff reported high, though typically unquantified, infant mortality in the years after the turn of the century. Such reports culminated in a circular that Commissioner of Indian Affairs Robert G. Valentine distributed in 1912, calling on OIA employees to "take immediate emergency measures to greatly reduce infant mortality. Save the babies."[21] The commissioner's directive marked the start of the OIA's Save the Babies campaign, as well as the start of the office's concerted effort to scientifically determine the scope of infant mortality on reservations. Valentine, a consummate progressive, recognized the utility of IMRs in securing much-needed funding for Indian health services.[22] In a special message to Congress in 1912, President William Howard Taft singled out infant mortality despite the lack of precision that surrounded the issue. "No exact figures are yet available for infant mortality among Indians," Taft declared, "but field studies now being made show that while proportionately more Indian babies than white babies are born, very many more Indian babies die."[23] The intensive focus on acquiring data on infant mortality stands in contrast to the lack of statistical data on Native maternal mortality in these years and throughout the decade.[24] This omission is striking given the fact that by 1916, child welfare advocates at the Children's Bureau argued that "maternal mortality is a part of the problem of infant mortality."[25]

Exact figures on infant mortality remained difficult to come by, as reservation-level data were spotty at best. After a visit to the Crow Reservation, for example, Supervisor of Field Matrons Elsie Newton reported, "The figures for infant mortality are not readily obtainable and are unreliable." The reports on many reservations remained speculative rather than statistical.[26] Field matrons began compiling mortality statistics—with varying reliability—as part of their official responsibilities in 1914.[27] By mid-decade, Assistant Medical Supervisor Ferdinand Shoemaker reported startling mortality rates on many reservations. On the Cheyenne River Reservation in South Dakota, Shoemaker cited the mortality rate for infants and young children under three years of age as 150 per 1,000 births. Immediately north of Cheyenne River, families on the Standing Rock Reservation endured still greater losses, as Shoemaker alleged that the mortality rate for the same demographic was 596 per 1,000.[28] A year earlier, the National Center for Health Statistics had estimated that the national IMR was 92.8 per 1,000 for whites and 149.7 for nonwhites.[29] These rates cannot be compared directly with Shoemaker's figures because the National Center for Health Statistics measured deaths within the first year, while Shoemaker extended his scope to age three. One year was a common marker for infant mortality off reservations, but OIA officials and employees often used three or five years. Any explanation of this choice is necessarily speculative, but it may reflect some acknowledgment that trends in infant morbidity and mortality differed for white and Indian children; toddlerhood and early childhood proved as dangerous to the latter group as the first days or months of life.

Reservation-level surveys led Valentine's successor, Cato Sells, to the oft-repeated conclusion that "approximately three-fifths of the Indian infants die before the age of 5 years."[30] Sells's figure demands some skepticism given the inadequacy of available data, notable regional variation, and the utility of IMRs in securing funding and justifying the wide-ranging interventions described below. Nonetheless, the gravity of the situation on reservations ravaged by malnutrition, illness, decreased mobility, and the suppression of cultural practices is indisputable, and it is at least as plausible that infant deaths were underreported in some locations because of dispersed settlement and continued mobility. Human stories reveal the reality of Native infant mortality as powerfully as statistics. In the Southwest, a Pima woman named Molly Moore gave birth to eleven children in the decades surrounding the turn of the century. Only five survived childhood.[31] For Ojibwe women on the Lac Courte Oreilles Reservation in Wisconsin, the loss of multiple children was a common experience, and some families buried as many as six or seven infants.[32] For these and other Native women, the loss of an infant's life was a cause for grief and sorrow, emotions that were expressed differently in different communities. Such emotions are evoked, however, by one Euro-American observer who married a Native man and lived for a time on a reservation; she later vividly recalled hearing "the bitter wail across the night" when a mother lost a child.[33]

By mid-decade, Commissioner Sells had come to view the OIA's pronatal initiatives as a struggle for "the rescue of a race."[34] Between his appointment in 1913 and early 1916, Sells gradually expanded his predecessor's campaign.[35] He did so with the encouragement of Supervisor Newton, who recognized the potential of a baby-saving campaign to increase the professionalism of the field matron corps and the program's status within the OIA.[36] In a letter to all OIA employees in early 1916, Sells enumerated a central role for field matrons, whom he viewed as uniquely suited to the task owing to their "motherly solicitude."[37] Employees on many reservations followed the commissioner's lead. "The field matrons have charge of the Save the Babies campaign," a physician at Crow Agency reported the same year.[38] The field matron program had already been growing as a result of early twentieth-century health campaigns, and many reservations received their first field matron during Save the Babies. Yet other reservations, including Standing Rock, where more than half of all infants reportedly died before three years of age, had no field matron for years at a time in the 1910s, and the field matron's centrality to OIA pronatalism is arguably demonstrated more clearly by her absence than her presence. When Dr. Ferdinand Shoemaker visited Standing Rock at the height of the pronatal campaign, he reported that there was "no particular effort being made to control or reduce the high infant mortality rate." Shoemaker attributed this lackluster implementation to the absence of a woman who could earn reservation women's trust through intimate exchanges.[39]

The field matron program, created in 1890, exemplified the OIA's investment in maternalism. The program brought hundreds of Euro-American women into the federal bureaucracy to serve the government's interests by guiding Native women and children to civilization through instruction and example.[40] The earliest field matrons were charged with imparting lessons in "civilized" domesticity and Victorian gender norms. The program underwent two important changes in subsequent decades. First, while a handful of educated Native women worked as field matrons in the program's first years, some policy makers, social reformers, and reservation employees were skeptical of Native women's capacity for this civilizing work. Pessimism grew after the turn of the century, and Native women's participation in the program declined after 1905.[41] Thus, when Sells singled out "the field matron with her motherly solicitude" in 1916, he most likely took for granted that the field matron was a white woman.[42] Second, although field matrons' efforts to encourage "attractive homemaking" did not disappear after the turn of the century, in the midst of health crises and inadequate government medical services, many field matrons gradually shifted their focus to the provision of basic nursing care and lessons in sanitation and hygiene. This shift was institutionalized in 1911 when Commissioner Valentine moved the field matron program from the Industrial Division to the Medical Division.[43]

Building on this short history, during the Save the Babies campaign OIA officials charged field matrons with teaching Native women "the simplest rules of motherhood."[44] Commissioner Sells believed that ignorance of such rules was responsible for the many Indian infants "who annually fill untimely graves," and this conviction was echoed in the field. One field matron reported, "Ignorance on every hand was the prime factor in the piling up of infant mortalities."[45] This almost exclusive focus on maternal ignorance rather than structural factors was certainly self-serving, but it was also in keeping with prevailing opinion in infant welfare circles. By the 1910s, public health officials and others invested in the infant welfare movement had come to define infant mortality as "a problem of motherhood."[46] In an influential 1906 treatise entitled *Infant Mortality: A Social Problem*, the English physician George Newman argued that the "problem of infant mortality is not one of sanitation alone, or housing, or indeed poverty as such, *but it is mainly a question of motherhood*."[47] The allure of this diagnosis for progressive infant welfare advocates was both its all-encompassing nature—environmental surroundings, nutrition, even material conditions to some degree could be subsumed under the umbrella of maternal culpability—and the relatively simple prescription it presented of maternal education. The diagnosis and prescription had particular appeal for Valentine, Sells, and employees within the growing bureaucracy of Indian affairs because it diverted blame for IMRs from colonial processes and OIA policies to the bodies and behaviors of Indian mothers.

Throughout the 1910s, Native mothers and women of childbearing age who lived on a reservation with one or more field matrons could expect a female field employee to make regular visits to their homes, where the government representative would preach the gospel of "scientific motherhood." Where government field staff was lacking or inadequate, female missionaries often filled the gaps and promoted complementary messages. As Lisa Emmerich has defined it, scientific motherhood in this context "blended Euro-American gender ideology, family norms, and Westernized medical care."[48] Depending on the personalities of both parties and the field matron's tactics, such visits may have been experienced as intrusive, tolerable, or welcome. If a mother was interested, or if she simply wanted a social outlet, she might attend mothers' meetings organized by a field matron or female missionary or enter her infant in the baby shows the OIA sponsored at annual Indian agricultural fairs, where she would receive further instruction.

By mid-decade, state hygiene bureaus, the Children's Bureau, and private organizations had begun sponsoring baby contests, and Supervisor Newton and Commissioner Sells believed similar events on or near reservations presented an ideal opportunity to showcase the OIA's work in promoting assimilation and saving babies.[49] Just as off-reservation baby shows revealed linkages between the infant welfare and eugenics movements, the infants — or, more accurately, mothers — who received prizes at reservation baby shows displayed more than just healthfulness.[50] One superintendent proudly reported, for example, that the blue ribbon at a recent baby show had gone to the "prettiest, cleanest, neatest, fattest, and best behaved" infant.[51] As Lisa Emmerich and Mary Klann have both observed, physicians and other employees who served as judges favored mothers and babies who exhibited outward markers of assimilation.[52]

Armed with such iconic progressive texts as Luther Emmett Holt's *The Care and Feeding of Children* and the Children's Bureau's *Prenatal Care* and *Infant Care*, as well as the OIA's own publications regarding infant welfare, field matrons endeavored to transform Native women into "scientific mothers."[53] This required that Native women discard old customs, such as placing their children in cradleboards — or what one superintendent referred to as "tight bound native containers."[54] It also required that they eschew old sources of

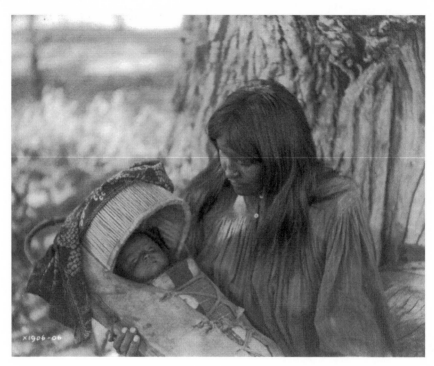

Mizheh and Babe, 1906. Field matrons generally disparaged the cradleboards this Apache mother and other Native women used to hold their infants. LC-USZ62–46949, Curtis Collection, Prints and Photographs Division, Library of Congress (Washington, D.C.).

reproductive knowledge, namely grandmothers and other female kin. In their place, mothers were to adopt "modern" methods of childrearing.

The translation of these constantly evolving modern ideas to rural reservations was sometimes confusing for all involved. Feeding practices offer a good example. On and off reservations, most physicians, public health authorities, and other vested parties generally agreed that "improper feeding" was a primary cause of infant mortality, but experts had not reached consensus as to what proper feeding in the first year of life entailed by the time the OIA launched Save the Babies.[55] Most physicians believed the mother's milk was, in Luther Emmett Holt's words, the "best infant food," but the apparent scientific precision offered by artificial feeding made it increasingly attractive to mothers and doctors alike. Many also conjectured that modernity placed pressures on the bodies of "civilized" women that made it necessary for them to supplement their milk with formula or cow's milk.[56] So-called primitive mothers were ostensibly free from such bodily strain, but some

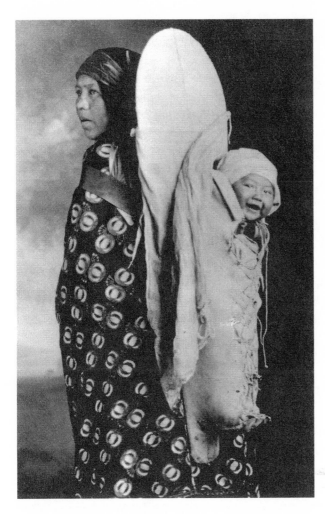

Ellen Kallowat Kenmille (Kootenai) carries her nephew Camille Kenmille in a cradleboard. The 1916 photograph underscores the active role played by aunts, as well as other female kin, in daily child care. Catalog number 955-490, Legacy Photograph Collection, Montana Historical Society (Helena, Montana).

field workers on reservations recognized that the ill health facing many Native women in the early twentieth century potentially compromised their capacity for lactation.[57] Field staff on many reservations first discouraged breastfeeding, which they presented as a backward and "barbaric" practice but quickly reversed course because of the difficulty of ensuring access to formula or cow's milk and adequate sanitation in its preparation.[58] In 1916, Ferdinand Shoemaker disapprovingly noted that many Lakota mothers artificially fed their babies. With little sense of irony, Shoemaker presented this as yet another "custom among the Indian women [that] should be combated in every possible way," as it was another means by which mothers brought "a great deal of harm" to their infants.[59]

Native women came under further scrutiny and criticism for the non-nuclear structure of their families and the "flexible childrearing" systems that allowed for shared maternal—and parental—labor in many societies. Despite the insistence of successive commissioners as well as many reservation employees that Indian mothers loved their children, the trope of the apathetic or indifferent mother undergirded allegations of maternal ignorance.[60] Reservation employees generally disregarded or attempted to undermine the grandmothers who often played a significant role in childrearing because grandmothers were viewed as obstacles to progress and their childrearing labor deviated from the ideal nuclear unit the OIA and social reformers promoted. The regular reports from the field describing government employees' efforts to instill maternal "interest" in the care of their babies attest to the OIA's continued disapproval of flexible childrearing and the office's view of the campaign as a tool for undermining it.[61] For Native families, however, some version of flexible childrearing remained as important as ever owing to economic pressures and high reservation morbidity and mortality, in which women of childbearing age were especially vulnerable.

To date, scholarship on Save the Babies has focused on home visits, mothers' clubs and meetings, and baby shows, and in all these activities, the field matron loomed large. Yet field matrons' centrality in the progressive campaign to combat infant mortality—and within the OIA more generally—was somewhat anomalous. Field matrons had no consistent training at a moment when the Indian Service was increasingly embracing professionalism and expertise.[62] For all her work with mothers and families within the home, perhaps no role the field matron performed was more important than the one Commissioner Valentine highlighted a year before the onset of Save the Babies: "The field matrons . . . prepare the way for physicians."[63] Maternalism paved the way for medicalization. Among the many messages field matrons imparted to Native women and mothers was the necessity of seeking the guidance of physicians, rather than Native healers or female kin, in matters regarding their own and their family's health. The OIA relied on field matrons to persuade mothers and other family members to accept a visit from a field physician or to journey to the reservation hospital when a young child was ill. It was often field matrons who organized and promoted baby shows, where infants were inspected and mothers evaluated by government physicians.

As the OIA's emphasis on infant welfare expanded to include prenatal care, the field matron played an important intermediary role here as well.

Field matrons offered pregnant women physician-approved advice on self-care and encouraged physician supervision of their pregnancies. Shortly after assuming office, Sells authorized all field employees, including field matrons, to arrange for the provision of additional rations, such as sweetened condensed milk, for parturient women and mothers with small children whom field staff believed would otherwise be insufficiently nourished. This provided some women with crucial nutritional support, and it offered field employees one means of ensuring physician supervision, as the extra rations came with significant strings attached. Sells specified that the rations should be contingent on the mothers "present[ing] themselves and their babies to the physician for examination, treatment and advice at each issuance of rations" and following the advice of government employees' child care instructions.[64] Finally, the OIA expected field matrons to urge all pregnant women to make proper arrangements for their deliveries, which typically meant securing a physician's assistance and increasingly meant entering a government hospital. Field matrons also sometimes served as intermediary birth attendants, "prepar[ing] the way" for women's acceptance of the physician's presence in their birthing spaces.[65]

Medicalizing Childbirth

By the mid-1910s, Commissioner Sells had come to believe that changing the social circumstances and location in which women gave birth was a critical step in saving Indian babies. Government physicians had been attending some reservation births since the turn of the century, but their reports affirm women's historians' observation that as long as birthing remained in the home, women and families maintained a significant degree of control over the process.[66] Physician-assisted birth, preferably in hospitals, became the OIA's official policy during the progressive pronatal campaign. Although the least-studied component of Save the Babies, the Indian Service's attempt to bring Native birthing under government purview was one of the campaign's most enduring legacies.

Sells began advocating hospital childbirth in late 1915 and enumerated his instructions to employees the following January.[67] The commissioner urged that "every Indian hospital bed not necessarily occupied with those suffering from disease or injury should be made available for the mother in childbirth." Before closing the letter, he circled back to this directive two more times, adding a few qualifications. Hospital childbirth should be arranged "if practicable," particularly when "the home surroundings are unfavourable."[68] When such arrangements were not possible, a physician or field matron should attend the birth. The commissioner's enthusiasm for hospital childbirth only grew in subsequent years, and qualifications and equivocations became fewer and farther between. The following spring, he chided employees, "I am sure . . . there are many beds available that could be used" for mothers during confinement. Shortly thereafter, he approvingly noted the "policy" of "bringing every possible case of confinement to the agency hospitals for the lying-in period."[69] As with other aspects of the Save the Babies campaign, Sells requested regular progress reports from the field, and employees often echoed their commissioner. In a typical example, after a visit to the Flathead Reservation in Montana, an OIA inspector reported that "expectant mothers are constantly being urged to accept hospital conveniences." Such prodding came from virtually every government employee with whom women came in contact.[70]

The OIA's concerted push for hospital childbirth would scarcely have been possible a decade earlier. In 1900, the federal government operated only five hospitals on reservations, but early twentieth-century health campaigns prompted a surge in construction. By 1911, the number of government-operated reservation hospitals had grown to fifty. That year, Congress appropriated funding specifically for Indian health services, and such appropriations continued in subsequent years. In 1918, the OIA operated eighty-seven Indian hospitals and employed twice as many physicians as it had two decades earlier.[71] The campaign to combat infant mortality helped grow the medical infrastructure on reservations. Not only did President Taft emphasize infant deaths in his special message to Congress; at the local level, OIA employees foregrounded infant and child welfare in their requests for hospitals and increased health services. In recommending the construction of a hospital on one reservation, Walter G. West, an OIA inspector, argued that "the infantile mortality would be reduced by half."[72]

The urgency with which Sells promoted the hospital as the ideal location for childbirth speaks to the institution's evolving image in early twentieth-century America. As the historian Charles Rosenberg has demonstrated, between the end of the Civil War and the first decades of the twentieth century, hospitals slowly but steadily gained broader acceptance in American society.[73] In the spring of 1916, S. A. M. Young, the superintendent in charge at the Navajo Agency in Arizona, sent a telegram to Sells boasting that three infants had been born at the agency hospital the previous night and that five women were in the hospital awaiting labor: "can you beat it[?]" Sells in fact could not beat it, replying with equal enthusiasm the following day, "This is splendid and foretells a happy awakening sure to accomplish gratifying results in preserving the health and lives of the mothers and babies."[74] The commissioner's response reveals his confidence that the hospital was a safer location for childbirth than a tent, tepee, or hogan.

He was likely genuine in this view, and he certainly was not alone. Middle-class white women began to embrace hospital childbirth in these years for the very same reasons, a trend that rapidly accelerated in subsequent decades.[75] Mary Mills West, the mother of five who authored the Children's Bureau's 1915 *Prenatal Care*, asserted, "There can be no doubt that it is safer."[76] While West pointed to the hospital's equipment and staff on hand in the event of an emergency as evidence of superior safety, growing awareness of germs and germ transmission led others, particularly physicians and public health officers, to favor the hospital for its ostensibly superior sanitation. Hospitals even began to market themselves in this way—as "a super-clean, germ-free place, safer than the home."[77] Sanitation-related arguments resonated among OIA personnel, who blamed insanitary surroundings, alongside Native ignorance, as the cause not only of infant morbidity and mortality but also of other poor health outcomes on reservations. Thus, Sells celebrated hospital childbirth as giving Indian children "a start in life that would have been impossible had their birth been consummated under the old unhygienic environments."[78] Faith in the hospital's superior sanitation and safety on and off reservations far surpassed demonstrated outcomes in these years, and physicians certainly had additional motivations for encouraging this transition. But such qualifications do not negate the very real power of this emerging consensus.[79]

The commissioner's reference to the Navajo mothers' "happy awakening" also hints at what he and others viewed as the hospital's potential for both marking and facilitating progress toward assimilation. Indian Service officials and employees almost universally agreed that Native healers—especially the "medicine man"—hindered assimilation, and one function of the new hospitals was to diminish their influence.[80] Recognizing the important role women played in the provision of their family's health care, Sells urged his employees to focus their efforts on convincing women of the value of hospital care for themselves and their children, and he believed that the lying-in period presented the best opportunity "to make an impression on the Indian mother and obtain her confidence."[81] He and others hoped that gaining a woman's confidence during such a pivotal event as her child's birth would have long-lasting consequences.

There were other lessons to be learned within hospital walls, and OIA officials and employees believed that the hospital's function as an educational setting was especially critical for childbearing women. From Sells's perspective, a woman who opted to give birth in a hospital rather than a tent already signaled her acceptance of science over the supernatural or superstitious. During her confinement, hospital staff provided further instruction in scientific motherhood. Nurses, matrons, and even physicians offered lectures and demonstrations in bathing and feeding infants, as well as admonitions to visit the hospital for exams and in the case of illness. In other words, they delivered messages regarding sanitation and child care that resembled those that field matrons and other employees imparted in women's homes. One superintendent emphasized the need for lengthy confinement periods, as he and the physicians on his reservation feared that ad hoc home instruction did little good. In the hospital, by contrast, mother and child were "under the personal direction of the Physician."[82]

Ultimately, OIA officials and employees expected that hospital childbirth would displace Native midwifery. Two decades earlier, Euro-American observers had commented favorably on the skill of Indian midwives, but positive assessments were expressed less frequently after the turn of the century.[83] Nationally, antimidwifery sentiment reached its zenith during the 1910s, the very years in which the OIA embarked on its multipronged campaign to combat infant mortality.[84] Outside reservation boundaries, physicians and especially obstetricians began to speak and write about "the midwife problem" in ways that resonated with a host of cultural anxieties.[85] Amid growing public concern regarding infant and maternal health, physicians and other social commentators placed the blame at the hands of the "uneducated," "ignorant" midwife, although this wholesale condemnation was generally not supported by available evidence.[86] Physicians' antipathy toward midwives also became intertwined with the medical community's ongoing antiabortion campaign. Although abortion had been criminalized decades earlier, women of all races and classes continued to terminate undesirable pregnancies, a trend that was particularly unsettling for those already disturbed by changing social and sexual mores. By alleging that midwives bore responsibility for the continued practice of abortion, antiabortionists downplayed physicians' complicity and presented midwives as dangerous not only for the nation's health but also for its morals.[87] Finally, the ignorant, immoral midwife who was evoked in Progressive Era medical literature and popular culture had a specific identity: she was almost always an immigrant. Reflecting rising anti-immigrant sentiment, the midwife's opponents further characterized her as "back-ward" and "un-American."[88]

Indian Service officials and employees were not isolated from these cultural trends. In fact, for the above reasons and more, antimidwifery sentiment proved alluring for those working in Indian affairs. Although the midwife's leading national critics hailed from urban centers and paid little attention to Native midwives on rural, predominantly western, reservations, their insistence that the midwife was "a remnant of barbaric times, a blot on our civilization" resonated powerfully among OIA personnel committed to an assimilationist mission.[89] Much like diagnoses of maternal ignorance, the trope of the ignorant or even nefarious midwife functioned to transform a complicated and very real problem into a matter of individual culpability. In reporting Cheyenne and Arapaho women's resistance to hospital childbirth, Superintendent W. W. Scott condemned local midwives, alleging that they were "responsible for deaths without number, among the children."[90] Scott was one of many employees in the field who felt that older women's authority in reproductive matters, much like their influence in family life more generally, hindered OIA objectives. Condemnation of Native midwives reverberates in the reports and correspondence of some, although not all, OIA employees, providing a sense of the messages many Native women received during home visits, baby shows, and other exchanges with government personnel.

Yet it is nonetheless notable that the official OIA messaging surrounding the Save the Babies campaign—in the form of circulars to employees and commissioner's speeches and reports—rarely mentioned Native midwifery or midwives directly. For all his emphasis on the trained physician "with his science" and the superiority of hospital childbirth, Commissioner Sells seldom singled out midwives for opprobrium.[91] This reticence is in stark contrast to the OIA's aggressive campaign in these years against male healers, or "medicine men," whose curative work was often more visible and diverged more sharply from Western medical practices. Government employees recognized the threat male healers posed to the OIA's religious objectives, while most overlooked or de-emphasized the spiritual component of female healers' and midwives' work. Since the 1890s, the campaign against medicine men had been formalized through regulations that criminalized the rites and rituals of these healers.[92] The OIA's growing concern about Native midwives after the turn of the century was dwarfed by the perceived urgent demand of combating the "evil" of the "superstitious" "fakers" who hindered their tribe's progress toward civilization.[93] When Commissioner Sells declared in

1916 that "the antipathy of the Indian woman to the white man's hospital is fast being overcome," the optimistic prediction that followed was that "the medicine man"—not the midwife—"will soon be only a memory."[94]

Sells and many of his employees recognized that the desired transformation in birthing would not—could not—happen immediately, if for no other reason than that the OIA lacked the necessary manpower, funding, and facilities to execute it. Even as Sells and others presented hospital childbirth as central to the OIA's pronatal agenda, the opportunity remained out of reach for many, likely most, Native women in the 1910s, regardless of their desires. The ongoing boon in hospital construction notwithstanding, many reservations remained without a viable hospital, despite repeated pleas by reservation employees and in many cases by Native peoples themselves.[95] Still others had hospitals that could not meet the needs of dispersed populations. In the Southwest, the forty-bed hospital at Fort Defiance, initially a school hospital, began serving the general Navajo population during the Save the Babies campaign. The institution's two-bed maternity ward could hope to serve only a small portion of women on such a large and populous reservation.[96] The hospital on the Turtle Mountain Reservation in northern North Dakota had been constructed for the use of tubercular patients, but in response to Sells's urging, the hospital staff set aside one room for birthing. The small maternity "ward" was in fact intended to serve as employee living quarters, but the employment of a husband and wife as laborer and cook freed up space and allowed this accommodation.[97]

Faced with a notable gap between the directives they received in OIA circulars and correspondence and the realities they encountered on the ground, some reservation employees devised localized—and explicitly temporary—solutions. Peter Paquette, superintendent of the Fort Defiance School and Agency during the Save the Babies campaign, experimented with an ad hoc training system that he viewed as a compromise measure. Paquette, a man of Ho-Chunk and French heritage, was ruthless in his condemnation and prosecution of Navajo medicine men but took a different approach toward birthing.[98] "Our Indians are such a large tribe and so widely scattered," he explained, "that for many years they will depend on midwives." Paquette believed that the best option was to facilitate better, more scientific midwifery: "In the camp," the superintendent argued, "the Indian girls learn the wrong way to care for labor cases." To "offset this training," Paquette arranged for some of the older female students to "attend and take care of a labor case under the Physician. This way they obtain a knowledge of the right way these cases should be managed." Similar efforts occurred informally in other locations; more than two decades later, field workers continued to deem it necessary to coordinate in various ways with Native midwives, particularly those who met employees' expectations of education or competence.[99]

Paquette's experiment mirrored more formalized efforts in other colonial contexts in these years. In British and other European colonies in Africa and the Pacific, colonizing governments and missionaries trained young Indigenous birth attendants, whom they hoped would displace older women's role in the birthing process. Indigenous communities often viewed such training programs with skepticism, at least initially. To receive training as a birthing attendant, young women typically had to leave their homes and communities to attend school. Furthermore, administrators' deliberate targeting of youth—women who in most cases had not given birth themselves—upset many societies' understandings of the social order surrounding childbirth.[100] On the Navajo Reservation, the very limited training efforts Paquette described represent a similar disruption in the generational hierarchies surrounding biological reproduction.

By and large, however, the fragmentary record that remains of government midwifery training at Fort Defiance represents a path not taken. In American colonies such as Guam, colonial administrators implemented training programs comparable to their European counterparts.[101] The OIA did not do so on reservations. Although a handful of Indian boarding schools established nurses' aide programs, and although in subsequent decades the Indian Service took limited steps to encourage Native women to become nurses, there is little evidence that boarding schools provided notable obstetrics training or that midwifery significantly factored into OIA attempts to incentivize nursing training. Nor did the OIA follow the footsteps of European colonial powers—or the U.S. Navy in the Pacific—in implementing licensing programs so that young and old midwives could be monitored, regulated, and, in some cases, disciplined.

On the U.S. mainland, policy makers' and social reformers' expectation that Native peoples would be culturally assimilated left many impatient with steps that would prolong the desired assimilation process. Furthermore, the growing medical apparatus on many reservations led policy makers and Indian Service officials to believe that the elimination of Native healing practices, including those surrounding biological reproduction, was not only feasible but inevitable. But the contrast in approaches to Indigenous midwifery also reflects divergent national trajectories. While European domestic policies generally encouraged the maintenance of an educated and regulated midwifery class, many American physicians and social commentators disapproved of any efforts that would prolong the midwife's abolition.[102] In the decade after the Save the Babies campaign, the Sheppard-Towner Act allowed for midwife education and licensing in some regions, but the program was short-lived and underfunded.[103]

At least one Euro-American observer believed that the Indian Service did not confront Native midwifery with enough urgency. Grace Coolidge, the white wife of an Arapaho Episcopal priest who lived for a time on the Wind River Reservation in Wyoming, felt so strongly about the need to eliminate Indian midwives that she advocated the passage of a law that required a "reputable" physician's attendance at childbirth. Coolidge argued that coercion was necessary in this case, just as she believed it was necessary for the Indian Service to compel Indian children to attend school.[104] The legality of midwifery—on and off reservations—indeed became murkier in the following years, as lawmakers passed legislation to regulate the practice on a state-by-state basis.[105] Through the duration of the Save the Babies campaign and beyond, however, Sells and his successors generally preferred that OIA employees rely on moral suasion and education. In the short term, the OIA's reliance on the art of persuasion invited a range of responses from Native women.

Resistance and Negotiation

Women's historians have revised earlier historical narratives that presented childbirth's gradual move into the hospital as an imposition by a male medical class determined to diminish women's control over their bodies and reproductive experiences.[106] Judith Walzer Leavitt, for example, has argued that the transition to hospital childbirth occurred because of the convergence of physicians' evolving preferences and middle- and upper-class white women's ongoing quest for safer and less painful birthing experiences.[107] There is no question that Native women experienced these trends differently than the women at the center of Leavitt's analysis. The coercive power of the federal government was a daily reality for women on reservations, and the steady pressure government employees exerted regarding the medicalization of pregnancy and childbirth had few parallels outside of Indian Country. Yet on the specific question of where and with whom they would deliver their babies, Native women made intentional and often creative decisions. As Anne Perez Hattori observed in her study of Chamorro peoples' engagement with U.S. hospitals and health services in Guam, "In between the poles of acceptance and resistance is a wide spectrum of possibilities."[108]

The size of many reservations, the dispersed populations, and the inadequacy of OIA infrastructure meant that most Native women continued to give birth under circumstances not unlike those of older female kin. Some women welcomed government employees into their birthing spaces. Paiute women on the Pyramid Lake Reservation in Nevada, for example, invited field matron Janette Woodruff "to be present at nearly all confinements." These women viewed Woodruff's presence as appropriate because of her gender; birthing remained an occasion "for women only." Yet Woodruff had no role to play in Paiute deliveries—"I was not trusted with the responsibility"—because older Paiute women performed all midwifery work.[109] Women on other reservations accepted or invited a more active role from field matrons. Southern Ute women in Colorado sought field matrons' assistance in childbirth in the 1910s. As Katherine M. B. Osburn explains, Ute women "received field matrons on Ute terms, accepting them in traditional female roles as healers and midwives."[110] Their receptiveness to field matrons stood in contrast to their resistance to male government doctors, whose presence laboring women refused until the late 1920s.[111]

Gendered restrictions surrounding childbirth in many Native societies loosened in the first decades of the century, and government physicians' persistent interest in reproductive matters contributed to but did not necessarily force this trend.[112] Women on some reservations accepted a physician's assistance in childbirth, or even invited his attendance, but many viewed this as a means of combining the physician's skill with that of the other women present, rather than simply embracing the physician's authority. In cases in which a woman refused to accept hospital childbirth as government employees urged, accepting a physician's presence in her birthing space represented a compromise of sorts.

With the surge in reservation hospital construction, the pressure on at least some Native women to accept medicalized childbirth increased, particularly after Sells began demanding progress reports from government employees in 1916. Growing pressure made women's resistance more visible, but most resistance followed long-established patterns. In one such pattern, pregnant women listened politely to employees' directives with little intention of following them.[113] The situation W. W. Scott described at the Cheyenne and Arapaho Agency hinted at a more overt struggle. Two years after hospital construction had been completed, Scott complained that despite his and his employees' best efforts, "we have never been able to get a maternity case into the hospital—the old women considering that service as their peculiar prerogative." The following year, Scott repeated this report almost verbatim, this time referring to midwifery as the older women's "inalienable prerogative."[114] Such overt standoffs were relatively rare in these years, but they nonetheless underscore the politics and generational dynamics implicit in struggles over birthing. On the Wind River Reservation, where Northern Arapahos shared a reservation with Shoshones, Grace Coolidge similarly viewed older women—the "old and doting grandmother"—as an unyielding obstacle that prevented younger women's acceptance of medicalized childbirth.[115]

Citing Coolidge's 1917 essay, at least one historian has argued that this component of the Save the Babies campaign was a failure. Echoing Coolidge's own conclusions, Diane T. Putney contended that "women stayed away from the hospitals, even the young women who had been educated at the government schools."[116] Indeed, hospital childbirth remained rare throughout and beyond the 1910s, and in some locations physician-assisted childbirth did as well. But Putney's assertion does not account for the fact that some Native women embraced hospital childbirth almost immediately, or for the fact that the medicalization of childbirth was arguably the most successful feature of the campaign when viewed from a few decades out.

Alongside pessimistic reports like W. W. Scott's, Commissioner Sells received more promising news. Government employees on the Crow Reservation, for example, began promoting hospital childbirth as soon as construction of an expanded hospital at Crow Agency was completed in the summer of 1916. They saw quick results. "The Indian women are now coming into the hospital for childbirth," two reservation physicians reported shortly after the hospital's completion. In the institution's first year of operation, approximately 15 percent of births occurred within hospital walls—a notable percentage in such a short time frame.[117] Furthermore, although an overwhelming majority of Navajo women continued to give birth "in a hogan, far away from a hospital," S. A. M. Young's enthusiastic telegram to Sells makes clear that in the midst of the Save the Babies campaign at least some women chose to take advantage of hospital services.[118] Even as Superintendent Paquette acknowledged that the transformation of childbirth would necessarily be a long-term effort requiring compromises and intermediary steps, he enthusiastically, if optimistically, reported that growing numbers of Navajo women were entering the hospital for confinement.[119] Navajo women gave birth to forty babies at the Fort Defiance hospital between 1913 and the summer of 1916. Fully half of these births had taken place over a five-month period in 1916, suggesting that Sells's increased emphasis on the issue was showing some results, even if the campaign's reach remained limited to those living in the vicinity of the agency.[120]

Employees on other reservations made similar and even more impressive reports. In Wisconsin, several Menominee women had given birth at the Keshena Agency Hospital by 1916, and within four years the physician reported that 40 percent of births occurred within the reservation hospital.[121] On the Rosebud Reservation in South Dakota, where some women had accepted the government physician's presence and even the employment of interventions such as forceps since the turn of the century, "a considerable number of Indian women" entered the hospital for confinement almost immediately after the opening of a "large modern hospital" on the reservation.[122] In all the above examples, the women who entered government hospitals for childbirth were a minority, as they would remain in subsequent years. It is notable, however, that in explaining this limited—though very real—progress, reservation employees were as likely to cite the inadequacies of staff or facilities as they were women's ignorance or the undesirable influence of midwives.[123]

What persuaded these women to enter a government hospital for childbirth? What motivated them to alter so drastically the circumstances in which they labored and delivered? They have left few records of these decisions, but Native peoples' relationship to government physicians and hospitals underwent notable change in this period. The first decades of the century witnessed the emergence of what the historian Mary-Ellen Kelm has labeled "medical pluralism" on some reservations. Kelm defines medical pluralism as "a continued acceptance of indigenous medicine alongside an ongoing struggle led by Native people to strip the overlays of cultural superiority from the provision of non-Native medicine."[124] As Native peoples came to accept some aspects of Western medicine and government health services, they engaged individually and collectively in negotiations regarding which services to solicit under what circumstances and how best to combine healing systems to suit their needs. Although women came to different conclusions, pregnancy and birthing fit somewhere within this equation.

The context of high infant mortality and morbidity is also crucial. Just as high Indigenous infant mortality spurred the OIA's growing emphasis on hospital childbirth, a mother's personal experience of the loss of one or more infants could make health workers' promise of safer births and healthier babies incredibly attractive. This was the case for Lucy Turns Back Plenty, a Crow mother who lost two of five children in infancy. Preparing for the birth of her sixth child in the early 1920s, Turns Back Plenty journeyed the approximately sixty miles from her home in the reservation's westernmost district to the hospital at Crow Agency. She did so—in the words of the female Baptist missionary who recorded the mother's story—in the hope that "the little one might have the best start possible." In this tragic case, however, birth in the hospital could not protect Turns Back Plenty's baby from subsequent ailment. Within six months, the infant succumbed to pneumonia, an illness that received limited attention in OIA literature on infant mortality. As she struggled to care for her ailing child, Turns Back Plenty discovered the frustrating limits of OIA medical services. There was no doctor in her district, and weather conditions prevented the physician at Crow Agency from making a home visit.[125]

Turns Back Plenty's story hints at the important though fraught role trust played in reservation women's childbearing and child-rearing decisions. On the one hand, Native women's close relationships with non-Native women could encourage them to accept these women's advice regarding their and their children's health and well-being. Turns Back Plenty had apparently developed some degree of trust in this female missionary; in other cases, Native women formed similar relationships with field matrons or government nurses. But infant mortality could also foster distrust in government health services. In her grief, Turns Back Plenty concluded that "it's because we're Indians, the doctor won't come."[126]

When the historian Maureen Lux interviewed Indigenous women in Canada about their early twentieth-century birthing experiences, she learned that some women who opted to give birth in a hospital simply wanted to have "their babies in the new way."[127] While novelty could be an attraction in and of itself, "the new way" evokes associations regarding social status and generation. In the United States, some reservation employees understood childbearing decisions to be closely linked to a woman's level of "assimilation." Such correlations were often tautological in nature. Employees observed that women they viewed as more acculturated were more likely to choose hospital childbirth, and they then read this choice as evidence of the woman's assimilation. The superintendent on the Cheyenne River Reservation in South Dakota reported that most obstetrical patients at the government hospital were women from "mixed-blood families," by which he alluded to cultural as well as ostensibly biological characteristics.[128]

On many reservations, younger women, particularly those who had received some boarding school education, were overrepresented among maternity patients. The generational divide was clear among Salish and Kootenai women on the Flathead Reservation, for example, as more and more young women called on the physician to attend deliveries in their homes, and some ventured into the hospital for childbirth. In contrast, an OIA bureaucrat reported that "the older women . . . still adhere to the old custom and depend upon some woman."[129] At boarding schools on and off reservations, through the gendered curriculum as well as extracurricular activities like "Little Mother's Clubs," young women received lessons in scientific motherhood, including the importance of Western medicine and trained physicians.[130]

Boarding school also separated students from their families, and historians have demonstrated that policy makers viewed this as one of the advantages, even objectives, of this educational system.[131] Separation had particular implications for female students. In an effort to "protect" young women from the perceived sexual immorality of their communities, administrators at many schools, including those on reservations, were adamant that female students remain in school until age eighteen — or marriage, if that came first. For a short period of time, the OIA officially required that Native women between the ages of twelve and eighteen attend boarding schools rather than day schools.[132] This meant that young women were separated from the older female kin who would otherwise have played an influential role in their reproductive development. "By the time I entered fifth grade," Irene Stewart (Navajo) later recalled, "I had forgotten about my grandmother and other relatives."[133] Boarding school further hindered Stewart's ability to follow ancestral teachings regarding the path toward Navajo womanhood. "The customary puberty ceremony [the Kinaaldá] was not made for me because I was in school at that age."[134] Removal to boarding school interrupted the intergenerational transmission of knowledge in ways that could but did not inevitably — or, in the 1910s, even usually — alter the way returned female students birthed their babies.

To understand why a minority of Native women on reservations throughout the West were willing to enter the hospital for childbirth, however, it is necessary to look past the image of reservation hospitals presented by Sells and others and instead consider how Native women and their families experienced these institutions in the first decades of the century. For some, certainly, the hospital was sterile, lonely, and frightening. It was often overcrowded and understaffed, and maternity patients were frequently in the minority, surrounded by illness and disease. Women's dissatisfaction with the hospital environment or its staff can be discerned from the trend, beginning in the 1910s and continuing for decades, of women entering a government hospital in anticipation of their estimated due date and leaving before the onset of labor.[135]

Yet a close look at the new Crow Agency Hospital in the first years after its completion hints at the potential for a different sort of experience and illustrates the degree to which Crows, like other Native peoples, endeavored to incorporate the colonial institution into their healing systems and social world.[136] The institution that is revealed through OIA correspondence and reports is not the ordered, hierarchical facility OIA officials envisioned but rather a space in which Crows wielded notable control. In early 1917, the non-Native head nurse, complaining of the various "evils endured at the hospital," characterized the institution as a "boarding and rooming house."[137] Crows visited patients at their leisure, coming and going with no regard for visiting hours. Family members expected to board and be fed at the hospital, especially when their loved ones were there for extended periods of time, such as a lying-in period. The disgruntled nurse's complaints, which the superintendent and an OIA inspector confirmed, make visible the possibility that some of the Crow women who entered the government hospital for confinement in the late 1910s did so in the company of trusted female kin, subverting the OIA's vision of an individual woman being under the physician's direct authority within the hospital.

Despite the nurse's opposition, Crows who expected to board at the hospital and who assumed authority within hospital walls by opening windows and arranging furniture to suit their needs could be reasonably confident that they would have the support of other hospital personnel. The hospital matron, for example, was an "Indian" woman, likely Crow, who had been educated at Carlisle Indian School. W. S. Coleman, a visiting inspector, described the hospital matron as possessing "characteristic Indian qualities" and scornfully reported that she "is not a graduate Nurse yet aspires to be head nurse in charge of the Crow Agency hospital." He viewed her as "a hindrance or an obstruction" to the maintenance of a disciplined institution.[138] Crows could also generally count on the support of Dr. Edward Lieurance, a white man who had worked on the reservation for eight years. Six years earlier, an OIA inspector had characterized Lieurance as "a young man of energy and ability," and the physician was highly regarded by tribal members.[139] Lieurance married a Crow woman in 1912, through which he became incorporated into kin networks and the obligations and reciprocity such relationships implied. The reviews of tribal leaders and patients remained exemplary, but reviews within the OIA began to wane. Inspector Coleman accused Lieurance of displaying excessive generosity toward patients and visitors and of "yielding to the requests of the Indians however ridiculous."[140]

This snapshot of the Crow Agency Hospital should not be understood as typical of early twentieth-century Indian Service hospitals. Even on the Crow Reservation, the moment was fleeting. After receiving Inspector Coleman's report, which characterized Lieurance as a "typical squaw man," Commissioner Sells concluded that the physician could not be trusted to practice medicine among his wife's people. Sells notified Lieurance that he would be transferred in May 1917, and the physician instead resigned from the Indian Service and enlisted in the Armed Forces as the United States prepared for World War I.[141] After the war, he briefly rejoined the Indian Service, reporting for duty on the Fort Belknap Reservation north of Crow before moving to Warm Springs, where he worked at Montana State Hospital until retirement. After Lieurance's departure, attendance at the Crow Agency Hospital declined, and government reports and correspondence offer none of the optimism that characterized mid-decade records.[142]

It is this documented decline in hospital usage, which seems to have extended temporarily to obstetrical cases, that points to an essential aspect of the federal government's medicalization agenda. In the first decades of the twentieth century, reservation employees relied primarily on the art of persuasion rather than overt coercion in their effort to promote hospital childbirth and prenatal and postnatal services. In this context, employees faced the challenge of making the reservation hospital at least somewhat attractive to Native women, and this frequently necessitated varying forms of accommodation. Even the disgruntled nurse whose complaints contributed to Lieurance's departure acknowledged that "in order to get the Indians to patronize the hospital they have to be humored to a considerable extent or likely they wouldn't come to the hospital at all." "To humor them," she explained, "is simply a means to an end."[143] Throughout Indian Country, Native women engaged in implicit and explicit negotiations with hospital staff regarding the presence of kin, the privacy and condition of their birthing rooms, and the duration of their lying-in period. The growing urgency with which Sells and other OIA officials promoted hospital childbirth created a limited space for women to shape the institution according to their needs and desires.

IN THE LATE 1910S, Commissioner Sells's attention — and OIA resources — shifted to the war effort. As other historians have demonstrated, Sells was either disingenuous or mistaken in the statistics he cited to proclaim a premature victory over Indian infant mortality, but there is evidence that infant deaths declined over the course of the pronatal campaign.[144] Not surprisingly, the campaign's success in fulfilling its primary objective of saving Indian babies varied from location to location. Infant mortality declined on the Southern Ute Reservation in Colorado, for example, but the campaign appears not to have made a dent in IMRs on the large and scattered Navajo Reservation, where mortality climbed in the first decades of the century and increased still more in the 1920s and 1930s.[145] The loss of infant life would remain an enduring feature of many Native women's reproductive lives in subsequent decades, and in contrast to Sells's optimism, some government employees increasingly approached the issue with a sense of fatalism or inevitability.

Rather than officially ending Save the Babies, Sells declared that the campaign's components had "become a regular feature of the reservation activities" and thus no longer needed the structure of a concerted initiative.[146] In the fall of 1918, Sells reminded superintendents of the OIA's wartime "policy of restricting our activities to [the] absolute[ly] essential" and advised them to consider canceling that year's Indian fair. He continued, however, "If you hold a fair, I am very anxious that a baby show be made an important and prominent part thereof, as in the past."[147] Indeed, baby shows continued, at least sporadically, in a few locations through World War II, but they lacked the consistent support and attention of the commissioner.[148] As the OIA's emphasis on health continued to grow in the decade after Save the Babies, the field matron—so central to 1910s pronatalism—appeared increasingly anachronistic, and Sells's successor Charles Burke began the process of replacing field matrons with field nurses in the mid-1920s.[149] Native women on many reservations continued to receive messages from government employees regarding nutrition, sanitation, housekeeping, and child care, but it was field nurses and, beginning in the 1930s, social workers and home extension agents who delivered them.

The premature waning of Save the Babies did not affect the OIA's promotion of hospital childbirth, which continued unabated. Mirroring and at times outpacing national trends, growing numbers of Native women entered the hospital for childbirth in the 1920s and 1930s, a majority on some reservations. Midwifery and hospital childbirth coexisted in Indian Country, sometimes uneasily, and in this context, Native women made intentional decisions about birthing. Returning to the Crow Reservation, the next chapter examines such decisions through the experiences of one Crow woman who gave birth within the reservation hospital and outside of it and attended other women's births as both a midwife and a hospital nurse.

CHAPTER THREE

Nurse, Mother, Midwife

Julia Lathrop, director of the U.S. Children's Bureau, appointed Lewis Meriam as the bureau's assistant chief just as the new federal agency was getting off the ground. Meriam thus spent much of the 1910s studying infant and maternal health outcomes throughout the United States.[1] Among Native American historians, however, Meriam is better known for a later investigation. In the 1920s, Secretary of the Interior Hubert Work appointed Meriam to investigate the administration of Indian affairs amid growing criticism of the Indian Service. Meriam and his nine-person survey team spent seven months in the field gathering data on almost one hundred Indian reservations before submitting a more than 800-page report to Work in early 1928. Officially entitled *The Problem of Indian Administration*, the report is closely associated with the identity of its lead author and became more commonly known as the Meriam Report. To contemporary observers and subsequent scholars, the Meriam Report reads as a damning indictment of both federal policies and congressional appropriations for Indian affairs. The Indian Medical Service came in for particular criticism, as Meriam and his staff emphasized the poor health conditions plaguing many reservations and characterized the service's efforts to combat tuberculosis and trachoma as inadequate. In contrast to Commissioner of Indian Affairs Cato Sells's optimism a decade earlier, the report's authors were also unimpressed by the Indian Bureau's efforts to prevent infant morbidity and mortality, a subject on which Meriam could speak with some authority.[2]

Meriam and his team did point to a high note, however modest: "Here and there some effective work is done in maternity cases." The report explained that this maternity work was "just about enough to demonstrate that competent, tactful physicians can induce a very considerable number of women to have professional care in childbirth and to advance beyond the crude, unsanitary, and at times, even brutal primitive practices."[3] In other words, the medicalization of childbirth, whether inside or outside a hospital, continued apace, as did the government's disparagement of Native midwives. The same report that took the quite radical position that an Indian should have the right "to remain an Indian and live according to his own culture" could not countenance Native midwifery as a cultural experience of any value to Native women.[4]

Less than a decade later, Robert Yellowtail articulated a similar theme in his annual reports as superintendent. Yellowtail was the first Native American to be appointed superintendent of his own reservation, and his appointment reflects some of the changes the Meriam Report had set in motion. In early 1936, Superintendent Yellowtail echoed Meriam and his staff's confidence in government physicians' skill in maternity work. He proclaimed, "We have . . . established through the ability of various physicians" that childbirth in a government hospital under the supervision of trained physicians was far preferable to "the old method." The superintendent characterized the old method as one in which "the mother was delivered in the Crow Camp where she was attended by women with no training and only trusted to good luck and nature to make a safe and proper delivery." Yellowtail contrasted this lack of sophistication to the obstetric prowess of government physicians at Crow Agency who had mastered even the "dangerous Caesarian section."[5] The Crow man did not use adjectives like "crude" or "brutal" to describe Crow midwifery, but he confidently relegated the work of Native midwives to the past.

This chapter explores the divide between the "old" and "new" childbirth methods presented so starkly in government records, as well as many anthropological studies, through the life story of one Crow woman: Susie Walking Bear Yellowtail, Robert's sister-in-law.[6] The first Crow registered nurse, Susie Yellowtail experienced the Crow Indian Hospital as both an employee and a patient. Her story offers one window into Crow and other Native women's creative—and sometimes mundane—decisions regarding pregnancy and childbirth during a transitional moment in which midwifery and medicalized biological reproduction coexisted, even intersected, on reservations. Robert Yellowtail's declarations notwithstanding, his sister-in-law's personal and professional experiences further demonstrate that Crow women did not necessarily view childbirth at the reservation hospital as the "safer" option in the 1930s. In fact, Susie Yellowtail and other Crow women came to fear the hospital because of the mistreatment they received there, including in some cases involuntary sterilization. The policies and practices at Crow in this decade reveal some of the implications of eugenic thinking on Indian reservations and underscore the need for further research into colonial eugenics. Through Yellowtail's story, the chapter also explores health, healing, and reproduction as sites of Crow women's activism and resistance.

A Nurse among Her People

Susie Yellowtail's life, like that of her brother-in-law Robert, can be read as an assimilationist success story, but this interpretation obscures a richer and more complicated history. For both Yellowtails, attributes that observers read as markers of assimilation did not preclude—and sometimes facilitated—a commitment to Crow identity and sovereignty. Susie Walking Bear (Yellowtail) was born in 1903 in Pryor, the reservation's westernmost district. Her mother, Jane White Horse, who was half Lakota, was a member of the Whistling Water clan, so relatives welcomed Susie into that clan at birth. As a child, the young Walking Bear attended the Catholic boarding school at Pryor, but her parents soon arranged her transfer to the government boarding school at Crow Agency. According to Yellowtail's descendants, she transferred to Crow because her parents learned that authorities at the Catholic school were sexually abusing their pupils, a violation that tragically occurred in a number of government and denominational Indian boarding schools.[7]

Jane White Horse died while her daughter was attending school. Yellowtail's descendants refer to her as an orphan after this point and contend that the experience of being orphaned inspired some of her activism later in life.[8] "Orphan" was a Western rather than an Indigenous concept, but adoption of the term did not necessarily reflect the same meaning.[9] The Crow practice of "flexible childrearing" meant that children without living biological parents generally had no shortage of extended kin willing to provide them with a home. As their predecessors had before them, white government employees regularly commented on flexible childrearing on the reservation. In the late 1920s, a physician stationed in Pryor reported that in cases of broken homes caused by death or separation, "caring for these children seems to be the least of their troubles." He emphasized that Crows recognized little distinction between biological and nonbiological children.[10] Calvin Asbury, superintendent at Crow Agency, disapprovingly reported that the "old custom" of giving away children to relatives continued to thrive even when the biological parents were alive and theoretically able to care for their children. In contrast to Samuel Reynolds's determination to eliminate the practice after the turn of the century, Asbury approached the issue with relative resignation: "I do not know just how this can be remedied."[11] In Yellowtail's case, an aunt assumed responsibility for her and her sister following their mother's death.[12]

In 1919, at the age of sixteen, Susie Yellowtail followed in the footsteps of Robert Yellowtail and several of his contemporaries when she left Montana to attend an off-reservation boarding school.[13] Bacone Indian School, a Baptist institution in Oklahoma, resembled the boarding schools Yellowtail had previously attended on the reservation in offering a gendered curriculum that combined academic study with vocational training. As Yellowtail's granddaughter Valerie Jackson put it, the schools trained female students "to be housemaids."[14] Yellowtail's relationship with a female missionary named Frances Shaw soon resulted in the young Crow woman journeying still farther from her reservation. In the early 1920s, Yellowtail accompanied the missionary, who had recently married, to the East Coast. Yellowtail worked as a maid and nanny in Shaw's home and enrolled at the Northfield Seminary for Young Ladies in Massachusetts. Unfortunately, Yellowtail's relationship with the missionary soured. She later recalled that Shaw "lost her missionary spirit somewhere along the way." The guardian made prejudicial remarks, practiced corporal punishment, and overworked her young maid.[15]

Perhaps as a way to escape this demeaning environment, Yellowtail decided to pursue a career as a nurse. With the assistance of other Baptist sponsors, she enrolled in the nursing program at Franklin County Memorial Hospital in Greenfield, Massachusetts, before going on to Boston City Hospital School of Nursing, one of the oldest and most prestigious nursing schools in the nation. By the 1910s and 1920s, East Coast nursing schools attracted applicants who, like Yellowtail, tended to hail from rural areas and to have been born in the United States. In contrast to Yellowtail, however, the overwhelming majority of students in these nursing schools were white. Nursing students served as an important labor force for growing eastern hospitals; students worked long hours and had no choice but to submit to rigid disciplinary standards. According to the historian Susan Reverby, the nursing school "looked more and more like a reformatory" in the 1920s.[16] Yellowtail's years in government and religious boarding schools, which also demanded military-like discipline, likely prepared her well for the experience.

When she graduated alongside her five classmates in 1927, Yellowtail became the first Crow registered nurse and one of the first Native American registered nurses.[17] A few Native women had received degrees from non-Indian schools, and a handful of Indian boarding schools offered some level of nursing training. In the early 1930s, Dr. Clarence Salsbury established the first fully accredited Indian school of nursing at Sage Memorial Hospital, a Presbyterian institution on the Navajo Reservation in Arizona. Salsbury recruited young Native women from throughout the West to his nursing program in the hope that graduates would then take their medical skill and Christian conviction back to their communities. In part as a response to this Presbyterian initiative, Commissioner of Indian Affairs John Collier secured funding for a nurse-training course at the Kiowa Indian Hospital in Oklahoma in 1935. Much to Collier's disappointment, the experimental course was somewhat of a failure, as it lacked accreditation and a formal curriculum and effectively prepared Native women to work as aides in government hospitals.[18] By 1941, 89 of the more than 800 nurses in the Indian Service were of Native descent.[19] Over the course of the preceding decade, the Indian Service's Indian-hiring preferences, as well as economic pressures caused by colonization and exacerbated by the Depression, encouraged growing numbers of Native women to seek careers in Western health care.

In 1927, however, Yellowtail was very much a trailblazer in the field of Native nursing. She joined the Indian Service a year after graduation, but it would be another year before she returned to her reservation. She first spent six months as a night nurse at the Fond du Lac Indian Hospital in Cloquet, Minnesota, and a few frustrating months attempting to find work as a private nurse in Billings, Montana. Like other Native Americans who attempted to find health-related work off reservations, Yellowtail found that her boarding school education and a nursing degree did not preclude discrimination on the part of hospital administrators or patients. She wound up back at Crow Agency, this time working as a supervisory nurse at the hospital.[20]

Crows had continued to incorporate government health services into their repertoire of healing options throughout the 1920s. By 1926, reservation employees reported that more than 90 percent of Crows accepted hospital care in at least some situations.[21] As growing numbers of Crow men and women visited the government hospital for a broader range of services, they became less likely to view the institution as "the sick peoples' lodge" from which one would not come out alive.[22] This increased familiarity with the hospital also helped buttress the Indian Service's promotion of hospital childbirth, which reservation employees had continued in the decade after the Save the Babies campaign. Shortly before Yellowtail came to work at the hospital, the district superintendent in charge praised the reservation's health workers for their success in bringing parturient Crow women into the hospital and favorably compared the situation with that on the nearby Northern Cheyenne Reservation, where, he claimed, the women "refuse hospitalization almost

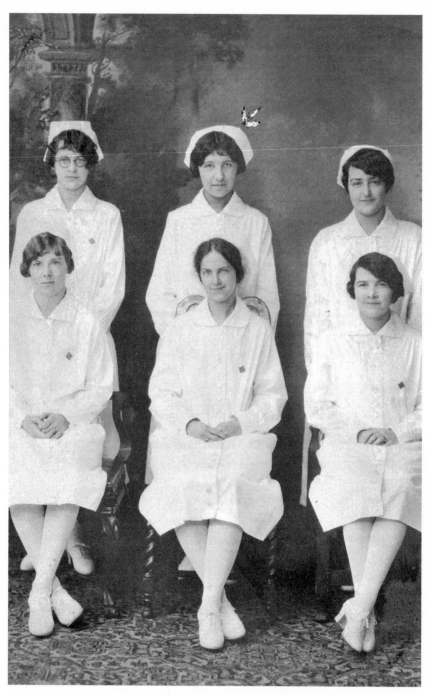

Susie Walking Bear (center, back row) graduated from Boston City Hospital School of Nursing in 1927. School officials insisted that she go by the surname Bear rather than Walking Bear while enrolled. Catalog number PAC 87-70, Legacy Photograph Collection, Montana Historical Society (Helena, Montana).

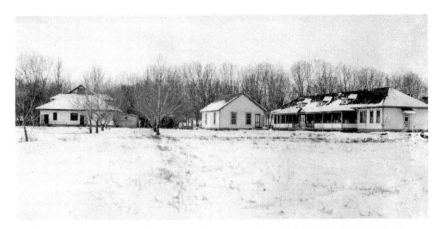

The Crow Agency Hospital (right) was located next to a small dispensary and the Crow Agency Office. By the time this photograph was taken in 1929, nearly half of Crow women gave birth in the reservation hospital. Decimal Correspondence Files, 1926–32, Accession 8NS-075-96–230, Crow Agency, Records of the BIA, RG75, NARA, Broomfield, Colo.

entirely upon this line."[23] The Northern Cheyenne hospital had opened in Lame Deer only one year earlier.

Crow women approached maternity services selectively, much as they did government health services more generally. Many women in Robert Yellowtail's family, despite his assured proclamations just a few years later, chose to give birth at home throughout the 1920s. At mid-decade, Robert's younger sister Agnes went to the hospital in anticipation of her delivery, but she "got scared and came back home." She gave birth with the assistance of two trusted women — her brother-in-law's mother and the "mother" who had adopted her into the Tobacco Society.[24] Robert's wife, Lillian Bullshows, chose to deliver the couple's first and only child outside the hospital a few years later. Robert and Lillian lived at Crow Agency at the time, but as the latter prepared for her impending labor, she informed her husband that she wanted to go stay with her mother in Pryor so that her mother could serve as midwife for the birth: "That's the way I want it." As she later recalled, Robert deferred to her judgment, replying, "I'll do your way. We'll go over there, live there."[25] These examples suggest that at least through the 1920s, some women in Robert's family continued to trust the midwives Robert would soon disparage. Robert's wife Lillian also made clear that she continued to view childbirth as a woman-centered event. Although Robert accompanied Lillian to Pryor, he was not in the log house when their daughter was born.[26]

In addition, logistical considerations continued to bar some women from giving birth at the reservation hospital, even had they wanted to do so. Owing to Montana's vast territory, rugged terrain, and harsh winters, midwife-assisted home birth remained a necessity for many non-Native rural women throughout the state until the 1940s.[27] On the Crow Reservation, the distance from Pryor to Crow Agency was about sixty miles, a journey some families would have made via horseback or wagon. Pryor's relative geographic isolation surely contributed to women's slower embrace of hospital maternity services, as compared, for example, with Lodge Grass, where field nurse Ethel Smith reported in the early 1930s that most of her "prenatals" desired a hospital birth.[28] The superintendent similarly remarked on the trend of hospital childbirth among those "within easy reach of the Agency."[29] "Easy reach of the Agency" connoted both logistical advantages in accessing the hospital and more frequent contact with government employees, who regularly urged hospital attendance. A field nurse on the Fort Peck Reservation to the northeast of Crow boasted of her success in persuading Assiniboine and Sioux women to enter the hospital for confinement. Some of these women "had been quite determined to have their babies at home," but the field nurse's persistence paid off when the women "finally consented."[30] Pryor residents, in contrast, did not consistently have a field nurse assigned to their district until 1940.

On the Crow Reservation and elsewhere, government records affirm that distance and poor traveling conditions could be prohibitive, but white field workers also frequently complained that Native women presented such excuses in order to evade government employees' efforts. This suggests that pregnant women's deference to logistics was sometimes an act of resistance. Field workers throughout Indian Country bemoaned women's attempts to hide their pregnancies and expressed frustration with women's false promises about their birthing plans. In an attempt to avoid conflict, pregnant women assured field nurses that they intended to give birth in the reservation hospital but did not always follow through.

The Ojibwe historian Brenda Child discovered that her grandmother "rebuffed the offer" of the government hospital on the Red Lake Reservation in Minnesota and instead gave birth with the assistance of her own grandmother—Child's great-great-grandmother. Child's grandmother was unmarried, and a home birth allowed her to deliver outside the paternalistic and judgmental gaze of hospital staff.[31] Field nurses at Crow and in other locations often conflated moral and medical objectives; some dedicated particular attention to the "problem" of "illegitimate" pregnancies, a matter of far less concern in many Native societies. Like Child's grandmother, many women resisted the services and advice of government employees, whom they viewed as sanctimonious or condescending.[32]

Crow women thus had many reasons to continue to birth outside the hospital, but by the late 1920s, other women found aspects of hospital obstetrics appealing. A year before Susie Yellowtail came to work at the hospital, employees estimated that approximately half of Crow women gave birth within hospital walls.[33] Four years after Robert Yellowtail had accompanied his wife Lillian to Pryor for the birth of their child, Yellowtail's third wife, Margaret Pickett, whom he married after he and Lillian separated, gave birth to their daughter Anita in the hospital at Crow Agency.[34] Proximity, familiarity, and the consistent urging of government employees each contributed to these women's decisions, as did a number of "situational" factors. Some women sought hospital care when they had reason to expect a difficult delivery; others were especially likely to accept hospital conveniences during harsh Northern Plains winters.[35] Crow patients continued to expect that the hospital would conform to their needs, but the institution was more regulated and regimented than it had been a decade earlier. In 1929 as in 1916, a maternity patient who entered the hospital accompanied by kin would have expected that her companions board and be fed at the hospital throughout her confinement.[36]

Susie Yellowtail assisted a number of women in childbirth during her brief and overwhelmingly negative employment at the Crow Agency Hospital, but she resigned following her marriage to Thomas Yellowtail after only a few months on the job. As she later made clear, this decision was prompted by her complete and total frustration with the hospital's white employees. Obstetrics exemplified the institution's inadequacies. Yellowtail later recalled one incident in which she and another nurse could not persuade the senior physician Ira Nelson, who had worked on the reservation for over a decade, to come to the hospital to deliver a baby. In the end, Yellowtail delivered the infant herself. She had gained obstetric experience by necessity during her tenure at the Ojibwe hospital in Minnesota, where the government physician had been equally unreliable.[37] One irony of Robert Yellowtail's and other government employees' emphasis on the superiority of the "trained physician" is that due to understaffing and/or apathy, it was not uncommon for Native women in the 1920s and 1930s to birth in a government hospital with no physician present.[38]

In the instance Yellowtail described, she reported that after Nelson finally showed up, he "was in a hurry and just cut the umbilical cord and left, didn't even look at me."[39] Yellowtail alleged that the physician cut the cord too short, causing the infant to bleed excessively. The Crow nurse was left to take extraordinary measures to save the child's life. Katherine Nova McCleary, a Little Shell Chippewa-Cree scholar who was raised on the Crow Reservation, speculates that this incident may have further unnerved Yellowtail because of Crow beliefs about the umbilical cord's significance for an individual's health and identity. Typically, Crow midwives saved the umbilical cord and presented it to the infant's parents for ritual use.[40] It did not take long for Yellowtail to conclude that Nelson "couldn't be depended on for anything."[41]

More generally, Susie Yellowtail's interlude as an "insider" convinced her of the mistreatment Crows endured as patients at the government hospital. She later recalled that she "went to bat" for mistreated patients: "I . . . would have it out with the doctors, trying to improve things. It was just really bad. I'd tell those doctors, 'Just because we're Indians, doesn't mean you can do this to us. You think you can get away with it, but finally somebody is here who knows what's going on.'"[42] The historian Cathleen Cahill has demonstrated that in contrast to the federal government's intentions and expectations, twentieth-century Native Americans turned positions within the Indian Service into "politicized sites of resistance."[43] Yellowtail's experience at the Crow Hospital provides an additional example of this process. Like so many of the Native men and women identified in Cahill's study of the Indian Service, Yellowtail was deemed a "troublemaker" by some of her superiors.[44] She was unable to secure health-related employment on the reservation throughout the 1930s, despite her brother-in-law's repeated efforts, and other Crow nurses later reported that the Bureau of Indian Affairs attempted to steer them away from their home reservations after their training.[45] For her part, Susie Yellowtail's resignation from the Crow Agency Hospital did not signal the end of her investment in Crow health and well-being, a commitment that would only increase in subsequent years.

Reservation Politics in the 1930s

Significant changes came to Indian Country and the Crow Reservation in the years after Susie Yellowtail left the hospital at Crow Agency. In 1933, President Franklin Roosevelt appointed John Collier, a social worker and vocal critic of the Indian Service, as commissioner of Indian affairs. Collier rejected many of the assumptions undergirding the government's assimilation agenda. As commissioner, he advocated greater respect for Native cul-

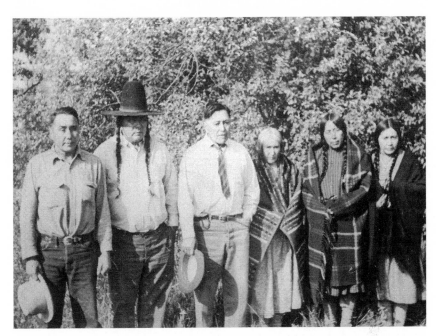

The Yellowtail family (left to right: Thomas, Carson, Robert, Lizzie, Amy, Agnes) around 1930. Thomas married Susie Walking Bear in 1929, and Robert became superintendent of the Crow Reservation in 1934. Archives and Special Collections, Mansfield Library, University of Montana, Fred Voget Papers, 318.VI.004.

tures and promised increased political autonomy for Native groups. Collier faced his first challenge regarding the Crow Reservation soon after his appointment when Robert Yellowtail and other Crow leaders waged a campaign to remove James Hyde, sitting superintendent and a career Indian Service administrator. The recently appointed commissioner viewed the campaign as an opportunity to put his commitment to tribal autonomy into practice. He approved Hyde's transfer and took the unprecedented step of appointing Robert Yellowtail to replace him.[46]

With Collier in Washington, D.C., and Robert Yellowtail in charge at Crow Agency, the 1930s was a decade of political and cultural resurgence on the reservation. With Robert's support, Crow leaders reintroduced the Sun Dance and revived the Crow Fair. Superintendent Samuel Reynolds had introduced the fair in the early 1900s to incentivize Crow agricultural production, but under Superintendent Yellowtail's watch, the Crow Fair was transformed into a vibrant social and cultural celebration.[47] For Susie Yellowtail, the timing was fortuitous. She spent the early 1930s re-embracing

Crow lifeways and readopting the Crow style of dress that she had given up in the years she spent away from the reservation.[48] Decades later, Crow women remembered Robert Yellowtail's appointment as portending a decisive change in reservation life. Robert's cousin Mae Takes Gun Childs, for example, recalled that Calvin Asbury, who had served as superintendent for more than a decade preceding Hyde's appointment, was "known . . . as a mean uncaring man who tried to force the Crows to give up some of the cultural events" and who did not hesitate to use police power to enforce his instructions. After "Robbie took over," Childs explained, "then the people could do as they pleased, they could have dances and celebrations, tobacco dances or anything else. They weren't afraid anymore."[49] Crow recollections often conflated the administrations of Asbury and Hyde, underscoring the turning point that Yellowtail's appointment represented.

Whites who lived on the reservation viewed the increase in Crow political and cultural consciousness with uneasiness. Reflecting broader trends, missionaries tended to blame Collier. In 1939, William Petzoldt, a Baptist missionary who had lived on the reservation for more than two decades and enjoyed a generally good relationship with the Yellowtails, expressed his "violent disaggreement [sic]" with the Crows' renewal of "old customs" — customs he had hoped had "died out" under previous commissioners. He explained that his opposition to "present Collier policy" stemmed in part from "the disturbance created in the mind of the Indian in telling him to recreate the days of old, which are def[initely?] gone forever."[50] Chester Bentley, another Baptist missionary who lived and worked on the reservation, echoed these sentiments. Bentley contended that Collier's policies represented "a step backward," serving only to create "a chaotic state of affairs where the mind and purpose of the Indian is concerned." He explained that "10 years ago the Indian was more 'submissive,' whereas today the Indian was rather *haughty, proud, conceited*."[51] Above all, Bentley lamented this change he believed he witnessed in Crow attitudes.

Like the missionaries, many government health workers were suspicious of Collier and the changes his appointment portended. They viewed his interest in social work and anthropology as impractical and feared his administration would reverse the progress employees had made in eliminating the influence of Native healers over the preceding decades.[52] The historian Wade Davies has cautioned that although Collier's attitude and policies represent a significant shift in federal Indian policy, progress was limited by the unwillingness of reservation employees, including many physicians and nurses, to accept his vision.[53] White health workers at Crow had reason to be wary of the spirited atmosphere that prevailed on the reservation in the 1930s. Observers noted a resurgence in Crow healing practices, and the agency hospital and government health services became visible sites in Crows' struggle for self-determination.[54]

Shortly after Robert Yellowtail's appointment, Crows voted against Collier's Indian Reorganization Act (IRA), much to the commissioner's frustration. Many tribal members were suspicious of a new round of government intervention, and at any rate, they viewed the legislation as unnecessary. The IRA established guidelines for tribal governments and constitutions, but most Crow leaders were satisfied with the tribal council that had developed over the past decade, and they did not want to see it replaced with a new political institution.[55] Throughout the decade, Crow men and women's complaints regarding hospital staff and policies were litigated through the tribal council. The complaints themselves were not necessarily new, but they now often had the support of the superintendent. Superintendent Yellowtail repeatedly called on physicians to attend council meetings to answer charges in person.

The Crow Tribal Council included all adult enrolled members of the tribe, but at least until the mid-1940s, council meetings tended to be dominated by men.[56] To some degree, this gendered political structure can be seen as an adaptation of pre-reservation practices. Alma Hogan Snell later explained that before the establishment of the reservation, when a Crow woman wanted to be heard by her band's council of warriors, she typically spoke through one of her male relatives.[57] The male-dominated council can also be read as a Western intrusion, however, as nineteenth-century Euro-American observers had commented on the frequency with which Crow women participated in deliberative councils.[58] Since the nineteenth century, a cornerstone of the colonial project had been the imposition of patriarchal relationships and structures of governance on Native peoples in the West. As the historian Jennifer Denetdale has argued, even the tribal nations that rejected the IRA were forced to operate within a Western model of government that viewed men rather than women as political leaders. Some Native women have further charged that sexism in tribal politics increased amid Collier's efforts to "recover" Native traditions, as male leaders, many of whom had been educated in government boarding schools, "attempted to define 'traditional' leadership as the exclusive domain of men."[59] As growing numbers of Crow women visited the hospital for prenatal care, delivered their babies in the hospital, and/or brought their infants in for care from the government physician, unsatisfactory experiences resulted in appeals to the tribal council, which pushed reproduction-related issues into the male-centric political sphere.

These gendered political dynamics are demonstrated even more starkly through the Crow health council. The council was formed in 1934, shortly after Robert Yellowtail's inauguration, at the behest of Charles Edward Nagel, a newly arrived government physician. Nagel envisioned the entity as a means of facilitating reservation health work and tempering patients' criticism. Frustrated with the politicized atmosphere of the general tribal council, the physician hoped that he could wield more control over a smaller body. The council consisted of two male delegates from each district and a handful of white government employees. While this iteration of the Crow health council would ultimately be short-lived, surviving minutes from the group's first meetings in early 1935 provide a fascinating window into the council's wide-ranging purview. At one such meeting, in response to a female hospital patient's complaint about being separated from her infant overnight, Crow men and the white government physician discussed the merits of Crow women's breastfeeding habits. The physician argued that Crow and other Native women breastfed incorrectly; in keeping with the medical community's increasing emphasis on the "science" of infant feeding, Nagel lamented that Crow women did not abide by a defined schedule. The minutes imply that the male delegates deferred to the physician's authority—rather than that of absent Crow mothers—on the matter, but the bureaucratic record provides no insight into their actual views.[60]

Robert Yellowtail's disparagement of Crow midwifery in his second annual report as superintendent one year later can also be interpreted in this vein. Indian Service officials would surely have appreciated his interest in Crow women's reproductive practices and his promotion of the government hospital. But the disconnect between Robert's bold proclamations and the experiences of Yellowtail women remains striking. As will be demonstrated below, multiple women in Robert's family practiced midwifery in the 1930s, a fact of which he would have been aware. This disconnect underscores the need for caution in interpreting Robert's promotion of hospital childbirth in his annual reports and serves as a reminder of the complexity of his location as a Crow superintendent. He was, after all, writing in the capacity of a government employee to his superiors. Robert Yellowtail's disparagement of Crow midwifery was unremarkable in his capacity of government employee but was notable for a Crow man, as it presented an erasure of the status of older women such as his aunt Mary Takes the Gun, whom many Crow women continued to hold in high regard.

Crow women were far from silent regarding health and politics in the 1930s. In fact, on the Crow Reservation as in other locations, the decade is characterized by Native women's increasing visibility in reservation affairs.[61] The historian Becky Matthews suggests that Crow women's involvement in reservation politics began in the 1920s, and this early activism prompted the establishment of the Crow Indian Women's Club in 1930.[62] Minnie Williams, a Crow woman born in 1879 and educated at Carlisle Indian School, was an active women's club member and officer. Williams later described the club's founding as an attempt to give women a voice in tribal politics that they had previously lacked.[63] The preamble of the Women's Club's constitution speaks to the group's ambitious objectives, including the preservation of "our cultural values" and "our rights under the Crow Indian treaties with the United States" and the promotion of "our common welfare."[64] "With the establishment of their Women's Club in 1930," Becky Matthews has argued, "some Crow women"—the group consisted of thirty to forty members over the next several years—"made it clear that they were moving from the edge to the center of Crow politics."[65]

Matthews may have overstated the case, which at most applied to a very small handful of women.[66] But especially on matters regarding health and education, the Crow Indian Women's Club displayed tremendous energy and commitment—despite women's exclusion from official bodies like the tribal health council and despite opposition from some government employees. Club members promoted maternal and infant health on Crow terms, advocating in 1934 for the establishment of a course for young women and mothers on prenatal and early infant care. Kate Stewart, the group's president, proposed that the course be taught by Alice Other Medicine, a Crow woman who had followed in Susie Yellowtail's footsteps in becoming a registered nurse. In this case, the Office of Indian Affairs (OIA) rejected club women's attempt at greater involvement in women's health initiatives on the reservation, citing financial concerns and satisfaction with field nurses' existing program.[67] The Crow Indian Women's Club achieved more success in its demands for a new hospital, which would open in the late 1930s, and the hiring of more registered nurses, ultimately including Crow and other Native nurses.[68]

Obstetrics and Gynecology on the Reservation

Susie Yellowtail does not seem to have been involved with club work in the 1930s, although she was active in countless other ways. After leaving her job at the hospital, Susie and her husband, Thomas, settled on a ranch in

Wyola, the reservation's southernmost district. Wyola was approximately thirty-five miles from Crow Agency, the hub of club work in these years. The newlyweds busied themselves ranching and starting a family, but the nurse's brief tenure at the Crow Hospital had nonetheless been transformative. Yellowtail's later recollections suggest that she witnessed physicians performing unethical sterilizations during her stint at the hospital, and the emotional distress she endured in the aftermath of her departure certainly supports her recollection. Marina Brown Weatherly, a family friend of the Yellowtails who recorded Susie's story in the final year of the Crow woman's life, concluded that what Yellowtail observed in the hospital placed her on a trajectory of lifelong activism.[69] In the short term, her experiences within the hospital influenced how Yellowtail approached the births of her children.

Susie Yellowtail gave birth to her first child in 1930, a year after her departure from the Crow Agency Hospital and around the time the Crow Indian Women's Club was founded. Yellowtail delivered her daughter Virjama at a hospital—but not at the institution in which she had worked. She hoped to avoid the reservation hospital because she "had seen so much mistreatment of Indian women in that place." During her pregnancy, Yellowtail sought prenatal care at a hospital in Sheridan, Wyoming, and during a checkup hospital staff urged her to deliver there because they anticipated a difficult delivery.[70] Sheridan and Crow Agency are roughly equidistant from the Yellowtails' ranch in Wyola, so it is not clear whether the senior physician at Crow approved of these arrangements. Crows could obtain health care off the reservation at government expense only with the authorization of the government physician.[71] The following year, Yellowtail journeyed to Crow Agency for the birth of her second child. Given her apparent satisfaction with her experience at the Sheridan hospital, as well as her concerns about the government institution, Yellowtail's 1931 delivery at Crow lends credence to the hypothesis that Thomas and Susie had paid for the birth of their first child out-of-pocket but were not able to do so for a second. It is also possible that the senior physician, relatively new to the reservation during Susie's first pregnancy, had become less willing to authorize outside care in the intervening year and a half.

According to Yellowtail, the delivery of her son Bruce was a "nightmare."[72] She was familiar with the setting, as it was the same building in which she had recently worked, but Crow patients and government employees alike were well aware of the hospital's deficiencies. Visiting OIA inspectors regularly commented on the hospital's "very poor state of repair," and a senior physician more memorably characterized the building as "at best . . . a horrible wreck." He complained that the Crow Agency Hospital was "unsuitable and unfit for the purpose used and most certainly should not bear the title of Hospital."[73] The space was suited for twelve beds, but regularly operated at an eighteen-, twenty-, even thirty-bed capacity.[74] Successive superintendents' practice of using the hospital as a jail for women deemed guilty of various moral and/or criminal infractions—a practice staunchly condemned and disavowed by the commissioner of Indian affairs—only exacerbated overcrowding.[75] Physicians consistently lamented that the hospital did not have "proper facilities for obstetrical work," such as a separate delivery room, and Crow Indian Women's Club members were among the many patients who complained of the lack of isolation wards, which placed maternity patients in unsettling proximity to patients with tuberculosis and other communicable diseases.[76]

In Yellowtail's case, however, her "nightmare" had less to do with her physical surroundings and more with the doctor who attended her delivery. As she had observed so many times as a nurse, "the doctor was in such a hurry [that] he didn't do too well by me . . . and I almost died."[77] Yellowtail did not mention this doctor by name, but it is likely that Charles Buren, the senior physician who succeeded Ira Nelson, delivered her second child. Two months before Bruce Yellowtail's birth, the district medical director had visited Crow for an inspection, and he was not impressed with the quality of doctors at Crow. He noted that Dr. Buren was "a graduate of the old P. & S. [Physicians and Surgeons] Medical School of St. Louis, which was always a low grade school and in its later years was a diploma mill." Equally troubling, Buren was apparently "badly handicapped by some affliction of one eye, which is believed to be entirely useless to him."[78] Bruce Yellowtail was one of the last babies Buren delivered at Crow. The physician was dismissed from the Indian Service in early 1932 due largely to his inability to get along with colleagues.[79]

In stark contrast to Robert Yellowtail's declaration that "the ability of various physicians" had "established" the superiority of obstetric services at the government hospital, his sister-in-law's experience as a patient at Crow Agency led her to pledge that she "wouldn't have any more children in that hospital."[80] Instead, when Susie Yellowtail prepared for the birth of her third child in the summer of 1934, she made plans to deliver at home with the assistance of trusted women in her family. In other words, she placed her faith in the "old method" of Crow birthing. Yellowtail may not have viewed old and new methods as incompatible. She apparently requested that a government physician or field nurse attend her home birth in addition to her Crow attendants. While the specific nature of her request is unclear, it was not uncommon for field staff on many reservations to attend home births in these years or for families to send for a government physician in the event of a prolonged labor.

In this case, however, the senior physician Charles Nagel, who had transferred to the reservation a few months earlier, responded with an unequivocal refusal. Nagel condemned the expecting mother's "selfish" request, proclaiming, "You have been offered the services of the Hospital. . . . You are therefore not entitled to receive the courtesy of the Field Service." He informed Yellowtail that he was ordering reservation field workers "not to render you assistance." The physician closed his letter by declaring that "service by a Non-Service Doctor will be at your expense," as he would not authorize payment for medical bills associated with her confinement.[81] The hostile tone of Nagel's letter suggests that he may have been aware of Susie Yellowtail's reputation as a "troublemaker" with regard to government health services on the reservation and of her prior connection to the hospital. Nagel had previously been in the army; Robert Yellowtail later characterized him as a "military man" who demanded discipline.[82] He did not countenance dissent from individual patients, the tribal council, or his own staff. Fern Rumsey, a non-Native nurse at the hospital, noted—with admiration—his "explosiveness" when faced with patient complaints, which the nurse believed were "only too numerous."[83]

At any rate, Nagel's letter could not have influenced Yellowtail's ultimate decision regarding her third delivery. The letter was dated a week after Constance (Connie) Joy Yellowtail's birth. Yellowtail gave birth to her second daughter at home with the assistance of Robert and Thomas's aunt Mary Takes the Gun. Susie's mother-in-law, Elizabeth (Lizzie) Yellowtail, was likely present for the birth as well. Takes the Gun was an experienced midwife and in fact had attended Lizzie Yellowtail's last delivery more than two decades earlier. Susie Yellowtail recalled that Thomas's aunt was "a good medicine woman, and she knew just what to do."[84]

Part of Takes the Gun's birthing knowledge included the use of peyote. Susie and Thomas did not belong to the Native American Church, but some Crows had begun incorporating peyote into their spiritual and healing systems decades earlier.[85] When Takes the Gun recognized that Susie would have a difficult delivery, she instructed her to eat two peyote buttons. "After that," Yellowtail recalled, "it was really wonderful. I felt no labor pains and was wide awake for the whole delivery. It was such a joy to go through childbirth with no pain."[86] Women's historians have demonstrated that the prospect of pain relief drew many women to the hospital in the interwar period.[87] Crow sources seldom mention pain medication in their discussion of hospital birthing in these years, despite the fact that physicians employed obstetric anesthesia at least for difficult deliveries by the 1930s.[88] These sources do, however, demonstrate that many women took pain relief into their own hands, utilizing peyote during home births or finding ways to ingest peyote during hospital deliveries, yet another means of asserting some control over hospital childbirth. In addition to the practical benefit of pain relief, many women believed that peyote improved outcomes for both mother and baby.[89]

In the months following her home birth, Susie Yellowtail began experiencing "terrible pains in my lower belly."[90] Nagel's letter had not affected the Crow woman's birthing plans, but the physician's threats about the financial consequences may have contributed to Yellowtail's decision to go to the Crow Agency Hospital for her abdominal pain rather than to Sheridan. The "new doctor" who examined her was almost certainly Nagel, and the senior physician told Yellowtail that she needed an operation to remove a cyst on her ovary. Out of fear, Yellowtail put off the surgery until she could no longer handle the pain. Unfortunately, the delay may have caused her condition to worsen. "They were just supposed to remove the cyst," she later recalled, "but that doctor in Crow ended up sterilizing me and I didn't even know it until he was through. He said, 'Three is all you want and three is all you're going to get.' I was so upset."[91] During the surgery, Nagel may have determined that he could not remove the cyst without the ovary, but he apparently had not discussed this possibility with Yellowtail, who felt violated and outraged.

Yellowtail further alleged that her trauma was not unique. The sterilization of Crow women "without consent," she later argued, was "routine practice"; it was "common government procedure back in those days." While Nagel sterilized Yellowtail in the midst of a gynecological procedure, she reported that in other situations physicians "would go in and operate right after childbirth. Just tie up their tubes without even asking permission." Yellowtail's allegations add an unsettling layer of meaning to her brother-in-law's reference to the "dangerous" cesarean section. She explained that most of the women "didn't know what was going on and didn't realize they couldn't have any more kids until long after the operation. A lot of them would be so puzzled why they weren't getting pregnant." Aware of her medical knowledge and nursing background, frustrated women sometimes came to Yellowtail, and she would have to explain what had likely caused their sterility.[92] The circumstances Yellowtail described resemble the "Mississippi appendectomies" black women in the South would report in the 1950s.[93]

Yellowtail singled out Nagel specifically, and government records created by Nagel confirm a high sterilization rate during his brief tenure at Crow. In a letter to Superintendent Yellowtail in the spring of 1935, Nagel indicated that thirteen "Gynecological Operations, such as Salpingo-oophorectomies," had been performed at the hospital from 1933 through the first months of 1935, as well as one hysterectomy and salpingectomy.[94] A salpingo-oophorectomy, which entails the removal of the fallopian tubes and ovaries, is a somewhat more complicated surgery than a salpingectomy, which involves only the fallopian tubes. According to Harry Laughlin, assistant director of the Eugenics Record Office in Cold Springs Harbor, New York, the operation was used "primarily for eugenical purposes," although he noted that the surgery frequently resulted from mixed motives. "Oftentimes," Laughlin explained in his magnum opus *Eugenical Sterilization in the United States*, "surgeons in opening the abdominal cavity for the eugenical purpose of removing a section of the Fallopian tube find the conditions such that in their judgement, it is pathologically or physiologically advisable to remove both the ovaries and the entire tubes. This operation is thus looked upon as a surgical incident in eugenical sterilizations."[95] Nagel's use of "Gynecological Operations" is frustratingly vague, but if most were in fact procedures comparable to a salpingo-oophorectomy, this would amount to approximately one such operation for every 6.5 hospital births during this two-year period—on a reservation with a total population of fewer than 2,000 people.[96]

Any explanation of these numbers must take into account Nagel's attitude and objectives, as well as the troubling discretionary authority he and his peers throughout Indian Country wielded as senior physicians in reservation hospitals. Collier had transferred Nagel to Crow Agency from the Fort Belknap Reservation in part because Robert Yellowtail and his political ally James Carpenter had been vocal about the need for a physician with surgical capabilities on the reservation. From the two men's perspective, this was simply a matter of the federal government meeting its obligations to the Crow people. Native leaders throughout the West argued that tribal members should have access to the same health services as a white person living off the reservation, and that included surgical operations.[97] Without question, Crow men and women benefited from Nagel's surgical prowess. In 1935, for example, Carpenter praised the physician in front of the tribal council, insisting that an operation Nagel had recently performed had saved his life.[98] But the recorded sterilization numbers raise concerns about Nagel's professional incentives to perform such operations. Shortly after his arrival at Crow, Nagel made clear to Collier that he hoped "to have as many surgical cases as possible in order that [he] might qualify with the American College of Surgeons."[99] Collier was untroubled by Nagel's ambitions, which he did not view as unusual. But these individual and bureaucratic circumstances did not exist in a vacuum. Rather, they must be considered in light of national trends in American eugenics.

Eugenics and Native Women's Reproductive Autonomy

Early twentieth-century eugenics was premised on the notion that the human race, and more specifically the Anglo-Saxon race, could be improved by discouraging the reproduction of individuals whom eugenicists believed to possess undesirable traits while encouraging reproduction of "fit" individuals and families. The eugenic sterilization movement that began in the first years of the century experienced a resurgence in the 1920s. A host of states passed eugenic sterilization statutes in these years, and in 1927 the Supreme Court upheld the constitutionality of such laws in *Buck v. Bell*, encouraging the passage of new laws in other states.[100] Despite growing criticism from geneticists and social scientists, eugenics flourished throughout the 1930s, and the decade witnessed the height of eugenic sterilizations. Historians have explained these developments by pointing to changes within the movement as well as to economic factors. Eugenicists broadened their purview to emphasize environmental rather than strictly biological factors in these years, and new professional classes such as social workers embraced eugenics in the decade preceding World War II. In the midst of the Great Depression, proponents of eugenics presented sterilization as a means of reducing welfare costs, and New Deal federal spending provided a new source of funding for eugenic programs.[101] Prevailing anxieties regarding degeneracy, delinquency, and dependence should raise important questions about how and to what extent eugenic thought functioned on Indian reservations.

Most scholarship on early twentieth-century eugenics, however, either ignores American Indians entirely or explicitly argues that Native women and men "fell outside" these campaigns.[102] The most notable exceptions to this generalization focus on eastern states. For example, Vermont began a eugenics survey in 1925 that resulted in the eugenic institutionalization and sterilization of Abenaki men and women. Abenaki leaders argue that the eugenics survey "forced Abenaki families to conceal their identity, leave their ancestral homeland, or relinquish their language, religion, and customs."[103] Scholars have demonstrated that "eugenics-informed policy" facilitated Indigenous removal and erasure in the Southeast as well.[104] In Virginia, eugenics informed and buttressed Jim Crow segregation. Eugenicists became concerned with Indians in this period because of perceptions of Indians' impure "blood" based on real and imagined histories of "race-mixing" with African Americans. Given that the state's sterilization law targeted people of mixed-race ancestry, the historian Rose Stremlau emphasizes Native peoples' vulnerability to eugenic sterilization in Virginia.[105]

In the East as in the West, historians face archival and conceptual obstacles in studying and documenting these histories. To write about Native peoples in the eastern United States is to work against the archival grain, as state-level administrators endeavored to erase Indians from bureaucratic records by reclassifying them as "colored" or "black." Native peoples in the West also faced pressures of bureaucratic as well as physical erasure, but through the first decades of the twentieth century, the federal government's dominant policy objective on western reservations was erasure through cultural assimilation. Eugenicists' emphasis on heredity seems contrary to the prevailing assimilation agenda, but ideas about biology and culture had long coexisted uneasily in Indian affairs, and eugenicists' embrace of environmental factors in the 1930s can be viewed as closing the gap between potentially divergent perspectives. That eugenic sterilizations in these years tended to be institution-based—that is, performed in state asylums, mental hospitals, or schools for the "feebleminded"—also diverts scholarly attention away from reservations, as does leading eugenicists' persistent emphasis on southern and eastern European immigrants and working-class whites more generally. Indeed, the most prominent voices in the American eugenics movement, such as the California-based eugenics popularizer Paul Popenoe, remained satisfied that natural selection would continue to decrease the Native American population until its eventual extinction.[106]

Yet eugenics-informed policies, practices, and programs played out not at the national level but at the local and state levels. Furthermore, the question is not so much whether Native people were explicitly targeted in eugenic campaigns but how colonization had created the conditions that allowed Native women and men to become caught up in these processes. On the Crow Reservation, government reports and correspondence reveal that reservation employees utilized eugenic language and drew on eugenic logic in their assessments of social and economic problems on the reservation. A letter that Superintendent James Hyde wrote to District Medical Director O. M. Spencer in the summer of 1932—after Susie Yellowtail quit her job at the hospital but before Robert's appointment as superintendent and Nagel's transfer to the reservation—provides an especially explicit and extensive example of this phenomenon. The purpose of Hyde's letter was to inquire about sterilization arrangements for a twenty-three-year-old Crow woman. In making his case that "action must be taken," Hyde cited a laundry list of deficiencies, beginning with the fact that the woman had given birth to two illegitimate children (one of whom had died in infancy) and that she was "sub-normal although not really feebleminded."[107] Other reservation employees, including Nagel, regularly employed the intentionally vague label of "subnormal" as well.

Hyde went on to highlight both environmental and economic factors. He charged that the woman in question "has none of the accomplishments of a housewife and is unable to cook or sew or carry on her other household duties." Here, Hyde emphasized the young woman's distance from the middle-class gendered ideal of the homemaker that informed the government's assimilation agenda and in doing so implied that the mother's living child and any future children would not be raised in a suitable environment. He reported disapprovingly that the woman and child lived with the child's grandmother, and that the woman's mother assumed much of the child care responsibilities, without noting that it was common for Crow grandmothers to play a large role in providing daily child care. Hyde argued that the unwed mother and illegitimate child would be a financial burden to the rest of the family, if not the government, a matter of elevated concern in the context of the Great Depression. That the woman in question was allegedly prone to "dizzy spells" and showed "other symptoms of a nervous disturbance" seemed for Hyde to seal the deal.[108]

The superintendent stressed that he wished to remain in accordance with state law. He explained that he had encountered "a similar case" at his previous reservation and had found that the Indian Office was "favorable to the procedure, if carried out with strict conformity to State law on the subject."[109] Montana had passed a compulsory eugenic sterilization law in 1923, although in practice eugenic sterilizations in the state were rarely carried out without the consent of the patient or his or her guardian.[110] Hyde told Spencer that the field nurse had referred the case to him, and that he had sent her back to obtain consent from the woman and her mother. Montana's statute also specified that eugenic sterilization required that the individual in question be an inmate of a state institution, typically the Montana State Training School (often referred to as the School for the Feebleminded) in Boulder or the Montana State Mental Hospital in Warm Springs. Government employees and occasionally tribal judges or law enforcement sent Crow men and women to these institutions, which suggests that they may have been included in the more than 250 sterilizations legally performed on inmates of these institutions. It is not clear whether the sterilization Hyde recommended in this case ever occurred.

The Meriam Report had advocated the use of social work methods on Indian reservations, and the Indian Service began assigning trained social workers to some reservations around the time Hyde penned his above letter.[111] These new employees assumed responsibility for fulfilling the liaison role—among Native families, reservation staff, and county and state authorities—that Hyde had informally assigned to the field nurse at Crow. Social workers favored an individual case work approach, so their activities varied widely by location, but a review of Indian Service social worker reports in the 1930s and early 1940s suggests that some social workers became actively involved in arranging for the eugenic institutionalization and/or sterilization of Native women and, less frequently, men.[112]

In making such arrangements, social workers were required to conform to a range of state laws and procedures, and their reports and correspondence underscore the capriciousness of federal and state power over Native women's bodies. Social workers on the Consolidated Chippewa Agency in Minnesota, for example, were relatively active in following procedures for the eugenic sterilization of Ojibwes—securing familial consent, scheduling the required examinations for feeblemindedness, and making logistical arrangements for transportation and child care. In December 1936, one social worker reported that she had successfully secured "consents" for the sterilization of two women: "a feebleminded mother of seven" and "a girl who was transferred from the Home for Girls at Sauk Center to the Feebleminded Institute at Faribault."[113]

Much to the frustration of the social worker Mary Kirkland, however, state and county authorities did not believe that the state's sterilization statute applied to the Red Lake Band of Ojibwes. Tribal leaders at Red Lake had successfully resisted allotment and in other ways staunchly defended the nation's sovereignty in the decades surrounding the turn of the century. The State Board of Control as well as county officials believed Red Lake Indians, as "ward Indians living on an unallotted reservation," to be "wholly federal responsibilities."[114] Kirkland and Superintendent Raymond Bitney believed that feeblemindedness, female delinquency, and illegitimacy were urgent problems on the reservation, and both expended significant energy in advocating for "legislation" that would allow the eugenic sterilization of Red Lake Indians.[115] In the meantime, the agency paid for the institutionalization of a handful of delinquent and/or feebleminded women at the School for the Feebleminded at Faribault. Unable to accept a sterilization operation as a condition of their release, as "whites and allotted Indians" were sometimes able to do, these young women were detained away from home indefinitely, often despite familial opposition.[116] Reflecting on the different protocols that prevailed at the Consolidated Chippewa Agency versus those at Red Lake, the historian Molly Ladd-Taylor observed that "while federal jurisdiction 'protected' some Ojibwe women from unwanted sterilization, it did not protect others."[117]

The complexity of federal protection extended far beyond Minnesota. Lumbee women and other members of tribal nations that lacked federal status may have been particularly vulnerable to eugenic sterilization, for example.[118] Yet for Susie Yellowtail and other Crow women, it was precisely their status as "wards" of the federal government that seems to have facilitated their unwanted procedures. While the surgical abilities of reservation physicians varied widely, government physicians on underresourced and often isolated reservations who were so inclined were well positioned to blur the lines between "therapeutic" and "eugenic" sterilizations. Scholars have documented instances in which physicians working off reservations proved "flexible" in their definitions of "medical necessity," particularly when it came to women, and some physicians appear to have been especially proactive about operating on women who had been infected with a venereal disease.[119]

Feminist historians have emphasized that even in less than ideal circumstances, women have exerted agency in controlling their reproductive lives, and sometimes this has meant opting for a sterilization operation.[120] In the 1930s, Native American women had limited birth control options. Some Crow and other Native women continued to utilize herbal methods for pre- and postcoital contraception, but Crows reported at the end of the decade that abortion had significantly decreased because women feared the legal repercussions of terminating a pregnancy.[121] On many reservations, poverty, combined with the discrimination Native women faced in New Deal welfare programming, exacerbated the pressures facing women and mothers. In some cases, it seems that social workers genuinely believed that their Native clients, particularly those who already had several children, desired a sterilization procedure. In such cases, the surgery may have been a relief to mothers. The consent process must nevertheless be examined critically. Whether consent was sought by a field nurse, a social worker, or another government employee, the process, even when it occurred well before the procedure, raises concerns about language and cultural barriers and the potential for government employees to exploit Native women's dependence on them for other services. Finally, it must be emphasized that in Yellowtail's case, and in her description of other women's experiences at the Crow Agency Hospital, even these minimal standards of consent were not met. In some instances, Crow women apparently did not have full knowledge of their situation.

Decades later, health workers, activists, and government investigators exposed a new wave of sterilization abuses that occurred in government and contract hospitals in the 1970s. In this context, many Native women and men charged that the government's actions constituted "genocide."[122] Reflecting on earlier abuses in the midst of this later activism, Susie Yellowtail argued that "to sterilize our women was to kill us." Her words position the sterilization of herself and other Crow women in the 1930s squarely in its colonial context—as an assault on Native women and the important role they played as life givers, an assault on Native families, and an assault on the continuation of Native peoples.[123] The circumstances Yellowtail related must be read in part as a particularly blatant form of the "elimination" that the theorist Patrick Wolfe has argued is central to the settler colonial project.[124] As would be the case in the more extensively studied later period, the 1930s were characterized not only by political and cultural resurgence but also by the peak of successive decades of population growth.[125] That Robert Yellowtail's historic inauguration as superintendent of the Crow Reservation coincided so closely with his sister-in-law's and other Crow women's sterilizations speaks to the need for nuanced and gendered analyses of sovereignty and self-determination.

Susie Yellowtail, Crow Nurse and Midwife

Perhaps more than any other injustice, it was the sterilization of Crow women that propelled Susie Yellowtail's activism in the 1930s. She joined other tribal members in successfully advocating for the removal of two of the "worst doctors."[126] It is likely that Yellowtail was involved in the opposition to Nagel, which culminated in the physician's resignation in December 1935. Among the many issues that spurred some tribal members' opposition to Nagel was his tactlessness in policing venereal disease, his employment of interventionist techniques in childbirth, and Crow women's contention that the physician ignored their maternal rights in the hospital.[127] Turnover at the Crow Hospital was high in the late 1920s and 1930s, as Crow men and women like Yellowtail demanded personnel who respected their rights and wishes.

Considering the many health- and hospital-related complaints addressed in tribal council meetings throughout the decade, it is noteworthy that extant meeting minutes do not explicitly reference sterilization. The incomplete nature of surviving records presents one possible explanation, as does Crow men's continued dominance in meetings. But the most significant reason for the absence of references to sterilization in council meetings likely stemmed from the intimate and painful nature of the issue. In societies that celebrated women's role as life givers and mothers, the elimination of a woman's procreative capacity was an emotional event that provoked anger, and sometimes shame and guilt. As activists would discover in the 1970s, Native women who had been sterilized sometimes did not want their own families to know, not to mention their entire tribe.[128] Even as she protested coercive sterilization at the Crow Agency Hospital, Yellowtail apparently rarely discussed her own sterilization, at least until the end of her life.

In the years after she left her job at the hospital, Yellowtail began another type of work, which amounted to a form of political activism outside formal channels: she began serving as a midwife for women in Wyola and throughout the Little Bighorn Valley.[129] She had delivered a number of babies during her employment at Indian Service hospitals, and after 1930, she had also given birth herself, which many Crows still viewed as a prerequisite for midwifery. She combined her Western medical training with birthing knowledge she had learned from women in the Yellowtail family, in order to provide women with safe childbirth experiences outside the government hospital. According to Yellowtail, by mid-decade, many women avoided the hospital out of fear of the doctors and of Nagel specifically.[130] Not all Crow women who avoided the reservation hospital turned to a midwife. Some called on outside physicians to assist their home births, and others found ways to give birth at off-reservation hospitals, as Yellowtail did for the birth of her first child.[131]

For her part, Susie Yellowtail practiced midwifery from the 1930s into the 1950s, and she was not alone in her work. Matilda Roundface, for example, acted as a midwife for women in the Pryor district until midcentury. Geneva Whiteman, born in Pryor during Robert Yellowtail's tenure as superintendent, remembers that the women in her community had complete faith in Roundface. As they prepared for labor, pregnant women kept checking to be sure that Matilda would be home to assist them. Roundface's midwifery practice differed from Yellowtail's in that the former did not have a nursing degree. At some point, reservation employees apparently attempted to persuade Roundface to leave the reservation to obtain formal nursing training, but Whiteman explains that Matilda "wouldn't leave, and her family wouldn't allow her to go."[132] Like Yellowtail, however, Roundface had worked at the hospital before her marriage, and a field nurse in the 1940s deemed Round-face competent and knowledgeable enough to serve as her "unofficial assistant."[133] For women like Yellowtail and Roundface, and for many of the women who requested their services, the gulf between "old" and "new" childbirth methods was not always as vast as it appeared in government reports.

DURING THE 1930s, a decade in which the percentage of women who gave birth at the reservation hospital grew but likely did not surpass 60 percent, the factors contributing to women's childbirth decisions were complex. Despite—indeed, arguably because of—the gradual trend toward hospital childbirth at Crow Agency and on other reservations, Susie Yellowtail's story underscores the necessity of presenting a history of Crow midwifery that continues beyond the point at which government sources relegated the practice to the past. The relegation of Native midwives in government records in the 1930s and 1940s obscures the gendered politics at work in their erasure and distracts from the unethical practices and inadequate care that encouraged some women to choose a Native midwife or practice midwifery. Furthermore, women's choices were not strictly between midwifery and physician-assisted childbirth, as Crow women went to great lengths to give birth under circumstances that met their needs, sometimes traveling off the reservation to give birth at an off-reservation hospital at their own expense.

The ethically questionable and sometimes outright coercive sterilizations to which Yellowtail called attention had apparently declined at Crow Agency by the early 1940s. With the onset of World War II, the Indian Medical Service found itself spread thin, as manpower, resources, and attention were redirected to the war effort. Eugenic sterilizations also declined nationally in this decade; wartime production ended the Great Depression, and many Americans reacted in horror to Nazi atrocities. The tireless work of women like Yellowtail as agitators and watchdogs cannot be discounted as an additional factor in limiting sterilizations in government hospitals. Some Native women of childbearing age would face new challenges in the 1940s and 1950s, however. After decades of encouraging women to give birth in government hospitals, the federal government began closing some of these facilities in the years after World War II. Government officials simultaneously promoted the migration of Native men and women to urban centers far from their extended kin networks and the government health services that had been established for their use. The next chapter considers the experiences of Crow and other Native women who spent at least part of their reproductive years away from the reservation.

CHAPTER FOUR

Relocating Reproduction

Albert and Harriet Brown[1] (Crow) were among the thousands of Native men and women who moved from reservations to cities in the decades after World War II. As participants in the federal government's relocation program, the Browns received assistance in coordinating their journey from the Crow Reservation to California, and a Bureau of Indian Affairs (BIA) employee helped the couple secure housing and Albert find employment in East Los Angeles upon their arrival. The Browns' case file offers little indication of the couple's unique motivations and aspirations for their urban migration, but federal objectives were clear: policy makers and most BIA employees hoped that the Browns' resettlement would be permanent and that it would result in their assimilation into urban American society.

The Browns arrived in Los Angeles in August 1957. Within a month, the couple's prospects for a long-term relocation had declined owing to unexpected complications. From the perspective of the field relocation officer (FRO) George Felshaw, the unexpected complication was the birth of a child. Harriet gave birth to a son at a local hospital within two weeks of arriving in Los Angeles, but Felshaw had not been aware of her pregnancy. According to BIA policy, Albert Brown's application for relocation should have been rejected or delayed on account of his wife's advanced pregnancy, but this aspect of the couple's situation had slipped through the bureaucratic cracks. From the Browns' perspective, the unanticipated complication was the significant expense associated with their child's delivery. After welcoming their son into the world, the couple was presented with bills from both the hospital and the doctor, a situation that they would not have encountered had Harriet given birth in the government hospital at Crow Agency. The Browns paid what they could of the hospital bill but were left with a debt of $110. In subsequent months, the couple's maternity-related debt produced a paper trail that involved the BIA, the Public Health Service (PHS), and tribal representatives, but the balance remained unpaid. In February, the doctor who had delivered the Browns' child attempted to collect payment through Albert's employer and threatened to transfer the couple's debt to a collection agency. In the end, a BIA staff member contacted the doctor, who agreed not to turn the bill over to a collection agency as long as the

99

Browns made a small payment each month. Harriet was reportedly relieved by this resolution.[2]

Harriet Brown's experience of giving birth so soon after arriving in the city was unusual, but the questions she faced regarding where to give birth and how to pay for it were shared by many Native women who moved to cities during and after World War II. Pregnancy, childbirth, and motherhood were not the only means by which Native women experienced the city, but by foregrounding reproductive matters, this chapter adds a crucial layer to historical narratives of relocation and postwar Indian urbanization. BIA officials believed that the success of the relocation program depended on the migration of women as well as men, and the migration of large numbers of women of childbearing age resulted in accommodations, however inadequate, in relocation policy. In cities, Native women navigated, in many cases for the first time, the bureaucracy of health insurance. For many women and families, however, long-term health insurance was out of reach, and they relied on their own ingenuity and the support of familial and social networks both on and off reservations in their attempt to obtain adequate prenatal, obstetric, and postnatal care. This chapter demonstrates the changing geography of Indigenous communities with respect to reproduction and mothering in postwar decades and the centrality of reproduction in motivating Indian mobility to and from reservations and cities.

Native Women in the City

Native women's presence in cities was not a postwar development. As the historian Nicholas Rosenthal has demonstrated, Native Americans have traded, worked, and lived in American cities since the nation's founding.[3] In the late nineteenth and early twentieth centuries, the economic underdevelopment of reservations led some Native men and women to migrate to cities, temporarily or permanently. Lewis Meriam and his staff highlighted this trend in their 1928 report on the administration of Indian affairs, and John Collier implicitly acknowledged this reality by instituting a short-lived placement program to facilitate Native employment in border towns and urban centers.[4] Despite a long-standing Euro-American misconception that Indigeneity and urbanity are antithetical, the growing urban Indian population after World War II was a fact of scale, not a new phenomenon.

Anna Moore Shaw (Pima) offers a useful example of interwar migration. Anna married Ross Shaw in 1920. Shortly thereafter, the newlyweds moved from the Salt River Reservation to nearby Phoenix, Arizona. The city offered better employment prospects for Ross, who found work with the American Railway Express Company.[5] Cities such as Minneapolis and Albuquerque similarly attracted migrants from nearby reservations.[6] In Anna Shaw's case, Phoenix was a familiar setting because both she and her husband had attended Phoenix Indian School. Other female boarding school graduates also journeyed to cities. Facing limited employment opportunities on reservations, some young women pursued wage work in urban centers. Government employees and boarding school administrators often encouraged this urban migration through outing programs that placed young Indian women as domestic servants in white homes.[7]

The United States' entry into World War II pulled thousands of men and women away from their home reservations. About 25,000 Native men joined the armed forces, and some women enlisted as well.[8] Hannah Fixico (Lakota), for example, joined a U.S. Naval Reserve unit called Women Accepted for Voluntary Emergency Service, through which she received clerical training.[9] In the armed forces, men and women traveled through and were stationed in cities throughout the United States and the world. For her part, Fixico traveled to New York City for her training, was stationed in Hawaii during the war, and was discharged in San Francisco after the war's conclusion. Others left reservations to take jobs in war-related industries, paralleling national trends of rural to urban migration. Native women embraced wartime economic opportunities, migrating to cities with husbands, family members, friends, or on their own.[10] Ignatia Broker (Ojibwe) moved to the Twin Cities the year Japan bombed Pearl Harbor. The twenty-two-year-old woman immediately secured employment in a defense plant and also began taking night classes.[11]

World War II proved to be a significant turning point in Native urbanization. Although many veterans and defense-industry employees returned to reservations after the war, they had been exposed to, and in some cases became attracted to, city life, and some found the poor economic prospects and continued federal paternalism they encountered on the reservation frustrating.[12] For others, the wartime transition to urban life became permanent. Broker, for example, married and raised two children in the city.[13] Native men and women's wartime contributions influenced policy makers' perceptions as well, and some began to argue that the war had demonstrated that Indians were finally ready to assimilate into American society once and for all.[14]

This was the context for the emergence of the federal relocation program, which promoted the urban migration of Native individuals and families and provided basic assistance to facilitate the process. The program was one piece of a broader effort by policy makers to "get out of the Indian business" in postwar decades, an effort that will be discussed more fully in the next chapter.[15] In the dozen years following the end of World War II, approximately 25,000 American Indians moved to urban centers with BIA encouragement and assistance, and this number continued to climb into the 1970s.[16] Thousands more—a majority of postwar migrants—"self-relocated," meaning that they migrated to cities with no assistance from the new federal program.[17] The program's reach nonetheless extended beyond the number of participants. The BIA distributed promotional materials touting the perks of city life, and many men and women who moved without government assistance joined relatives on relocation.

The federal government first experimented with urban relocation in 1947, when it relocated Navajos and Hopis who hoped to escape a devastating blizzard that left tribal members with inadequate food and other resources.[18] The BIA expanded the burgeoning program beyond the Southwest in the early 1950s. Commissioner of Indian Affairs Dillon Myer, who had overseen Japanese internment and resettlement as director of the War Relocation Authority, established a new Branch of Placement and Relocation within the BIA. This branch established field offices in major cities throughout the West and Midwest, including Chicago, Denver, Cleveland, Dallas, Los Angeles, San Francisco, and San Jose, California, among other destinations.[19] Yet congressional ambivalence remained, and the program's budget stagnated after 1952. Hindered by inadequate resources, the BIA's new initiative faced criticism in its early years. From the vantage point of the 1960s, one of Commissioner Myer's successors characterized his predecessor's program as "essentially a one-way bus ticket from rural to urban poverty."[20] In response to this type of criticism, congressional appropriations increased in 1956, and the BIA began placing increased emphasis and resources on vocational training for relocatees.[21]

From the program's origins until its conclusion in the 1970s, the federal government's official line was that the program was entirely voluntary, a contention that scholars and Native participants alike have debated from the outset. There is no question that government employees attempted to "sell" relocation through promotional literature and interpersonal interactions on the reservation, leading relocatees who became dissatisfied with urban life to conclude that they had been sold on false promises.[22] Among the messages Native women and men received was that they could have no real future on the reservation—indeed, that there was no future for reservations at all. Relocation officers stationed on reservations felt pressure to maintain high numbers for the program, and rumors of quotas regularly circulated in Native communities.[23] In his 1969 manifesto *Custer Died for Your Sins*, the Native intellectual Vine Deloria Jr. described government employees' persuasive efforts as follows: "Considerable pressure was put on reservation Indians to move into the cities. Reservation people were continually harassed by bureau officials until they agreed to enter the program."[24] Wilma Mankiller (Cherokee), a young girl in the 1950s, recalled that her father had initially opposed relocation but acquiesced after repeated home visits from the "BIA people."[25]

It is also clear that many women and men sought relocation services for themselves. The BIA received more applications than it approved, and thousands of reservation residents opted not to deal with the federal bureaucracy at all in planning and executing a cross-country move. Postwar migrants moved to cities for a variety of reasons, including work, freedom, and adventure.[26] Debbie Clark (Cheyenne), who relocated to Los Angeles with her husband and children in the late 1950s, later recalled feeling stifled by rural life on the reservation. "I couldn't stand it anymore. It was so hard for me. I had four kids, and we lived kind of in a rural area, and we had no water, we had no toilet. . . . It was just overwhelming for me." Clark talked her husband into leaving the reservation: "I said, 'I feel like I'm being buried alive. We have to do something. We have to get out of here.' . . . So I coaxed him into going on relocation."[27] In contrast, when John and Lois Knifechief (Pawnee) relocated from Oklahoma to Los Angeles around the same time, it was John who persuaded his wife to move. More than a decade later, Lois remained dissatisfied with life in the city. "I'd rather live there," she said, "but he prefers to live here and he says that he can get a job here, and that's another thing that we were taught, that you go where your husband goes, where his work takes him. That's where he can provide you a living, that's where you go."[28] John Knifechief was not alone in being drawn to the city by economic opportunities; work was among the most frequently cited motivations for relocatees.[29]

The Knifechiefs also reflected the BIA's expectations regarding gender and work. As the historian Nicholas Rosenthal has emphasized, reservation employees and relocation office staff "favored men as primary breadwinners."[30] The BIA categorized relocatees in "units" consisting of a family, a single man, or a single woman. Families made up more than 40 percent of all units recorded in relocation documents between 1952 and 1959.[31] In such cases, the BIA required that the male head of household submit the application, and it was husbands—not wives—who received vocational training.[32] When Debbie

Clark and her family arrived in Los Angeles, the BIA helped her husband find a job, but she was left to make her own arrangements for the practical nursing classes she wished to take, for which she and her husband paid without government assistance.[33]

Unmarried women also pursued work opportunities in cities. The historian James LaGrand estimates that women made up one-fourth of all single relocatees in Chicago, and as much as 30 percent of all single relocatees in the program's first years.[34] In contrast to married women, single women were eligible to receive training in gender-appropriate vocations such as cosmetology, clerical work, and practical nursing.[35] Unmarried women with children, however, frequently found the BIA to be unsupportive of their ambitions. One BIA staff member explained his decision to deny three unmarried mothers' applications by insisting that the women in question had not "considered the problems involved in providing care for the children during working hours." Nor, he continued, did the women have any experience with "paying rent, utilities and or [sic] other miscellaneous expenses in the upkeep of a home," limitations that surely were not unique to these three women, or to unmarried mothers more generally.[36] Another relocation officer concurred that women with children "had more problems than [could] be adequately met" and discouraged the provision of relocation services in such cases.[37] The rule was not absolute, however. Perhaps because of her wartime service, which had provided her with a trade, BIA staff assisted Hannah Fixico when she moved to Los Angeles with a young child.[38]

Whether married or single, women had noneconomic reasons for moving to cities as well. As the historian Margaret Jacobs has demonstrated, young Native women had been drawn to modern urban leisure culture since the first decades of the twentieth century. For some recent boarding school graduates, the city offered a level of freedom that had been unavailable to them in the tightly regimented institutions in which they had spent their adolescence.[39] Some women viewed the city as an escape from federal paternalism and the scrutiny of government employees on reservations.[40] Others migrated for "personal reasons." Cornelia Penn (Lakota) relocated from the Rosebud Reservation in South Dakota "to begin a new life" after separating from her husband.[41] Hannah Fixico also relocated after a divorce. She was confident that she could make it in the city because she "had already been through all that" while in the Naval Reserves.[42]

When women like Hannah Fixico and families like the Browns went "on relocation," they did so with promises of BIA support and assistance. In the early years, such support was largely limited to a short-term stipend and the location of housing and employment for the head of household, and relocatees regularly complained of the inadequacy of these services. By the late 1950s, the BIA placed more emphasis and resources on job training for relocatees, as well as on orienting arrivals to their new home. As the relocation program expanded, the BIA also responded to Native demands by providing rudimentary financial and logistical assistance in accessing urban health services. Ultimately, urban health services did not meet the needs of many Native residents, a failure that would be left for Native leaders and activists to address in the 1960s and 1970s. In the short term, however, the BIA found that it could not ignore women's reproduction-related needs and demands.

Bureaucracy and Birthing

Although the male Indian laborer was especially visible in relocation records and rhetoric, the federal relocation program by definition involved coordinating the migration of large numbers of women of childbearing age. Policy makers and BIA employees believed women to be key to a unit's "successful" relocation, as well as the success of the federal program. Relocation officers concluded that male relocatees adjusted more smoothly to urban life when accompanied by a wife; they believed married relocatees to be more "stable" and more likely to remain in the city.[43] The promotional materials that Native women and men regularly encountered on reservations thus featured large, shiny photographs of happy Indian families.[44] The BIA's desired outcome of relocating women alongside men, as well as women's own agency in pursuing relocation, caused BIA staff to devise—belatedly and haphazardly—a set of policies governing Native biological reproduction during relocatees' transition to urban living.

The BIA relocated families with small children, and policy makers and relocation officers expected that most married women would bear children in cities, but BIA staff discouraged the relocation of pregnant women, especially in the latter half of a pregnancy. Anna and Tyler Begay (Navajo) confronted this restriction repeatedly. The couple first applied to relocate to Denver in January 1956. The Begays made plans to move later that spring, but Anna was pregnant, and BIA staff determined that their departure should be delayed. Tyler Begay submitted another application in early 1957, but another pregnancy resulted in another delay. Finally, in January 1958, Tyler and Anna, who was seven or eight months pregnant, visited the local relocation office and made arrangements to depart for Denver shortly after the birth of their third child.[45] Relocation staff on the reservation may have found the Begays'

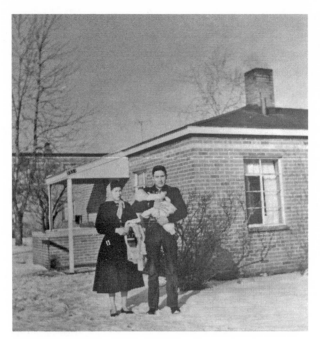

BIA officials believed that the long-term success of relocation depended on the migration of families and women of childbearing age. As a result, the BIA took modest though inadequate steps to accommodate women's reproductive needs. BIA Relocation Records, Newberry Library (Chicago, Illinois).

situation as frustrating as did the couple. The family of five boarded a bus for Denver less than three weeks after the new infant's birth, while in other cases the BIA insisted that a child be two months old before his or her family could relocate.[46]

The BIA's rationale for delaying the relocation of pregnant married women like Anna Begay was largely bureaucratic. Through an arrangement between the BIA and Blue Cross and Blue Shield, all relocatees were covered by a temporary health insurance plan. Typical of restrictions for maternity-related services in midcentury health insurance plans, relocatees' plans did not cover maternity services until after a woman had resided in the city for ninety days.[47] Most relocatees could not afford to pay for a hospital delivery out of pocket, so the BIA recognized that an ill-timed delivery could threaten a family's prospects for a permanent location. As George Felshaw explained to one reservation superintendent, if a family "were to arrive and immediately become indebted for doctor and hospital bills, plus the daily living costs . . . it is doubtful that they could become financially solvent."[48] This was the very situation that threatened the Browns' relocation. The insurance-based restrictions were further codified in 1958, the year the Begays finally relocated to Denver, by a federal rule that disqualified all pregnant women from relocation.[49]

When a head of household applied for relocation, reservation staff arranged for a doctor to perform a physical examination of each individual at BIA expense. The resulting Form 5–442, Indian Family Health Certificate, then became part of the unit's application. In reviewing the Family Health Certificate, relocation officers had two primary and very gendered concerns: (1) did the physical examination reveal anything that might compromise the male head of household's employment prospects? and (2) was the wife pregnant? This examination represents a particularly intimate iteration of government employees' scrutiny of Native women's bodies, which their predecessors had carried out in various ways since at least the turn of the century. Relocation officers later concluded that the physician who examined Harriet Brown before her relocation had somehow erred in stating "very plainly . . . that no pregnancy existed," and that this unfortunate mistake had allowed Brown's pregnancy to have gone undetected by the BIA staff who arranged the family's relocation.[50] Pregnancies went undetected in physical examinations frequently enough that it was not unusual for FROs to complain about the quality of physicians that the BIA employed for this work. It also hints at the possibility that some women who wished to relocate may have deliberately concealed a pregnancy—defying government surveillance—so as not to derail their plans.

Insurance restrictions demanded that the applications of unmarried women in the latter stages of pregnancy be denied or delayed as well, but BIA staff had additional reasons for discouraging such relocations, even before the 1958 rule. As demonstrated above, relocation officers were skeptical that unmarried mothers could achieve self-sufficiency in the city, as they would be burdened by the double demands of wage earning and child care. Furthermore, an unwed pregnant woman, or an unwed woman with an infant, defied the gendered familial model that the BIA intended to promote, and government employees sometimes used relocation procedures to pressure women into nuclear family units. For example, the historian Nicholas Rosenthal describes the case of a Spokane woman who learned that she was pregnant during her physical examination. The relocation officer denied the single woman's application and urged her to get married so that her husband could apply for their relocation as a familial unit.[51]

Native peoples on reservations were no strangers to bureaucracy, but because they received health services from the government—first via the BIA and after 1955 via PHS—most families who migrated to cities had no previous experience with health insurance. At least in theory, this was the subject of intensive counseling before relocatees departed the reservation and after they arrived at their destination.[52] The bureaucracy of health insurance was new not only to relocatees; postwar arrivals entered a rapidly changing urban health landscape. A Dallas hospital had pioneered the first prepayment plan for hospital services in 1929, and hospitals throughout the country followed suit, ultimately forming the Blue Cross network. State medical societies introduced comparable plans for physicians' services in the 1930s, which collectively became known as Blue Shield.[53] Both Blue Cross and Blue Shield organized as nonprofits, but commercial insurance companies soon entered the fray, offering their own plans. The health insurance market exploded in the 1940s and 1950s, the historical moment in which Native individuals and families began migrating to cities in significant numbers. According to the economist Melissa Thomasson, 12.3 million Americans had health insurance in 1940; two decades later, that number had grown to 122.5 million. Among the factors contributing to this growth was rising hospital costs for all Americans.[54]

Health insurance, then, potentially served an assimilationist function. As Great Britain and Canada moved toward nationwide health programs at midcentury, private health insurance, typically obtained through one's employer, was increasingly the "American Way."[55] Government-funded and government-managed health care for Indians on reservations was anomalous in American society, matched only by the veterans' health service.[56] For decades, BIA officials and employees had hoped that the use of government hospitals on reservations, staffed by trained physicians and nurses, would promote assimilation, but by midcentury, some policy makers feared that these reservation-based institutions, which exclusively served Indians, actually impeded assimilationist progress. Through short-term insurance plans for relocatees, Native women and men at least temporarily joined the growing numbers of Americans with health insurance coverage, and this coverage meant that Native women, men, and children could visit the same doctors and enter the same hospitals as other insurance-holding urban residents. Because BIA staff favored applications from young, able-bodied persons, the most urgent health need for many relocated families was prenatal, obstetric, and postnatal care.

Even with insurance, however, women transitioning from reservation health services often found their options frustratingly limited or prohibitively expensive. Blue Cross and Blue Shield offered bundled plans by midcentury, but despite steps toward standardization in the 1950s, Blue Shield plans remained decentralized.[57] This meant that a woman who relocated from a reservation to Chicago might have had different coverage than a sister who relocated to Dallas or Los Angeles, a source of confusion for relocatees and relocation staff alike. One woman living in Denver discovered that her temporary insurance plan did not cover the pre- and postnatal care that FROs and other government employees insisted was so important. This woman, like many others, discovered the unexpected gap in coverage too late, after she had made and kept the appointments BIA staff had urged, leaving her with a debt of approximately $50.[58] In contrast, an FRO in California urged a mother of four who was expecting her fifth child to visit a physician for prenatal care, explaining that the cost of such visits was covered by insurance.[59] Yet Mary Carson (Crow), who also relocated to California, found her coverage wanting. Carson visited two physicians during a 1958 pregnancy. It is unclear why Carson chose to change physicians, but her attempt to find a satisfactory practitioner resulted in bills that far exceeded the amount covered by her insurance plan. Carson owed $115 more than a year after her delivery, and her second physician reported her case to a credit agency.[60]

Relocatees' correspondence with BIA employees is littered with such complaints. Relocation records reveal these women's commitment to balancing their reproductive and financial needs in cities, and they provide a counterpoint to some contemporary government employees' and social scientists' characterization of Native women as apathetic about prenatal care and obstetrical arrangements. Far from uniquely Native frustrations, the historian Christy Ford Chapin points to a series of "media exposés" in the 1950s that recounted similar tales of individuals whose paltry insurance benefits left policyholders with medical bills they had not expected and in some cases could not afford. Indeed, consumer pressure was among the forces behind a steady expansion of coverage and benefits in these years.[61] So, too, for relocatees. Urban Indian women, alongside men, were vocal in highlighting the inadequacy of the BIA's short-term approach to insurance coverage. In the program's early years, if a relocatee received any health insurance, the plan might extend from several weeks to a few months, a situation that quickly proved insufficient for a population that included so many women of childbearing age. Individuals and organizations alike advocated for extended coverage. In 1956, the Los Angeles Indian Center passed a resolution recommending that relocatees receive long-term health insurance, and other Indian centers echoed this call.[62] The BIA responded to such demands by extending health coverage for up to one year.[63]

Despite this extension, in the end many, perhaps most, urban Indians found themselves left out of the national trend toward health coverage. "After one year," Inez Running Bear Denison (Rosebud Sioux), who relocated to

Chicago, recalled, "you were to pay your own expenses."[64] The historian Beatrix Hoffman has observed that the "workplace-based insurance system" that coalesced at midcentury "rationed coverage by occupation."[65] The low- and unskilled positions into which the BIA funneled Native men were among the least likely to offer affordable health insurance plans. Women were even less likely to receive health coverage through their employer. As late as the 1970s, even after the advent of Medicaid, a survey of Native mothers in the Bay Area found that almost half of the families in the study's sample did not have hospital or medical insurance.[66] In the recollection of Father Peter Powell, a non-Native Episcopalian minister who worked closely with Chicago's Native population, virtually none of the Native individuals with whom he came in contact had health insurance.[67] Thus, thousands of Native women navigated the urban health system without health insurance, and as the historian Myla Vicenti Carpio has explained, many of these women found themselves in a jurisdictional bind. After relocatees' first months in the city, the federal government assumed minimal responsibility for their care, but state and local governments proved equally stingy; each entity believed another bore responsibility.[68]

Some of these women skimped on medical prenatal care, an expense they felt that they could not afford, and when they gave birth in the city, many delivered in a public county hospital.[69] By the late 1950s and early 1960s, most Indians in Chicago had settled in the Uptown neighborhood. Native women living in Uptown without insurance generally avoided nearby private hospitals such as Illinois Masonic and Rice Memorial, where they knew they might be turned away or presented with a hefty bill, and instead made the longer trek to Cook County Hospital.[70] The county hospital was reputed to have quality practitioners, but Native patients were often frustrated by their experiences, complaining of overcrowded facilities and long wait times — complaints that ironically echo the frustrations their counterparts on reservations expressed about government hospitals in these same years.[71] Women in other cities expressed similar frustrations with county hospitals, including the insensitivity of physicians and "problems of paperwork, of referral, of not knowing the 'system.'"[72]

To the extent that hospital birthing and urban hospital services more generally had an assimilationist function as policy makers anticipated, the urban residents with whom many Native women shared reproductive experiences were typically poor, working-class, or otherwise marginalized communities of color. For her part, Debbie Clark was perfectly satisfied with her three deliveries at a county hospital in Los Angeles. She remembered it as being similar to the reservation hospital in which she had previously delivered four children—a hospital "was a hospital," she explained—except for the demographic makeup of the hospital's patients, which she recalled as a mix of black, Mexican American, and Asian American.[73] This trend extended to the postnatal care many Native women and their children received at free or inexpensive well-baby clinics. Margaret Mattson (Navajo), a mother in Denver, took each of her three children to the free baby clinic in the city "for regular supervision when they were small, and for immunization as they grew older."[74] Inez Running Bear Denison later recalled the great lengths to which she went to take her children to a well-baby clinic in Chicago. Denison regularly loaded her children on a bus that they rode across town because she had been told that she could not attend the clinic in her own neighborhood, likely due to her inability to pay for the services.[75] These women, like so many others, relied on their own resourcefulness in obtaining necessary care.

Reproduction on Relocation and the Reservation

In recent decades, scholars have eschewed binaries of "failure" and "success" that characterized some early studies of relocation and Indian urbanization. Historians such as Douglas K. Miller have instead proffered nuanced analyses that allow for Native agency and for the diversity of Native experiences of urban life.[76] Native biological reproduction in postwar cities merits the same approach. For some women, urban health services, including obstetric and gynecological care, were among the city's most attractive features. For others, the experience of bearing children in the city made women profoundly aware of the deficiencies of available care and contributed to return migrations. Whether Native women were on relocation or had self-relocated, they generally navigated pregnancy and childbirth with minimal assistance from the federal government. In many cases, they did so in ways that strengthened rather than diminished ties with reservations.

Elsie Burns (Navajo) was among the women who believed health care to be one of the city's advantages. After spending her adolescence in an Indian boarding school, Burns relocated to Denver at the age of eighteen and soon married a Navajo man who was also on relocation. Burns preferred city life to life on the reservation. She and many other Native women believed they received superior care in cities, and they appreciated their proximity to hospitals and clinics, an advantage that was especially appealing to women who had migrated from large reservations like the Navajo Nation.[77] When these women became pregnant in the city, the idea of giving birth in an urban hospital was not as jarring as it had been for some of the women of Anna Moore Shaw's generation. As will be addressed more fully in the next chapter, by the 1950s, most Native women delivered their children in reservation hospitals, and by mid-decade this trend extended to the Southwest, where women had been slower to accept hospital childbirth.[78] For Burns, as well as for women like Debbie Clark, the challenge was in determining where to go and how to pay for reproductive services.

Some relocatees received guidance from relocation officers, but government assistance was short-lived and often inadequate. Lois Knifechief relocated with her husband, John, and four young children from Pawnee, Oklahoma, to Los Angeles in 1957. The federal relocation program was five years old by that time, but Knifechief later remembered her family as "one of the first families that came out under the Bureau of Indian Affairs Program of relocating Indian families." Her recollection of the program's novelty resulted from the rudimentary assistance she and her husband received from the federal government. Instead, Lois Knifechief navigated the urban medical landscape with the assistance of her neighbors: "I asked where the nearest hospital was, the nearest doctor was," and so forth. Yet she speculated that this adjustment process was even more difficult for other relocatees, as the Knifechiefs did things "on our own that a lot of the Indian people don't do because they're too shy."[79]

For many postwar arrivals, other Indians filled the gaps. As scholars have demonstrated, the increased migration of Indians from reservations to cities after World War II prompted the establishment of urban Indian centers. While a few cities had boasted small Indian centers before the war, the American Indian Center of Chicago and the Intertribal Friendship House in Oakland, California, founded in 1953 and 1955, respectively, are representative of these postwar institutions. Indians in other cities quickly followed suit.[80] Urban Indian centers became hubs for Indian advocacy, and they also offered tangible assistance, medical and otherwise, to women and men in the city. As social centers, institutions like the Intertribal Friendship House also connected newly arrived Native women with more settled women who had experience birthing and mothering in the city. Native women in Seattle successfully formalized these networks when they founded the American Indian Women's Service League in 1958. Beginning in 1960, a Native woman arriving in Seattle from a reservation may have gone to the Indian center the Service League established that year for assistance in arranging for her prenatal care or delivery. Had she arrived a year earlier, someone may have directed her to a member of the Service League, or one of the Service League members may have shown up on her doorstep to offer support and guidance.[81]

In the early 1960s, a second Indian center opened its doors in the Uptown neighborhood of Chicago. St. Augustine's Center for American Indians was not an Indian-run center, although it employed Native staff and shifted to all-Indian administration by the end of its first decade. The city's second Indian center was founded and directed by Father Peter John Powell, a non-Native Episcopalian priest with a long history of working with Native peoples.[82] A Chicago resident in the postwar years, Powell became a fierce critic of the federal relocation program, which he believed was failing Native families and individuals. He envisioned St. Augustine's, part social services center and part religious community, as an institution that would compensate for the relocation program's inadequacies. St. Augustine's proved especially valuable to young Native women and mothers in Chicago, as staff members told clients about the local well-baby clinic, as well as how to use hospital facilities. Powell and his staff also gave women rides to and from prenatal, postnatal, and other appointments, a valued service considering Inez Running Bear Denison's frustratingly long commutes via public transportation. St. Augustine's also sponsored baby showers for expecting women, replicating the social and material support the women may have received had they experienced their pregnancy on the reservation.[83]

In addition to Indian centers and other urban institutions, women turned to kin. Although policy makers and many government bureaucrats envisioned relocation as a means of severing extended kinship ties and promoting the nuclear family, kinship networks proved critical to many new arrivals' adjustment to city life. This was especially true for women in their childbearing years. Because Native women, men, and families often chose to migrate to cities in which they already had family, newly arrived women turned to sisters, aunts, cousins, and in-laws for advice in navigating urban health services.[84] Family members' assistance was not always confined to city boundaries, as the experience of a Haudenosaunee woman living in postwar Detroit demonstrates. The woman had lived in the city for many years when she suffered severe nausea during a pregnancy. She appealed to her family for help, and her father responded by driving to a New York reservation to purchase what the historian Edmund Jefferson Danziger Jr. described as "Indian medicine."[85] The parturient woman's symptoms were alleviated, and her pregnancy resulted in a healthy baby.

Women also relied on female kin during confinement. The most pressing need for those who already had children was for someone to assume responsibility for child care when they went to the hospital to give birth. Some women did not feel that they could rely on their husbands to fulfill these child-care responsibilities, but more frequently husbands were not able to take time away from work. In these years, a woman might be expected to remain in the hospital for a recuperation period of five or more days.[86] One woman who had relocated with her husband and young child to a California suburb was fortunate to have a sister living in a nearby town, who cared for her son during her confinement.[87] Many who did not benefit from such proximity could nonetheless rely on this kind of familial support, as mothers and sisters left reservations to reside temporarily with expecting and new mothers in cities.[88] Indeed, the mobility that scholars of urban Indian migration have emphasized extended in many directions. Those without kin living nearby or able to make the sometimes-long journey to the city created fictive kin networks with Native or non-Native women. The early conversations initiated by women like Lois Knifechief sometimes evolved into trusting relationships. Debbie Clark and Mary Reese (Navajo), for example, each had an African American neighbor with whom they bartered services. In both cases, this neighbor cared for the women's children when they went into the hospital to give birth.[89]

These creative strategies notwithstanding, not all women who migrated to the city remained there, and reproduction played a prominent, if complicated, role in influencing women's (and men's) decisions regarding residency. Scholars continue to debate rates of return migration. BIA records suggest that between 28 percent and 35 percent of relocatees returned to their reservation in the program's early years, but some area offices reported higher figures throughout the decade.[90] The program's critics cited a much higher return rate, with some alleging that as many as three-quarters of relocatees did not remain in the city. The BIA stopped keeping formal statistics in 1959, in large part because these data had become fodder for criticism.[91] At any rate, competing numbers is not the only challenge in assessing return rates. These rates do not account adequately for the many individuals and families who went on relocation two or more times. Grace Shafer (Navajo) and her husband, for example, relocated to Los Angeles shortly after their marriage but soon returned to their reservation in Arizona. After two years and the birth of a child, the Shafers relocated once again, this time to Denver. Susie Yellowtail's son and daughter-in-law relocated to California, returned to Crow, and relocated again to Chicago before returning once again to the Crow Reservation.[92] Furthermore, an overemphasis on the relocation program's contested statistics obscures the migration patterns of the thousands of women and men who moved to and from cities without government assistance or oversight.

Rose Maney (Ho-Chunk) provides an early example of an individual who moved back and forth between the reservation and the city, in her case without government assistance. Maney and her husband left their Nebraska reservation to begin a new life in Chicago in the late 1930s. When she became pregnant during World War II, the couple decided to return to the Winnebago Reservation so that Maney could give birth there. Maney's motivation does not seem to have been primarily financial. She had previously given birth to one child on the reservation and two children in the city, and she later recalled without elaboration that she "wanted my baby to be born in Winnebago hospital."[93] The Maney family returned to Chicago by 1946, well before the official start of the federal relocation program.

Maney's desire to give birth on her reservation was not unusual. Throughout the relocation era, childbirth became an occasion for brief sojourns to reservations, and women's reproductive histories underscore the connections many relocated individuals maintained with reservation communities, spaces, and institutions.[94] As explained in earlier chapters, before the transition to hospital birthing, if a pregnant woman's mother did not live nearby, it was common for the woman to go stay with her mother in anticipation of delivery and remain a few weeks postpartum. Although not a universal practice, an iteration of this pattern emerged in the postwar years that transcended reservation borders. In a typical example, a woman who had relocated from the Fort Belknap Reservation returned to Montana in late January or early February 1959 to stay with her parents in anticipation of a March delivery. As the expecting mother planned to return to California after giving birth, her husband remained in the Los Angeles area during her absence.[95] Such arrangements occurred frequently enough that relocation officers sometimes noted exceptions. The file of one relocated husband and wife includes a BIA staff member's observation that the couple "did not even return [to the Northern Cheyenne Reservation] for the birth of their baby."[96] Citing Rose Maney's experience, James LaGrand has suggested that "most Indians thought that the beginning . . . of life could not be marked appropriately in a foreign land of noise and skyscrapers."[97] LaGrand's characterization is exaggerated and romanticized, and Indians did not inevitably view urban spaces as "foreign." Nonetheless, it is true that some women felt drawn to the support of reservation-based kin when preparing for childbirth, as well as to reservation homelands. Navajos, for example, recognize a powerful connection between place, an individual, and his or her umbilical cord. Some urban women remained committed to honoring the ancestral teaching of burying their child's umbilical cord in a special location on the reservation because they believed that this act solidified their child's bonds with Navajo homelands, even if the child would spend most of childhood and adolescence away from the reservation.[98]

Native women were as likely to cite extremely practical factors to explain their reproductive journeys. For relocated parents who hoped to maintain their children's connection to the reservation and to their Indian identity, the politics and bureaucracy surrounding tribal enrollment sometimes encouraged a temporary return. Some Native nations required that a child be born on the reservation in order to be eligible for tribal enrollment. In other cases, an off-reservation birth delayed enrollment because the new parents had to navigate the process from a distance. A parent's desire to enroll his or her child may have been personal, political, cultural, or social, and it was also sometimes financial, as the profits from tribal resources and any payments from the federal government were distributed among enrolled tribal members. In most cases, the motivation to pursue enrollment stemmed from some combination of these factors.[99]

Financial pressures motivated women's reproductive decisions in other ways as well. As late as the 1970s, Native and non-Native researchers reported instances of women and families leaving cities because of "difficulty in obtaining and paying for medical care."[100] The Anderson family relocated to Decoto, California, in 1957 but returned to the reservation within months. Like Harriet Brown, Joy Anderson (Assiniboine) relocated in the latter stages of pregnancy, another apparent oversight on the part of BIA staff on the reservation. When the Andersons learned that Joy would not yet be eligible for maternity services through her insurance due to the ninety-day waiting period, they decided to leave Decoto.[101] Although it is unclear from available records whether the Andersons remained on the reservation long term, it would not have been unusual for the family to apply for a second relocation after the arrival of their new addition.

For women who did not want to return to the reservation permanently, urban living was sometimes made sustainable by obtaining reproductive and other medical services on reservations. The federal government's decision that in most cases Native people would have to return to reservations to receive government health services resulted in temporary returns that relocation officers and other BIA employees generally had no choice but to accept.

When discussing health services in Los Angeles, Lois Knifechief emphasized that even the county hospital was not free.[102] Margaret Mattson, a mother in Denver, strongly preferred life in the city and had no intention of moving back to the Navajo Reservation, where she anticipated a life of hardship. Like Elsie Burns, Mattson appreciated the quality and proximity of health services in Denver. Yet when Mattson was pregnant with her first child, she traveled to the reservation to give birth. According to Romola Mae McSwain, a graduate student who recorded Mattson's story in the early 1960s, this reproductive journey "was not on account of any sentimental or traditionally ingrained feeling about the benefit of having one's baby born there." Rather, as Mattson herself explained, "it's free down there. . . . I didn't have any money, any insurance, and went down there and had my baby."[103] Mattson and her husband estimated that it would have cost $200 for her to deliver in Denver, so for them the financial calculation was simple. By the time Mattson gave birth to the couple's second child, the family had achieved some economic stability, and this child as well as the next was born in Denver.[104]

Like Margaret Mattson, Diane Nez and May Tsosie considered returning temporarily to the Navajo Reservation for childbirth. Echoing Mattson, Nez explained that the appeal of a reservation delivery was that "we don't have to pay our hospital bills there."[105] Neither Nez nor Tsosie ended up following through with this plan, however. Nez did not make the necessary transportation and logistical arrangements until it was "too late," and Tsosie and her husband had "so many bills" at the time that she "didn't have money to go back on." Tsosie visited a doctor for prenatal care in the final months of her pregnancy, and both women birthed in the city, likely in a public county hospital.[106]

In recalling their early reproductive experiences in the city, Nez and Tsosie revealed some of the dynamics of their decision-making processes. Each woman's husband expressed strong opinions about where she should deliver. While Nez hoped to give birth on the reservation for financial reasons, her husband, also Navajo, preferred that his wife deliver in the city, perhaps because he expected that she and their child would receive superior care. Tsosie's Navajo husband, in contrast, wanted her to return to the Navajo Nation for childbirth; "financial benefits apart," Tsosie herself was content to avoid the stress of a long journey and remain in Denver.[107] This small sample of two families offers no conclusions about the relative authority of fathers and mothers regarding Native biological reproduction in postwar cities. In Nez's case, her husband's desires prevailed, while in Tsosie's, her preferences carried the day.

It was not necessarily new to the postwar period or unique to an urban setting for a Native man to participate in his partner's childbearing decisions, but at least two features of urban living increased the likelihood of this situation. First, although the transition was far from absolute, urban families were more nuclear than families on reservations, which made it more likely that a woman navigated pregnancy and childbirth decisions without the close guidance of female kin. In some but certainly not all families, husbands or boyfriends stepped in to fill some part of this role. Second, the financial cost associated with reproductive services in cities meant that decisions about where to seek which reproductive services could have a significant effect on the family's budget. Male wage earners sometimes weighed in accordingly. Norma Hoskie (Navajo) did not seek prenatal care for her second pregnancy, for example, because her husband discouraged her from doing so. He was worried about acquiring more debt, as the family had not paid off the hospital bill for the birth of the couple's first child.[108] These dynamics regarding family and finances, which proved so influential in shaping women's parturition and obstetric experiences in the city, continued to shape women's experiences as urban Indian mothers.

Urban Indian Motherhood

What did it mean for recently relocated women to raise children in the city? Native mothers forged their own answers to this question. For many, urban motherhood meant forming new social ties within urban Indian institutions and advocating for their children in white-dominant or heavily minority spaces. For some, urban motherhood required the maintenance of their family's connection with relatives and homelands. As the Navajo poet Esther Belin writes, mothers "organized weekend road trips back to the rez / Back to the rez where we all came from / and where we need to return / to heal our wounds."[109] After more than a decade in Los Angeles, Lois Knifechief explained, "We've taken the kids back [to Pawnee, Oklahoma] every year because we want them to know their people."[110] Lena Haberman (Kiowa) and her children made a similar annual journey to Oklahoma.[111] While some maternal practices necessarily changed in the city, others—shored up by regular migrations and the Native "hubs" about which the Indigenous feminist scholar Renya Ramirez has written—showed little regard for reservation boundaries.[112]

Despite the BIA's ongoing pressure on Native families to embrace the nuclear family unit and the gender roles that familial model implied, and despite policy makers' expectation that relocation would facilitate this process, many families continued to rely on the inherently expansive practice of "flexible childrearing" at midcentury. This trend included many relocatees, and in fact flexible childrearing made relocation possible for some married couples and individuals. When Susie Yellowtail's son and daughter-in-law moved to Chicago for vocational training in the late 1950s, they left their older children on the reservation in the care of their grandparents.[113] A husband and wife who departed for Denver around the same time migrated with two children, leaving their youngest child with relatives on the reservation.[114] Flexible childrearing could also be a strategy for survival in the city, a means of weathering new challenges or periods of instability. In Flagstaff, where Navajo and Hopi women benefited from proximity to their respective reservations, the scholar Joyce Griffen observed a "pattern of fluid residence" among the Navajo children in her sample. Of the twenty-two mothers she interviewed, only three did not report one or more of their children having spent stretches of time with relatives, typically on the reservation.[115] Flexible childrearing extended into cities when mothers relied on sisters or in-laws who lived in proximity to assist in childrearing, as well as when a woman's mother, sibling, or cousin left the reservation to reside temporarily with urban kin and provide daily child care. By 1975, a study by the Native American Research Group found that urban Indian families were "more extended than most nuclear families."[116]

These kinship and child-rearing practices facilitated women's employment as wage workers, a necessity for many urban Indian families. Adult Native women, including biological mothers, had long performed necessary productive labor in their communities, and especially since the 1930s, women had begun working for wages, often on a temporary or flexible basis that accommodated their responsibilities at home.[117] In cities, single mothers in almost all cases worked for wages as soon as they were able to find employment, but married women, whose families generally entered cities at the lower rungs of the urban class structure, frequently pursued work outside the home as well. Nationally, the proportion of American mothers with small children who worked for wages grew by one-third in the 1950s.[118] To some degree, the BIA recognized these national trends, as well as Native families' economic needs. While Nicholas Rosenthal is certainly correct that the BIA favored male breadwinners, his related assertion that relocatees "were held to notions of gender and family that . . . limited married women to serving as housewives" requires qualification.[119] Relocation officers sometimes advised married women, including mothers, about day-care options "in case the mother wishes to go to work to augment the family income."[120] An FRO in Denver urged a reservation superintendent to reject one family's application to relocate to that city, adding, "If this family does insist on coming to Denver, we want to make it clear that it is *absolutely necessary* that [the mother and daughter] contribute continuously to the support of the family."[121] In this case, a married mother's employment was not a matter of her own choice or her family's perception of their needs but rather a precondition for the approval of the head of household's application for relocation.

Further research is needed regarding how urban Indian mothers handled what the historian Margaret Jacobs refers to as "the very modern dilemma" of balancing wage work and motherhood in cities.[122] Flexible childrearing provides a partial explanation, and new friends and fictive kin were gradually incorporated into these networks, but the fact remains that for many women, migration to the city meant a physical separation from kinship networks. For some, the solution was straightforward: Margaret Mattson and Hannah Fixico hired babysitters for their children, while other mothers dropped their kids off at a day-care service.[123] Other women employed more creative and less costly strategies. Fannie Johnson (Creek), mother of nine, worked the night shift in a factory so that she could be at home during the day.[124] Debbie Clark's situation was similar; she stayed home with her children during the day and attended night classes when her husband returned home from work.[125] May Tsosie provided domestic service in another woman's home, a common occupation for urban Indian women. To accommodate her domestic responsibilities, Tsosie arranged to alternate weeks with a Native friend. When it was Tsosie's week to work, she took her son with her.[126]

Although some Native women believed the city presented several advantages over midcentury reservations, urban life also presented new constraints. In a period in which family planning options and societal attitudes about birth control were changing, evidence suggests that the realities of urban living may have gradually altered some women's perspectives regarding their own reproductive labor and ideal family size. Women living in cities were exposed and sometimes had access to family planning methods before the Indian Health Service began providing these services on reservations. Navajo women living in Denver in the early 1960s, for example, learned about family planning options through friends, hospital staff, and visiting nurses.[127] For her part, Margaret Mattson embraced the opportunity and began using artificial contraception after the birth of her third child. Others displayed tepid interest but also hesitation. Elsie Burns's four young children kept her very busy, and she did not want another pregnancy in the short term, but the researcher Romola Mae McSwain reported that Burns did "not really know what she feels about taking advantage of [family planning methods]."[128] By the 1970s, studies conducted by medical researchers and social scientists suggested a correlation between women's wage work and their interest in using fertility control methods and also demonstrated that urban Indian women were more likely than their counterparts on reservations to utilize family planning services, although this tendency was not universal.[129]

Regardless of how many children one had, the experience of mothering—in a biological or social sense—in the city ultimately led many women to take on new roles or to adapt roles they might otherwise have occupied on reservations. Not only were women integral to the establishment and staffing of postwar urban Indian centers and organizations; they supported urban Indian community life by attending powwows and other social events in an attempt to maintain their children's connection with their cultural identity.[130] As urban Indian militancy gradually coalesced over the course of the termination and relocation era, mothers' experience with housing discrimination and their growing awareness of the discrimination their children faced in public city schools inspired and informed women-led activist agendas.[131] Men and women alike typically agreed that health care was among the most urgent issues facing urban Indian communities.[132] Recognizing that neither the BIA nor PHS would meet these needs adequately, Lois Knifechief in Los Angeles, Ignatia Broker in the Twin Cities, and countless others in cities throughout the country ultimately helped create the urban Indian health centers from which a subsequent generation of Native women would receive reproductive health services.[133]

ACCELERATING PREVIOUS TRENDS, more than 100,000 Native Americans moved from reservations to cities between the 1940s and the 1960s.[134] Many post–World War II migrants came "on relocation," part of a federal program that policy makers and BIA officials at least initially hoped would result in the permanent resettlement of Native individuals and families. Whether they moved with or without assistance from the federal government, however, when women left reservations they left behind the government health services and much of the familial and social network to which they would otherwise have turned for their reproductive health needs. The BIA desired the migration of women of childbearing age, particularly those who migrated in nuclear family units, and accordingly took basic steps to accommodate women's reproductive needs in the first months of their relocation. Due to the program's mismanagement as well as deliberate decisions by policy makers and government officials, however, most women found government assistance inadequate in this regard. In cities, many women had their first experience with health insurance but out of necessity more frequently obtained health services from public institutions and programs than from private medical institutions. For a variety of reasons, some women, even those who were satisfied with urban living overall, avoided urban medical institutions entirely when making childbirth arrangements and instead returned to reservations. Through reproduction and mothering, Native women modeled an expansive and fluid conceptualization of "Indian Country."[135]

Women relocated from reservations for wide-ranging reasons, but all did so at a historical moment in which reservation residents faced significant economic and political pressures, as policy makers sought to minimize and ultimately eradicate federal responsibility for Indian affairs. Some women who moved to cities during and after World War II, including Knifechief and Broker, remained there permanently, but others returned to reservations in the 1950s and early 1960s, bringing their experience of city living with them. These women returned not only to kin but to a medical infrastructure designed to provide health care to reservation residents. Many returning migrants quickly learned, however, that terminationist pressures on their reservations had not ceased in their absence. In some locations, including the Crow Reservation, returning women discovered that reservation health services were under threat, a potential casualty of the same motivation to "get out of the Indian business" that had propelled many policy makers' and government officials' enthusiasm for relocation in the first place.

CHAPTER FIVE
Our Crow Indian Hospital

In the spring of 1951, Susie Yellowtail, now a grandmother in her late forties, penned a letter to an old friend from her days at Northfield Mount Herman School for Ladies in Massachusetts. Land was on her mind, and she was angry. At the time of her writing, the Crow Nation awaited settlement of a claim that the tribe's lawyers had submitted to the Indian Claims Commission, a judicial body created after World War II to arbitrate disputes between Native nations and the federal government regarding broken treaties and Native land loss. "This claim we have is for millions of acres that 'Unky Sam' decided he could take away from the Crow Indians & use it for homesteads," Yellowtail explained, "& now he's going to have to pay for all those homesteads he handed out to people who wanted them."[1] Yellowtail expressed confidence that the tribe would win the case but doubted they would receive a fair settlement. She then shifted to more recent land struggles, recounting the federal government's ongoing efforts to persuade Crows to sell more land for the construction of a dam. Like many tribal members, Yellowtail opposed the sale. She suspected that the end result would be yet another case in which the Crows' non-Native neighbors would disproportionately benefit from tribal resources.[2]

Susie Yellowtail's casual letter to an old friend underscores the Crow woman's avid interest in the political and economic issues facing her people at midcentury, issues that few tribal members could ignore. As suggested in chapter 4, the post–World War II years brought policy changes and intensified pressures to Indian Country, as a handful of committed policy makers dedicated themselves to eliminating federal services that benefited only Indians. These policy makers envisioned the dissolution of the BIA and the termination of tribal members' political status as "American Indian." Prescient in many ways, Yellowtail could not fully predict the decade's developments from her vantage point in 1951. The following year, the Bureau of Indian Affairs (BIA) expanded the voluntary relocation program that resulted in her son Bruce leaving the Crow Reservation multiple times throughout the decade. The year after that, Congress passed House Concurrent Resolution 108 (HCR 108), a document that clearly articulated policy makers' intention to assimilate Native peoples "as rapidly as possible."[3] In

HCR 108's wake, Congress passed a series of acts that terminated the federal status of more than one hundred tribal nations.[4] By focusing on the Crow Reservation during these years, this chapter explores how the era's pressures and disruptions extended to groups that were not directly targeted by these explicitly terminationist acts, as well as how the members of one such nation dealt with the uncertainties of this period.

This chapter views termination as a host of policies and practices—not limited to the dissolution of a tribe's political status—that affected virtually every aspect of reservation life. Already a highly respected nurse and midwife, Susie Yellowtail assumed new health-related roles in the years following her above letter. Tracing her trajectory, alongside those of other Crow women, reveals termination's reach into the realm of health, healing, and birthing, as health care was among the services that some policy makers hoped to eliminate. After a half century of federal policies and practices encouraging Native women to seek reproductive health care from government health workers and give birth in reservation hospitals, Crow and other Native women faced the looming threat that the health services on which they and their families had eagerly or reluctantly come to rely would be a casualty of termination. While scholars readily acknowledge the poor health consequences that termination posed for Native nations, they rarely foreground health in their analyses of how tribal leaders navigated the termination era. At Crow, Yellowtail and a small group of women, many of whom had been galvanized by the political battles of the termination era, emerged as leaders in the community's effort to protect the reservation hospital and to reform the colonial institution to meet the evolving needs of Crow people. Displaying the same fighting spirit that she revealed in her 1951 letter, Yellowtail, along with her peers, presented comprehensive health services, and particularly maternal and infant welfare, as a federal obligation and a matter of Indian treaty rights.

The Hospital Habit

Native childbirth moved into the hospital at midcentury. As demonstrated in chapter 2, some Crow women had given birth in the reservation hospital as early as the 1910s, and hospital birthing rates had gradually, if not always linearly, increased in subsequent decades. By the late 1940s and early 1950s, approximately 90 percent of Crow births took place in the hospital. Of the remaining births, a few took place outside the hospital but with a private or, rarely, government physician in attendance.[5] Hospital birthing rates at Crow slightly outpaced the national average for Native women. Eighty-eight percent of all Native women gave birth in hospitals in 1955, and this figure would rise to 98 percent in the 1960s.[6] This trend is even evident in the Southwest, where the transition to hospital birthing occurred more slowly. Before 1929, for example, Navajo women in Tuba City, on the western end of the Navajo Nation, did not deliver any infants in the hospital. Four decades later, nearly all women did so, with the most significant leap occurring around midcentury.[7]

When Susie Yellowtail penned her letter to an old classmate, she still occasionally attended neighboring women's deliveries, but midwifery had notably waned on the reservation. Fewer than one in ten infants—6.2 percent, according to government figures—were born into the hands of midwives in those years.[8] Midwife-assisted births disproportionately occurred in Pryor, the reservation's westernmost district. Pryor residents recall that women continued to seek Matilda Roundface's assistance in the 1950s. Her practice seems to have slowed in this decade, due in part to "old age," and her daughters did not pick up their mother's trade.[9] As in previous generations, the decline of midwifery did not mean that Crow women viewed the midwife's expertise as obsolete. Crow midwives and female healers continued to pass down gynecological and pediatric knowledge after they stopped attending home births. One Crow midwife did not deliver babies after World War II, but at some point, she offered to teach a granddaughter how to terminate pregnancies. In this case, the granddaughter demurred.[10] This same midwife found that younger kin were more eager to learn her methods for treating colic, a skill for which Crow midwives were particularly renowned. Pretty Shield, Matilda Roundface, and others passed down their own practices for dealing with colic, and to this day Crow parents are as likely to take their infants and small children to *akbaawasée*, or baby doctors, as they are to government physicians.[11]

In oral history interviews, twenty-first-century Crow women are quick to praise Susie Yellowtail's and Matilda Roundface's birthing and healing skills.[12] That these and other midwives were held in such high regard leaves Native women's final embrace of hospital childbirth at midcentury unexplained. In fact, this shift in birthing locations can be attributed to a confluence of forces, many of which were long under way. By the late 1940s, Minnie Williams, a Crow woman in her sixties, approvingly observed that young mothers had been "educated to the idea that [hospital childbirth] is best for her and her baby."[13] Here, Williams referred to the subtle and less-than-subtle messages Native women had for decades received in schools, at reservation hospitals, and through regular interactions with field workers and missionaries. Women's historians have demonstrated, however, that it was not until mid-century that the hospital began to realize its long-standing promise as the "best" birthing location in terms of maternal and infant health care outcomes. On as well as off the reservation, the routinization of hospital procedures and medical advancements such as the development of antibiotics dramatically improved the safety of the hospital as an institution.[14] The medical sociologist Stephen Kunitz thus offers a simple explanation for the documented increase in hospital childbirth among Navajo women in these years: "Hospital utilization increased . . . because hospitals became safer places in which to have babies."[15]

Crow sources reveal additional factors. Not surprisingly, logistics remained crucial. During and after World War II, the reservation experienced its own rural to urban migration, as families moved from their allotments to reservation towns, including Crow Agency.[16] This placed more women "within easy reach"—in the words of an earlier superintendent—of the hospital.[17] Crows often cited increased mobility to explain increased hospital utilization. Dorothy Spotted Bear, whose mother sometimes assisted Matilda Roundface in delivering babies at Pryor, emphasized that by the 1950s tribal members had "better vehicles, better transportation."[18] Some point to less benign forces, most notably government employees' use of coercion in suppressing Native midwifery. One Crow elder reports that a government physician threatened a midwife in the Reno District with legal action after she assisted in the birth of her grandchild in 1947. She never attended another home birth again.[19] Former midwives on other reservations report similar experiences.[20] Even setting immediate legal threats aside, however, Native women faced intensive assimilationist pressures at midcentury, as will be demonstrated below, and such pressures further encouraged women to utilize hospital obstetric services.

Generally speaking, the immediate postwar years brought continuity rather than change in Crows' relationship with government health services and the reservation hospital. Health ways on the reservation continued to be characterized by "medical pluralism," and many Crows viewed Western medicine as complementary with a range of Crow healing practices.[21] Tribal members remained as committed as ever to exerting authority within hospital walls and regularly protested dissatisfactory policies and procedures, particularly those that restricted the presence of visitors. By the 1940s, former midwives were among the visitors whom patients expected to board and be fed at the hospital. After a government physician warned the Reno midwife to stop attending births, the midwife refused one woman's request to assist in the delivery of her third child, even though she had attended the women's earlier births. But the older woman agreed to the pregnant mother's request that she be present at her hospital delivery.[22] Other prominent midwives, including Mary Takes the Gun, who had attended Susie Yellowtail's third delivery in the early 1930s, also accompanied their daughters, nieces, granddaughters, and neighbors into the hospital during and after the war.[23] Within hospital walls, these women occupied an informal role as birth coach and sometimes patient advocate.

As had been the case for Yellowtail two decades earlier, the Crow Agency Hospital was also a more formal workplace for some Crow women. By the late 1940s, Alice Other Medicine was employed as a registered nurse at the institution.[24] One Crow elder vividly recalls interacting with Other Medicine—or "Mrs. O"—when she visited the hospital as a child. Although the elder admits to having been a bit afraid of Other Medicine, who "would really get after us about taking care of ourselves," she ultimately became a nurse herself and views Other Medicine as having been an important role model.[25] Other Crow women, including Cordelia Big Man and Pretty Shield's granddaughter Alma Hogan (Snell), worked as "nurses' aides with no training."[26] Hogan began working at the hospital during what she later described as "a bad time in my life." She was pregnant as the result of rape and still mourning her grandmother Pretty Shield's death. Hogan later recalled that the senior physician Theodore Crabbe—whom Hogan described as a "good Christian doctor"—had said, "Put her to work, or she will have a breakdown."[27] If the tragic circumstances leading to Hogan's hospital employment were somewhat unusual, Hogan in other ways represents a trend that emerged at midcentury and continued in subsequent decades: the female descendants of highly respected Crow midwives frequently gravitated toward nursing or nurses' aide positions, where they cared for patients and assisted birthing women under new circumstances.[28]

Other Medicine's position, although subordinate to the white head nurse, was something of an exception, while Hogan's and Big Man's situations were more typical. As Mary Jane Logan McCallum has found in Canada's Indian hospitals, Native people occupied "the least well-paid, the least secure, and the least autonomous positions" in midcentury government hospitals.[29] Much as Robert Yellowtail had done in the 1930s, tribal leaders consistently advocated that Crow women be employed as health workers on the reservation, but the BIA met these demands with some ambivalence. The bureau's official line promoted Indian preference for reservation employment. As one government official explained to Crow leaders, "The Health Division agrees with and generally follows the practice of assigning local persons to positions provided they are fully qualified to meet the requirements of the position and render satisfactory service on the job."[30] Yet federal officials recognized that Native nurses did not always abide by hospital hierarchies and could be disruptive forces, as demonstrated by Yellowtail's brief employment at the Crow Agency Hospital and as would once again be affirmed in the resurgence of Native activism in the 1970s. In practice, BIA officials responded to tribal leaders' request for the employment of Crow nurses by suggesting that the tribal council send young women from the community to the government's nurses' aide training program in Oklahoma. This response, which the official acknowledged offered only a "partial solution," affirmed rather than challenged hospital hierarchies.[31] Cordelia Big Man did receive certification as a licensed practical nurse at some point, but Crow women who received nursing training in the postwar years continued to face obstacles in their attempt to use their training on their own reservation.[32]

Crows had adopted the "hospital habit" as BIA officials and employees had long urged, but tribal leaders, patients, and hospital employees alike remained committed to engaging with the institution on their own terms. During and after World War II, however, the most significant power struggles concerning the reservation hospital and government health services would be waged outside hospital walls, in the realm of the BIA's budget and the allocation of resources. As the historian Wade Davies has argued, Native peoples' increased integration of Western medicine into their healing systems came with a "serious catch": "The more American Indian people demanded Bureau of Indian Affairs medical care, the more reliant they were on Congressional appropriations, and the more affected they were by broad changes at the national and global levels."[33] This became painfully clear on many reservations during World War II, as the demands of the war effort left reservation hospitals woefully understaffed and lacking resources. The BIA closed five government hospitals on the Navajo Reservation during the war and replaced other hospitals, such as that serving the Klamath Tribes of Oregon, with dramatically scaled-down clinics.[34] Government health services did not necessarily become more reliable following the war; rather, they became subject to a new form of threat.

Terminating Indian Health

The Native intellectual and legal scholar Vine Deloria Jr. characterized the termination era as "the most traumatic period of Indian existence."[35] Scholars have documented the dislocations and grief that members of terminated tribes experienced as they found themselves stripped of federal protections, resources, community, and identity.[36] The era's pressures and disruptions extended throughout Indian Country. Members of many Native nations quite reasonably feared that they would be next, and reservations endured a frustrating mix of federal neglect and undesired intervention, of which the proposed dam construction that Susie Yellowtail lamented on the Crow Reservation was but one example. Cordelia Big Man, former hospital employee and president of the Crow Agency Women's Club, described the situation facing Crows and other Native peoples in the late 1950s: "What with several termination Bills now in the Congress of the United States to get rid of Indians, the phrase used, 'let them sink or swim,' seems now to become the policy."[37] By Big Man's writing, termination had become a consuming issue for the Crow Tribal Council as well as the Crow Agency Women's Club. As will be demonstrated below, Big Man was also well positioned to recognize the threat termination posed to Crow health.

As the legal scholar Charles Wilkinson emphasizes, the midcentury termination policies through which policy makers hoped to assimilate Native peoples once and for all were in keeping with long-standing federal objectives. "Termination," Wilkinson argues, "offered full and final relief from the centuries-old weariness with the refusal of Indians to abandon their political and cultural identity."[38] More immediately, termination was a backlash against John Collier's agenda, described in chapter 3, and terminationist sentiment was accelerated by the wartime developments recounted in chapter 4. Senator Arthur Watkins and other leading termination proponents embraced the language of the post–World War II era, including the progressive vision of "integration" and the anti-Communist rhetoric of the Cold War. Most pointedly, Watkins referred to termination as "the Indian freedom program," and he sold policy makers' emerging agenda as "freeing the Indian from wardship" and from federal paternalism.[39]

Aspects of this message appealed to some Crow men and women who had grown tired of federal paternalism and viewed the BIA as an obstacle to their progress. At a tribal council meeting toward the end of the war, Harry Whiteman criticized Commissioner Collier and his "regime," which he characterized as "ultra-paternal." Whiteman staunchly opposed the dissolution of the Indian Bureau, but he called for a "more liberal program" with less "red tape" and more "self-determination."[40] Five years later, Minnie Williams reiterated Whiteman's call for relief from "the system now ruling [Indians] like an iron hand." She, too, advocated more self-determination and "less interference" from reservation employees.[41] Susie Yellowtail echoed Williams when she complained that government employees on reservations "do all in their power to hold the Indians back."[42] The desire to escape federal paternalism and interference was of course the same impulse that led some Crow and other Native men and women to leave their reservations and migrate to cities after World War II.[43]

Despite signs of convergence between terminationists' rhetoric and Crow objectives, Native peoples throughout Indian Country found that as termination policies developed, tribal members had little control over the timeline or circumstances under which they would be implemented. Nineteen forty-seven was a pivotal year for policy makers' evolving termination agenda, and some of the year's developments were felt at Crow. That spring, under pressure from the Senate Civil Service Committee, Acting Commissioner William Zimmerman submitted a document that divided tribal nations into three groups based on his assessment of their relative preparedness for the withdrawal of federal supervision. Zimmerman placed Crows in his second group, which the historian Kenneth Philp characterizes as consisting of "semi-acculturated people . . . [who] functioned with minimal supervision." The threat of federal withdrawal was less urgent for Crows than it was for those tribes included in Zimmerman's first group, but the acting commissioner proposed a rapid timeline. He predicted that the federal government could withdraw from the Crow Reservation in as few as two years and certainly within ten.[44]

Montana's Native nations were far from passive in the face of this threat. In 1951, they founded the Montana Inter-Tribal Policy Board in part as a bulwark against coercive termination policies. Chaired by Robert Yellowtail, the former superintendent of the Crow Reservation, the Policy Board consisted of two representatives from each reservation and two representatives from the state's landless Indians. In his capacity as chair, Yellowtail sounded themes of self-determination that he had promoted since World War I. He did not universally oppose termination for all tribes, but he argued that each tribal nation should be able to make its own decision without threat or coercion. Suspicious of western congressmen and other interested parties, he staunchly opposed the abolition of the BIA, which he viewed as a real possibility, and warned that abolition would facilitate further abdication of treaties and more land loss.[45]

These were not abstract or theoretical issues for Yellowtail and other tribal leaders in the state. William Zimmerman had included the Flathead Reservation to the northwest of Crow, for example, in the first group of his 1947 list. By the Policy Board's founding, even before the passage of HCR 108, policy makers had made clear that they intended to follow through with the termination of the Consolidated Salish and Kootenai Tribes, who shared the reservation. Reservation leaders reluctantly began preparing for their coerced termination while continuing to resist policy makers' machinations. Remarkably, the Consolidated Salish and Kootenai Tribes, through a sophisticated tribal council and with the support of Montana congressmen, defeated termination in 1954.[46] Although the timing of Cordelia Big Man's letter demonstrates that the pressure of termination did not cease following the Flathead victory, Montana Indians surely breathed a collective sigh of relief. As the historian Jaakko Puisto has argued, "Were the Flathead Reservation terminated . . . the Crow and the Blackfeet Reservations with their considerable resources would have been next in line."[47]

For the Crow Nation and on many other reservations, however, health services were among the most immediate threats of the termination era. In 1947, the same year William Zimmerman composed his list, the federal government closed the hospital on the nearby Northern Cheyenne (then called Tongue River) Reservation. Officials insisted that continued operation of the hospital was "wholly uneconomical" and instructed the superintendent to send Cheyennes to the hospital at Crow Agency when they required care.[48] Beginning that spring and continuing in the years after the Northern Cheyenne closure, BIA officials repeatedly informed the Crow Tribal Council that their hospital would be closed as well, also owing to economic necessity. Superintendent L. C. Lippert, who was firmly opposed to the closure of the reservation hospital, explained to tribal leaders that the BIA would continue to operate health clinics if the hospital closed, but the tribal council rejected this plan: "We do not think these clinics would give the medical care we need."[49] Among other deficiencies, such clinics would not be equipped to handle childbirth. Cheyenne women's most vivid recollections of the period after the closure of their hospital included stories of women giving birth on their way to the more distant hospital. According to Belle Highwalking, "many babies," including one of her grandchildren, were "born on the way over to Crow Agency."[50]

The situation remained tenuous at Crow in the early 1950s. For one thing, the closure of the hospital on the neighboring reservation increased pressure on the Crow Agency Hospital in a material sense due to the added expense of an influx of non-Crow patients.[51] Furthermore, Dillon Myer, the new commissioner of Indian affairs, was an avid terminationist who believed Indian hospitals and clinics "stifled [Native peoples'] development toward independence.[52] The BIA closed eight hospitals in these years, and at least one of the closures would have hit close to home for Crow observers. In 1953, the BIA closed the Fort Washakie Hospital on the Wind River Reservation in Wyoming. Because Crows and Shoshones shared a common Sun Dance and traveled back and forth to participate in dances on both reservations, the former would have remained abreast of the latter's unsuccessful effort to reopen their hospital. Shoshones and the Arapahoes with whom they shared a reservation argued that they had not been consulted about the hospital closure and that they faced discrimination when seeking health services from the county. Less than a year after the hospital closed its doors, reservation leaders alleged that the BIA's decision had already had a devastating effect on reservation health.[53]

Government officials generally explained hospital closures—and threatened closures—in economic terms, as a fiscal necessity, when in fact they were quite clearly a matter of policy. In 1947 and again in 1948, Congress dramatically reduced appropriations for Indian affairs, contributing to, if not creating, the "lack of funds" that placed the Crow Agency Hospital in "serious danger" in these years.[54] In the early 1950s, Commissioner Myer requested and received additional congressional funding for the Indian Bureau, a significant proportion of which went to health, education, and welfare services. Increased funding at a time when terminationist fervor was reaching its height at first glance appears paradoxical, but Myer made clear that this short-term increase was in the service of the federal government's forthcoming withdrawal from Indian affairs.[55] The commissioner approached reservation health care first and foremost as a means of furthering the government's assimilation agenda and only secondarily as a matter of Indian health outcomes. In Myer's view, health services for Indians were ultimately a matter of federal discretion. Hospital closures continued despite increased funding because policy makers and other authorities remained committed to chipping away at these and other services. As Myer's successor Glenn Emmons explained, the elimination of Indian-only health services was "a direct step toward assimilation."[56]

Native peoples were astute in their assessment of midcentury policy developments. Crows resisted the closure of their reservation hospital for political as well as medical reasons, interpreting threatened reductions of government services as an ominous sign of future actions. Crow men and women were not alone. After representatives from more than twenty-five tribal nations testified before a congressional subcommittee in protest of the proposed closure of an Indian hospital in Oklahoma, a government bureaucrat surmised that the Native witnesses were ultimately motivated by "the well-grounded fear . . . that the closing of Shawnee [Indian Hospital] will mark the loss of another outpost of Indian rights, that the boundaries of their unique status will shrink much more under the relentless eroding action of the Federal bureaucracy."[57] The forced closure of clinics and hospitals in other locations had foreshadowed the termination bills that policy makers introduced almost immediately after the passage of HCR 108.[58] At the local level, had it not been for the engaged resistance of the Crow Tribal Council, which remained reasonably united on health matters despite intratribal divisions on other midcentury issues, Crows likely would have shared the fate of Northern Cheyennes, Shoshones, Arapahoes, and others who lost their reservation hospital in these years.

In 1954, Congress passed, and President Dwight Eisenhower signed, the Indian Health Transfer Act, which transferred responsibility for Indian health care from the BIA to the Public Health Service (PHS). The PHS established the Division of Indian Health, soon renamed the Indian Health Service (IHS), to accommodate its expanded obligations.[59] Many tribal governments and Native individuals resisted the transfer to PHS on political grounds, fearing that the change would function as some of its proponents, including Senator Arthur Watkins, intended: as a step toward termination. As Commissioner Glen Emmons observed, the legislation initiated "the biggest reduction of program responsibilities in the history of the Bureau."[60] For their part, Crow leaders displayed a characteristic distrust of change mandated from above. The BIA, for all its deficiencies, was a known entity for tribal members, and Crows had developed ways of ensuring that government health services met their needs. Opposition was not universal in Indian Country, however. The Intertribal Council of the Sioux Nation and the Navajo Tribal Council, for example, favored the transfer due to their frustrations with the BIA and their hope that PHS would produce better health outcomes.[61] PHS had more resources at its disposal, and the transfer resulted in more physicians and hospital beds on reservations.[62] The legislation at least promised Crows a brief reprieve from the threat that the reservation would lose its hospital; to quell fears regarding the transfer, the act included a one-year moratorium on hospital closures.[63]

The Indian Transfer Act went into effect July 1, 1955, and the months immediately following the transfer only intensified Crow concerns. Patients complained about PHS's inflexibility, the administration's insistence on operating on a "whole-sale basis," and what they interpreted as the privileging of rules over Crow lives. They quickly perceived that the transfer to PHS had come at the expense of Crow influence within hospital walls. Tribal members were, as one Crow-produced report on the situation put it, "almost in arms" over hospital conditions.[64] Nor were Crows alone in their frustrations. Overwhelmed by complaints at Crow and elsewhere, PHS officers advocated the establishment of health committees at every PHS facility to act as a "liaison" between PHS and tribal councils.[65] The Crow Tribal Council authorized the tribal chairman to appoint five tribal members to form the Crow Health Committee in the spring of 1956. Not surprisingly, Susie Yellowtail, the retired nurse and midwife, chaired the committee in its formative years.

Crow (Women's) Health Committee

Alongside Susie Yellowtail, tribal chairman Edward Posey Whiteman selected four tribal members to join the new health committee: Josephine Russell, Eloise Whitebear Pease, George Hogan Jr., and John Glenn.[66] The committee's two male members disappear almost immediately from the group's records. Glenn apparently never attended a meeting; Hogan attended meetings in April and May but had left the group by summer.[67] Yellowtail, Russell, and Pease, in contrast, served as officers and remained active committee members in the following years. Although the group's membership changed frequently, the Crow Health Committee consisted entirely of women after its first few months. Whether a cause or effect of the committee's gender makeup, the Crow Health Committee devoted particular—though by no means exclusive—attention to maternal, infant, and child welfare in its first years.

It was not inevitable that the Crow Health Committee would be a women's committee. Such was not the case on all reservations. Annie Wauneka (Navajo), who would become a dear friend of Susie Yellowtail's in the following decades, worked alongside men on the Navajo Tribal Health Committee, for example.[68] Furthermore, Edward Whiteman initially envisioned the committee as a coed entity. The tribal health committee that took shape in the postwar period represented a complete reversal of the gender makeup of the first reservation health committee that had existed briefly in the 1930s. Several factors may have contributed to this gender reversal. First, the earlier reservation health committee had emerged at the behest of a government physician who hoped that a designated group of educated leaders might stem patient complaints and facilitate health initiatives, and this physician had a heavy hand in shaping the group's composition and purpose. It was the physician who determined that the committee would consist of two delegates from each district, and government employees' expectation was that Native men should be responsible for matters of tribal governance.[69]

The committee's postwar iteration reflected Native women's increased prominence in tribal politics more generally.[70] Two decades earlier, Crow women had had minimal direct involvement in tribal politics, but in the years after World War II, women like Minnie Williams and Eloise Pease began appearing more frequently in tribal council meeting minutes.[71] These women had been galvanized by the political struggles Susie Yellowtail detailed in her 1951 letter, as well as other pressures of the termination era. By the mid-1950s, a handful of women, including Pease, had earned themselves positions on critical standing committees such as Land and Budget. Crow women's clubs—at Crow Agency and Lodge Grass—continued to facilitate women's political involvement. The Crow Agency Women's Club had disbanded during the war, but women revived the group in the late 1940s.[72] The reconstituted group dedicated itself to studying the political and economic questions facing the Crow Nation and presented its conclusions to the tribal council.[73] As Cordelia Big Man's letter to the president of the General Federation of Women's Clubs demonstrates, club women also stayed abreast of developments in federal policy.

Although Susie Yellowtail was an important exception, the Crow Health Committee can be viewed as a who's who of active women's club members and women who appear in the minutes of postwar tribal council meetings. These women's visibility in tribal politics did not go unquestioned, however. According to Crow Health Committee secretary and Lodge Grass Women's Club member Josephine Russell, older men resented women's participation in tribal affairs: they "object and make remarks about being 'run by skirts.'"[74] Olive Venne, who briefly served on the Crow Health Committee, concurred. Speaking with an ethnographer in the mid-1950s, Venne related a recent instance in which she had felt compelled to publicly challenge an older male tribal member who "had asked the women to stop talking at the council because they knew nothing."[75] Eloise Pease believed that the community generally expected that women work "behind the scenes," an expectation that was not necessarily incompatible with service on tribal committees.[76] Women's dominance of the health committee may reflect the community's perception of the gender-appropriate nature of women's work in health, education, and social welfare.

The women who served on the Crow Health Committee were well positioned to garner the respect of fellow tribal members. Most of these women had been born in the early 1900s or 1910s. In their forties or fifties at the time of their appointment, they had reached what Crows considered to be mature age; if not elders, respected older women. They were mothers, clan mothers, and in many cases grandmothers. Many came from prominent families and were in some way connected to the generation of boarding-school educated men who had garnered reputations as tribal leaders in the first decades of the century. They can also be viewed as members of a fluid and flexible "middle class" on the reservation.[77] The category was not strictly economic, but because the committee met on Tuesday afternoons, service on the health committee generally precluded regular wage work.[78] Committee members prided themselves on and were generally admired for their industriousness. Although they did not always meet the bar they set for themselves, these women aspired to modeling "clean bills of Health themselves, clean homes, and clean yards."[79]

Committee members were also particularly suited for the role of "liaison." About a decade after the committee's establishment, at a time when anthropologists were busy categorizing Native individuals according to their degree of "acculturation," the tribal historian Joseph Medicine Crow joked with a graduate student that scholars would have to invent an additional category in order to classify women like Susie Yellowtail. Medicine Crow explained that those in "the Susie Category" were characterized by their ability to "go back and forth . . . bridging the two cultures, so to speak."[80] The tribal historian observed that several Crows would fit in this proposed category, and although he did not mention anyone by name, Yellowtail's fellow committee members are likely candidates. Many of the women either had spent time off the reservation or had otherwise obtained notable experience interacting with white society. For example, Josephine Russell's experience with non-Native society began early. As a child, she was the only Crow student at her public school, and in the 1930s, she attended college in Oregon, becoming one of a handful of Crows to obtain a college degree.[81] As importantly, at least some committee members were equally known for their involvement in various realms of Crow cultural life. Medicine Crow noted, for example, that Susie Yellowtail gave lectures on health at reservation schools during the week and was also actively involved in the Sun Dance, which became open to female dancers around the time Yellowtail began her tenure as chair of the health committee.[82]

Fieldwork on the Wind River Reservation in the 1960s led the anthropologist Michelle Newman to conclude that some Shoshone women's ready engagement with non-Native institutions and society "may actually be the means by which assimilation can be resisted rather than achieved." Newman

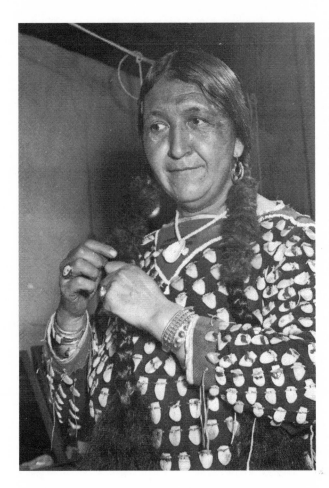

Susie Yellowtail was committed to educating non-Natives about Crow history and culture, and she traveled widely over the course of her life. This photograph was taken in the early 1950s when Yellowtail was in Europe as part of a Crow dance troupe. The Reginald and Gladys Laubin Collection, Spurlock Museum, University of Illinois at Urbana-Champaign.

argued that the women she studied believed that if they were to ward off the unrelenting threat of termination, "they must be able to deal effectively with the larger society, i.e., 'to play the game' according to the rules which predominate in the larger society."[83] Newman's observation provides a useful framework for interpreting the priorities and actions of the Crow Health Committee a decade before Newman visited Wind River. Recognizing the very real danger of the hospital becoming another termination casualty, committee members coordinated earnestly yet firmly with PHS officers not only to protect tribal health but also to maintain the Crow Agency Hospital as an Indian institution.

The committee's first written report reveals the group's attempt to display evenhandedness. After studying the health situation on the reservation, the committee reported that it had "found things to be remedied on both sides, the side of the Indian and on the part of Public Health." Regarding the latter, the report criticized the excessively bureaucratic nature of PHS health care, offering the simple yet profound conclusion that Native peoples must "insist that we are human-beings with human feelings and should be treated as such."[84] The report also acknowledged PHS administrators' concern that Crows used the hospital incorrectly. Just as their BIA predecessors in the first decades of the twentieth century lamented Crow and other Native patients' tendency to view reservation hospitals as dispensaries, PHS officers at midcentury complained that patients were too quick to visit the hospital for minor ailments that did not require hospital care, overburdening hospital staff. For committee members, the answer to this problem was more health education on the reservation. To that end, the committee requested the appointment of a trained health educator and pledged to be actively involved in all health education initiatives.[85]

Although not explicitly mentioned in the written report, committee members did not necessarily view the educational process as unidirectional. For her part, Yellowtail would later censure those who "make their living from us without ever making any effort to understand or get to know us." She argued that "whites who come to work on the reservation need to understand our religious and cultural background in order to work with my people."[86] Susie's granddaughter Jackie Yellowtail recalls her grandmother's efforts as chair of the Crow Health Committee to "acculturate" new doctors when they first moved to the reservation. Jackie, who lived with her grandparents as a child, recalls physicians visiting the family's home in Wyola, where Susie cooked for them and talked to them about "our culture, our ways."[87]

Yellowtail delivered the committee's first report to the tribal council in the summer of 1956. Her message was twofold. First, she urged tribal members to "use your hospital!"[88] Despite PHS officers' grievances regarding tribal members' overuse of the hospital for minor complaints, committee members recognized that in the context of prevailing termination pressures the more significant concern was that Crow patients would follow their long-established practice of registering dissatisfaction with hospital policies and personnel by avoiding the institution. Policy makers had justified the closing of the Fort Washakie Hospital, for example, based on inadequate use, even though Shoshone and Arapahoe leaders insisted that recent usage rates had been atypical, a reflection of the unpopularity of the current physician.[89] Yellowtail and her committee advanced an argument on behalf of the collective. If Crows who had the resources to do so chose to obtain private health services off the reservation, the politicians itching to reduce Indian services would interpret this as evidence that Crows no longer needed a reservation hospital or that tribal members could and should pay for their health care.

In their effort to persuade Crows to utilize the reservation hospital rather than securing health services off the reservation or eschewing Western medical care altogether, the committee emphasized "treaty rights" and the federal government's responsibility for Indian health. The medical sociologist Stephen Kunitz has argued that in the decades after the transfer to PHS, many Native men and women gradually came to view government health services in this way—as "something owed to Indians as a result of treaty rights and trust obligations"—but at Crow, these arguments were not new.[90] Robert Yellowtail had framed government health services in this way during his eleven years as superintendent, and the Crow Indian Women's Club advanced a similar argument in the 1930s. At midcentury, "treaty rights" was an especially powerful refrain in Native peoples' resistance to termination-related policy changes. The Consolidated Salish and Kootenai Tribes, for example, defeated termination in part by appealing to the Hell Gate Treaty of 1855, which had created the Flathead Reservation.[91] In the Crow Health Committee's first years, its female members insisted that treaty rights "guaranteed" to tribal members "better medical care" than they had been receiving.[92] They further contended that this care should be free. As one committee member informed a new physician several months after Yellowtail delivered the committee's first report to the tribal council, "All Crow people [feel] that as long as they [are] in a trust status they should not be required to pay regardless of income."[93] Finally, the Crow Health Committee used the language of treaty rights to underscore federal obligation and counter persistent and unsettling rumors that reservation health services were to be transferred to the state of Montana.[94]

In contrast to Salish and Kootenai appeals to the Hell Gate Treaty of 1855, however, the Crow women did not cite a specific treaty by name in claiming these rights. Only 12 percent of the 389 ratified treaties between the United States and tribal nations included health-related provisions, and most such provisions were limited by scope and time frame.[95] Yet government-supported health services had increased and expanded in the decades after 1871, when the federal government stopped signing treaties with Native groups. In these years, as the historian Cathleen Cahill has demonstrated, policy makers and social reformers began to ignore specific treaty provisions in favor of social programming that they believed would promote independence. They argued that programs related to land and education—and one could add health—would "uphold the spirit of the treaties."[96] While article

10 of the Crows' 1868 Fort Laramie Treaty included the promise of a government-supported physician, it was a 1904 congressional act establishing the terms for a further cession of Crow land that appropriated funding for the first Crow hospital. When the women on the Crow Health Committee emphasized "treaty rights" half a century later, they, too, evoked "the spirit of the treaties"—a history of land sales and land loss and of federal promises, broken promises, and shifting obligations.[97]

The second component of Susie Yellowtail's report to the tribal council was that if tribal members used the reservation hospital, they could be assured that the Crow Health Committee would hold PHS accountable for quality care. Committee members pledged to "battle the Public Health Department and secure fair and just treatment from them as we deserve." They promised to take the battle all the way to Washington, D.C., if necessary.[98] The committee advertised its meeting times and encouraged tribal members to take any grievances with the hospital or PHS staff to a committee member. They also circulated a flier in subsequent months that underscored this message. "USE YOUR HEALTH COMMITTEE," the flier instructed. All complaints should be registered with a committee member, and patients were further encouraged to have a committee member accompany them to the hospital. "This is important," the women intoned. "This is the only way you can be satisfied with the Crow Hospital."[99] Yellowtail and her committee stayed true to their word in investigating patient complaints and advocating on patients' behalf. Their persistence may have led PHS officers to wonder whether tribal health committees were worthwhile from PHS's standpoint.[100]

For the Women and Children

PHS officers did hope that committee women could be of assistance in matters relating to reproduction. Biological reproduction is difficult to locate in government or tribal sources in the midst of the political dramas of the postwar period, despite the fact that pregnancy, birthing, and childrearing remained at the forefront of many Crow women's lives. The birth rate per 1,000 women of childbearing age was 209.7 for Crow women compared with 128.4 for all races in the state.[101] Indeed, Montana was the state with the "highest reported Indian birth rates" in the nation when calculated per 1,000 women of childbearing age.[102] The minutes of Crow Health Committee meetings, in which committee members were usually joined by the senior physician and sometimes other health workers, offer one of the more explicit documented discussions of these issues in this period.

PHS physicians were reasonably satisfied with Crow women's use of the reservation hospital for childbirth in the years after the transfer. A small number continued to seek obstetric services off the reservation, but few saw home birth as a viable — or perhaps even desirable — option.[103] Susie Yellowtail stopped practicing midwifery when she became active on the health committee, depriving women in the Wyola district of yet another midwife, and the pressure health committee members exerted to persuade tribal members to use the hospital may have influenced women's obstetric decisions, though by this time they had few options.[104] PHS thus benefited from the success of the BIA's decades-long effort to move childbirth into government hospitals, as well as from the definitive nationwide trends in this direction.

The sometimes-sparse health committee meeting minutes contain minimal discussion of obstetric practices at the Crow Agency Hospital in the 1950s. In fact, women's experience giving birth at the reservation hospital in these years was shaped by a confluence of historical trends extending far beyond the reservation. Crow patients' experience of the transfer to PHS as a loss of influence within hospital walls in some sense mirrored American women's declining authority in hospital childbirth at midcentury. As the women's historian Jacqueline Wolf has argued, "Medical control of every stage of the birthing process became common countrywide."[105] In practice, this meant the routine use of drugs and anesthetics that effectively knocked women out for their deliveries and routine interventions such as forceps deliveries and episiotomies. The near-complete loss of control was symbolized by the common hospital practice of strapping women down during labor.[106]

Iris Black (Cheyenne) delivered four children at the Crow Agency Hospital in the 1950s. The birth of her first child preceded the transfer to PHS; the subsequent three followed it. Notably, it was during her later deliveries that Black recalls the sort of procedures described above. Black does not remember receiving any pain relief for the birth of her first child, but when she delivered her second, hospital staff gave her "a spinal block," regional anesthesia injected into the spinal area, which she believes had become routine practice at the hospital by that time. "They were doing it for everybody," she recalled."[107] Although anecdotal, the difference between Black's first and second births hints at how the transfer to PHS, a more standardized and better-resourced federal agency, could extend to obstetric practice. While some women — Native and non-Native alike — welcomed the promised pain relief of localized anesthesia, Black endured one of the procedure's common side effects: postpartum headaches. "I tell you what, I had a headache for about twenty years after that. I had a headache all the time."[108] Women who gave birth at the Crow Agency Hospital in the following years further report that hospital staff followed the increasingly common obstetric practice of strapping women down during labor and delivery.[109]

Childbirth had indeed changed in the half century since the BIA constructed the first hospital at Crow Agency. As Black's experience suggests, Cheyenne as well as Crow women had been affected by these changes. By the time of the transfer, approximately half of all hospital patients hailed from the neighboring reservation.[110] Intertribal tensions occasionally flared over this forced arrangement, and allegations of PHS favoritism flew in both directions, but there is no reason to believe that Cheyenne and Crow women's obstetric experiences within the hospital varied significantly.[111] While individual women resented some aspects of their experience, and women whose kin accompanied them were sometimes able to achieve minor accommodations to standard procedures, there is no evidence that the Crow Health Committee or any other tribal entity registered any formal challenge to obstetric protocols at midcentury. Black had two major complaints about her birthing experiences: the unquestioned use of the spinal anesthesia, a procedure that for her carried negative consequences, and the attitude of the non-Native hospital staff, whom she described as "mean as snakes."[112] The Crow Health Committee's insistence that patients at the reservation hospital be treated "as if they were paying-patients in a private room in a private hospital" led them to take up Black's latter concern—through their consistent demand for kinder, more sensitive treatment—while to some degree taking for granted the necessity of the former and related practices.[113]

The more immediate concern for PHS officers and the Crow Health Committee alike was infant mortality, as the BIA had been less successful in achieving the improvements in infant welfare that government employees had promised would accompany hospital childbirth. When the transfer to PHS went into effect, Native infant mortality more than doubled the national average, and similar trends prevailed more locally. The mortality rate for Crow infants under the age of one was 69.1 per 1,000 population compared with 26.9 for all racial groups in Montana. The situation at Northern Cheyenne was even worse, with 137.3 infant deaths per 1,000 population. In a reversal of trends for the United States as a whole, postneonatal mortality, occurring between twenty-eight days of life and one year, presented a greater threat to Native infants than did their first days of life; the postneonatal mortality rate for Native infants was six times that of all races.[114] Postneonatal mortality serves as an index of an infant's socioeconomic position as reflected in his or her home environment, and Native infant mortality would in fact decrease markedly in the decade and a half after the transfer, due in large part to PHS's investment in improvements to reservation sanitation, among other environmental factors.[115] The Crow Health Committee actively supported PHS sanitation efforts.

In early meetings with the Crow Health Committee, however, physicians intimated that the blame for poor infant health outcomes rested with Native mothers. In late 1956, for example, Dr. Fazly A. Melany alleged that "Crow mothers neglected" to abide by the prenatal program he prescribed, that "Crow mothers often neglect babies until he could weep with sorrow," and that "Crow mothers were very careless" about following his instructions to return to the hospital for postpartum examinations.[116] Although likely unconsciously, Melany followed a long-standing practice of generalizing, often negatively, about tribal women as a group, and he drew on a similarly entrenched trope of Native maternal neglect. Indeed, the physician's message could just as easily have been recorded in Save the Babies literature four decades earlier as in midcentury tribal health committee meeting minutes—but for the increased routinization of pre- and postnatal care in the intervening period.

The BIA had promoted prenatal and postnatal, or "well-baby," care in an ad hoc fashion through the bureau's Progressive Era pronatal campaign, but medical and popular enthusiasm for prenatal care grew after the passage of the Sheppard-Towner Act in the 1920s. In the 1930s and 1940s, routine prenatal care became an expected feature of pregnancy for most non-Native middle-class American women.[117] Years later, the BIA's capacity for providing prenatal examinations and related care still varied from reservation to reservation. A PHS report in 1957 lamented the "very incomplete service" pregnant women received in some locations.[118] On the Crow Reservation in the years after the transfer to PHS, medical officers held a prenatal and well-baby clinic one day a week. Doctors urged women to visit the prenatal clinic once a month during their pregnancies, increasing to twice a month in the final months of gestation.[119] In expressing his frustration that Crow mothers were not following these and other guidelines, Melany and other government physicians requested committee women's assistance in publicizing and promoting these clinics.

Committee members proved eager to promote maternal and infant welfare services on the reservation. Although there is no record of specific actions taken by the health committee in the months after Melany's visit, the notable increase in clinic attendance suggests that the committee was receptive to the physician's plea for assistance. By May, Melany's successor Dr. Lowell Edwards reported that in the previous month, sixty pregnant women had visited the clinic, and he and his staff had examined 128 newborn infants. He observed that clinic attendance as a whole in April was "close to a record."[120] Committee members also desired direct involvement in maternal and infant health education on the reservation. They proposed leading classes in which they would educate women and mothers on the benefits of prenatal and postnatal medical care and also provide basic instruction in the care of small children. Female leaders on other reservations engaged in similar efforts. In her capacity as chair of the Health and Welfare section of the Navajo Community Services Committee, for example, Annie Wauneka coordinated instructional clinics on infant care and other well-baby programming.[121] At Crow, however, committee members' ambitions were sometimes thwarted by PHS officers' insistence that the committee function as ancillary to the government health educator.[122]

These signs of the Crow Health Committee's support for PHS maternal and infant welfare efforts should not imply committee members' complete acceptance of the narrative of "neglect" that Melany and other PHS officers proffered. While Yellowtail and her fellow committee members largely concurred with PHS regarding the importance of medical prenatal care, they would also have been aware of the many other ways women cared for themselves during pregnancy. Crow women who bore children in the 1950s received advice from female kin that closely resembled the advice their mothers and grandmothers had received years earlier: "Eat right and walk a lot and . . . drink a lot of water . . . be exercising. . . . Don't be lazy and laying around."[123] One woman who lived in Pryor in these years recalled that the "whole family" would come together to ensure a pregnant woman was properly cared for.[124] Pregnant women chewed white clay because they believed it would ensure a smooth pregnancy, and they often asked a clan uncle or other relative to bestow blessings on the pregnancy.[125] Committee members thus likely viewed physicians' request to publicize and promote prenatal clinics as a matter of expanding the care pregnant women already received.

There is reason to believe that committee women were similarly skeptical of Melany's charge of neglect regarding the care of Crow children. More than two decades later, Susie Yellowtail would declare in an interview that "Indians may be poor, but they do love their children and take good care of them too."[126] Her insistence on this point speaks to the Crow woman's extensive experience defending Native women against charges of apathy and neglectfulness. Furthermore, during the Crow Health Committee's formative years, Susie and her husband, Thomas, were raising some of their grandchildren, and they had previously adopted and raised other children in their extended family.[127] Crow grandparents, aunts, uncles, and other kin remained active in the rearing of children, and, in contrast to Melany and most PHS officers, health committee members would have been unlikely to place exclusive responsibility for the care of small children on the shoulders of biological mothers.

As importantly, physicians' emphasis on maternal neglect obscured the concrete examples of federal neglect against which committee members struggled.[128] The Crow Health Committee countered Melany's blanket allegations of maternal apathy or carelessness with specific instances in which "panicky" mothers and fathers took ill infants to the hospital only to be turned away, either told to return the following day or that the infant's condition was not serious.[129] The cases that came to the committee's attention were those in which parents had been so concerned for their infant's health that they had felt compelled to procure health services off the reservation. Committee members insisted that Crow parents had a right to better, more reliable care than they received from PHS in the years immediately after the transfer. They also insisted that this care should be more accessible. Regarding women's attendance at prenatal and well-baby clinics, for example, the health committee charged that PHS clinics were limited and inconvenient. Committee members demanded that PHS extend clinic hours and hold clinics throughout the reservation, not only at Crow Agency.[130] In doing so, the Crow Health Committee effectively turned government physicians' messages on their head; routine medical prenatal, postnatal, and pediatric care were indeed important, and the federal government—via PHS—was obligated to ensure these needs were met for Crow women and children.

THE TERMINATION POLICIES of the post–World War II years threatened the political and cultural identity of Native peoples and also threatened to change the circumstances through which Crow women received health care, including reproductive health services. Decades later, the Mohawk activist Katsi Cook would contend that it was "in the 40's and 50's that [Native] women began going into the hospital" for childbirth, and she and others perceived that this trend was connected to termination.[131] At Crow as in many locations, the shift toward hospital birthing had begun years earlier, but several factors, including but not limited to the legal and assimilationist pressures of the termination era, accelerated and/or solidified the increased reliance on government obstetric services throughout Indian Country during these decades. As Native women experienced a narrowing of reproductive options in the postwar period, some also perceived a loss of control inside hospital walls. This resulted in part from the routinization of obstetric practice, which women's historians have argued consolidated physicians' authority in birthing. At Crow and elsewhere, it also resulted from the changes that accompanied the transfer of Indian health care from the BIA to PHS. The advantages PHS presented for Native peoples should not obscure the uncertainty and frustrations that patients and communities endured in this transition.

Like many Crow women and men, Cordelia Big Man deplored the prevailing policy that was geared toward forcing Indians to "sink or swim."[132] For her part, Big Man contested termination policies and pressures as president of the Crow Agency Women's Club and as a member of the Crow Health Committee. In the latter capacity, Big Man joined with a handful of other women in an effort not only to defend and protect the Crow Agency Hospital, where she had previously worked, but also to ensure the hospital remained an Indian institution. The story of the Crow Health Committee and the Crow Agency Hospital at midcentury is thus a microcosm of the larger story of termination spurring Native peoples' pursuit of self-determination. It is a story in which women, health, and reproduction are necessarily at the center.

The Crow Health Committee's very first report insisted on the need for Indians to band together to secure their health and welfare.[133] This vision was realized more fully in the 1960s, when the health committee regularly coordinated with tribal health committees throughout the region.[134] Susie Yellowtail, the health committee's first chair, gained a national platform during this decade, as she was invited to serve on federal committees and advisory boards. In the last decade of her life, Yellowtail was a founding member of a professional organization of American Indian and Alaska Native nurses.[135] Some of these nurses would go on to play pivotal roles in the highly politicized struggles over biological reproduction that emerged in the 1970s. Yellowtail, who died in 1981, thus provides a crucial link between Native women's local organizing at midcentury and the better-publicized and often more militant battles of subsequent decades.

CHAPTER SIX

Self-Determination Begins in the Womb

In 1977, elders and young activists from the Six Nations of the Haudeno-saunee Confederacy met in Loon Lake, New York, to discuss the meaning of sovereignty. John Mohawk, a Seneca scholar and activist in his early thirties, laid out a five-part definition of sovereignty, in which he identified "control of reproduction" as one of sovereignty's "essential elements."[1] This struck a chord with Katsi Cook, a young Mohawk mother who attended the meeting. Five years earlier, Cook had left Dartmouth College in New Hampshire to dedicate herself to activism. In 1975, despite many logistical challenges, she had insisted on giving birth to her first child at home, much as her mother had done two decades earlier. The meeting at Loon Lake intensified Cook's emerging mission to reclaim control of Native reproduction, and she soon took these ideas west. By the fall of 1978, Cook wound up in the Great Plains, where she became involved with the newly established Women of All Red Nations, or WARN.[2]

In the group's first years, WARN leaders articulated an agenda that should be viewed as an early vision of Native reproductive justice.[3] Like many Native men and women, WARN members were outraged over allegations regarding coercive sterilizations in government and contract hospitals, as well as various other challenges to Native women's procreative capacity and maternal rights. As activists throughout the country struggled for sovereignty and survival, WARN and other women presented reproductive control as inextricably linked to these efforts. Cook advocated expanded conceptions of sovereignty—"personal sovereignty" alongside tribal sovereignty—and she called on women to exercise "sovereignty over our own bodies."[4] Activists argued that the survival of Native peoples physically and "as Indians" now more than ever depended on women's reproductive labor and autonomy.[5] WARN's message paralleled and at times intersected with that of non-Native feminists who fought for "reproductive self-determination," as well as that of women involved in the burgeoning women's health and modern midwifery movements.[6] Yet WARN women understood their reproductive agendas to be rooted in their historical and ongoing experiences as targets of colonial-ism and, for them, reproductive control could not be defined narrowly. It had as much to do with spiritual freedom and environmental justice as it did with the legality of and an individual's access to any given reproductive technology.

This chapter explores Native women's quest for control of reproduction from the late 1960s through the early 1980s. Years before WARN's founding, Native women as patients, health workers, and activists navigated the web of evolving, often contradictory, and sometimes coercive family planning policies and practices that they encountered through the Indian Health Service (IHS). They negotiated tensions involving individual women's needs, bureaucratic procedures, and collective struggles. By the late 1970s, some Native women embraced Katsi Cook's call for a return to Native midwifery, while greater numbers of women pursued a vision of reproductive control that demanded new types of practitioners, a change in their own attitudes about reproduction, and/or greater authority in clinics and birthing rooms. WARN's founding emerged from a longer and broader history of Native women's reproductive organizing, and the group's influence extended beyond women who viewed themselves as militants or even activists.[7]

Federal Family Planning Policies and Politics

IHS began offering family planning services, excluding abortion and sterilization, in 1965 as part of an expanded commitment to family planning by the Department of Health, Education, and Welfare (HEW). The historian Donald Critchlow has argued that between 1965 and 1974, the federal government's role in family planning shifted "from nonintervention to active involvement."[8] Two postwar political movements—one promoting women's right to safe, legal birth control and one promoting population control—facilitated the government's attempt to bring family planning more squarely under its purview. Both movements foregrounded the issue of "control," but the different uses proved telling. As women's historians have demonstrated, artificial contraception could be liberating for women, but it was not inherently so, and many advocates of federal family planning had little interest in women's health, bodily autonomy, or sexual freedom.[9] Rather, population control advocates were motivated primarily by fears of global overpopulation and an expanding domestic welfare state. These concerns are similarly evident in early studies of IHS family planning services.[10]

As with so much of federal Indian policy, the implementation of family planning services varied by location, and the attitudes of government health workers often shaped Native women's options. Some physicians and nurses refused to provide women with contraceptives or contraceptive information due to moral or religious objections. Other physicians showed little interest in family planning because they viewed the work as less glamorous than other aspects of the job or because they found the consultation process awkward. Still others apparently pushed the issue quite aggressively.[11] Native women's reactions to government family planning services were similarly mixed. When a team of social scientists surveyed Omaha women in 1972, they found a strong preference for high fertility, which the researchers explained in part by pointing to "Omaha experience retained in tribal memory."[12] The historical experiences the investigators described—epidemics, drastic population loss, and the extraordinarily high birth rates that had been necessary to ensure survival—would have been familiar to men and women throughout Indian Country. Although the history the investigators narrated effectively stopped at 1900, more recent experiences figured prominently in collective memory among Omahas and in other Native communities. A physician who spent two years on the Navajo Reservation observed that as long as Native infant mortality doubled national rates, government officials would have to temper their expectations for family planning. "After all," he argued, "there can be no planning if the patient cannot also plan on his [or her] children's likely survival."[13]

A preference for high fertility did not necessarily mean an outright refusal of family planning services, but health workers in some locations did encounter staunch resistance. Often, this resistance reflected distrust of the federal government at least as much as it reflected rejection of birth control technologies. Past violations engendered ongoing suspicion, as was the case on one reservation where, according to a 1971 government report, "an overzealous physician allegedly performed so many unnecessary tubal ligations" that local women shunned all family planning services.[14] Mary Brave Bird, a Lakota activist involved with the American Indian Movement, later recalled, "Birth control went against our beliefs. We felt there were not enough Indians left to suit us."[15] Brave Bird, as well as other politically engaged women, viewed federal family planning as the latest manifestation of the government's long-standing effort to wipe out Native populations.

Non-Native observers believed that Native men were more likely than women to oppose family planning programs.[16] Physicians and other government officials generally attributed the hostility of male political activists and the disapproval of many husbands to either militancy or social conservatism, but in fact the gendered dynamics surrounding reproduction can be located in earlier colonial processes and policies. One of policy makers' and social reformers' objectives in promoting the allotment of tribal land at the turn of the twentieth century, a process that occurred to varying degrees on many, though not all, reservations, was to instill in Native men a proprietary interest in their wives' sexual and reproductive practices. In some locations, as on the Crow Reservation, government employees pursued this objective blatantly and explicitly, urging Native men to intervene in women's reproductive decisions and contending that high fertility—rather than any structural or policy changes—was the key to tribal survival.

Despite this relatively recent history, male (and some female) critics of family planning occasionally framed their opposition as a commitment to "traditional" practices. "Tradition" was a negotiated and contested concept in this politically charged historical moment, however. To underscore this point, Katsi Cook often added quotation marks to the word when she wrote about gender, reproduction, and related topics.[17] As early as the 1960s, a group of respected female elders known as the "Lakota grandmas" invoked tradition in their efforts to present birth control as a maternal and infant health measure. Before colonization, they argued, large families had not been "the Lakota way."[18] Suspicion of the U.S. government notwithstanding, spacing births or otherwise limiting fertility was a familiar concept to many Native women and a familiar practice to some. In many communities, elders if not younger generations remembered how their mothers, aunts, and grandmothers had relied on breastfeeding and other practices to space births, and in some locations, especially the Southwest, women continued to utilize herbal teas that they obtained from healers or older female kin for family planning purposes.[19]

Many Native women demonstrated that they were open to federal family planning services when the circumstances suited them. Contemporary studies suggest that somewhere between one-third and one-half of Native women of childbearing age used some form of artificial contraception in the late 1960s and early 1970s, and women reported their perception that many women in their communities used birth control.[20] In some IHS service areas, including Alaska, Oklahoma, and Billings, Montana, health workers reported acceptance rates of at least 70 percent.[21] A Lakota woman who worked at a free Indian clinic in the Los Angeles area estimated that about 80–85 percent of the young women who came through the clinic used artificial contraception: "And they are really for it. . . . They practice it faithfully."[22]

There was a politics to the provision and availability of birth control methods. The two most frequently prescribed methods were oral contraceptives, more commonly known as "the Pill," which had been available in the United

States since 1960, and the recently redesigned intrauterine device (IUD), which was available by mid-decade. Physicians tended to prefer the latter method, and by 1970 IHS employees prescribed IUDs with more frequency than the Pill.[23] IUDs placed reproductive control in the hands of the physician rather than the woman. The physician inserted and removed the device, while the Pill required women's diligence in ingesting it every day. Some physicians had little faith in the capacity of patients of color to use oral contraceptives successfully.

The high discontinuation rates on many reservations increased their concern. In the Billings area, almost half of the women who had accepted family planning services discontinued such services in a fifteen-month period.[24] Discontinuation rates included many women whom health workers labeled "lost to follow-up," indicating that the woman had not returned for subsequent appointments as instructed. In one government study, health workers speculated that reasons for high dropout rates included family disapproval, miscommunication, transportation difficulties, and migration. Other likely factors included disagreeable side effects, the woman having felt pressure to accept the doctor's recommendation in the first place, and the possibility that some women had only intended to use any given birth control method on a short-term basis.[25] At any rate, physicians recognized that a woman who had been prescribed oral contraceptives and failed to follow up was susceptible to pregnancy, while a woman who had agreed to the insertion of an IUD had some protection from an unplanned pregnancy.[26]

High dropout rates, physicians' concerns about women's capabilities and reliability, and the speed with which IUDs surpassed birth control pills in IHS family planning raise the possibility of coercion. The historian Virginia Espino has documented the "considerable pressure" physicians placed on Mexican American women to accept the insertion of an IUD at a Los Angeles county hospital in these years. In one extreme case, hospital personnel allegedly held a woman at the clinic against her will for hours until she "consented."[27] Yet coercion was not inevitable, and its potential does not discount the enthusiasm some women showed for the reproductive technology. One Native woman who gave birth to three children in the 1970s recalled that she kept getting pregnant even though she was taking an oral contraceptive: "Then they introduced IUDs. . . . They told us that that was something new, so I used it, and I never got pregnant after that." She later reflected, "I'm glad I did it, you know. If I didn't, I think I would have had ten kids by now." This woman further expressed appreciation that her reservation hospital had the same technologies that were available to non-Native women at the time.[28]

For other women, IUDs proved less reliable, leaving them with limited options in the event of an undesirable pregnancy. Native women reported becoming pregnant while using an IUD, but abortion was not always accessible. Before the Supreme Court's *Roe v. Wade* decision in 1973, abortion was illegal at the federal level and in most states.[29] After *Roe*, Native women obtained abortions at some government hospitals, but the judicial decision made no guarantees regarding availability.[30] Surveys by the Alan Guttmacher Institute and Centers for Disease Control, for example, revealed that "eight out of 10 public hospitals" provided no abortion services after *Roe*.[31]

In 1976, Congress passed the Hyde Amendment, which eliminated public funding for abortion. The legislation hinders the ability of all low-income women to terminate a pregnancy and disproportionately affects women of color, but Native activists charge that the act discriminates against them specifically because they receive their health care from a federal agency.[32] The amendment did not affect all Native women immediately, however. Until early 1982, IHS was the only Department of Health and Human Services (DHHS) program that did not follow the amendment's restrictions, and instead abortion decisions were "left to the doctor and patient." Under this policy, IHS performed 638 abortions in 1980—fewer, as will be demonstrated below, than the tubal ligations performed annually in the 1970s. The new abortion restrictions brought IHS in line with other DHHS programs and followed the Supreme Court's upholding of the Hyde Amendment in *Harris v. McRae*.[33]

The termination of pregnancies garnered more opposition in Native communities than other family planning services, although this reaction was not universal. In surveys of Omaha and Seminole women, researchers found that the "great majority" approved of abortion only in the limited circumstances of rape or endangerment to the woman's health, or if there was something wrong with the fetus.[34] It is worth noting, however, that the surveys in question were conducted in 1972, when abortion remained illegal at the federal level; this reality may have shaped women's perception of the issue as well as what they were willing to tell academic researchers. For her part, Mary Brave Bird explained her decision to carry her fifth pregnancy to term despite her poor health as owing to the "subconscious urge to reproduce" felt by her and many other Native women, whose communities had been the target of various campaigns for elimination. Brave Bird argued that "Indian feminists . . . think that abortion is all right for everyone else, but not for us."[35] Many women simply felt that abortion was not especially relevant in Native communities because of the persistence of "flexible childrearing." These women believed that if the biological mother were unable or unwilling to raise a child, one of the child's many relatives would step in to care for him or her.[36]

Yet women's attitudes toward abortion frequently reflected an unwillingness to meddle in others' affairs, a social norm in many Native societies. Navajo women who gave birth at the Gallup Indian Medical Center in New Mexico in the early 1970s displayed a noninterventionist attitude toward family planning more broadly. When asked their thoughts about other women's family planning choices, the women's responses included "I don't know," "Whatever they want," and "It's their business."[37] In Montana, an older Crow woman showed similar reticence when an anthropologist solicited her opinion on the liberalization of abortion laws in some states. When asked whether she thought women should be able to procure an abortion in a doctor's office, the Crow grandmother simply stated, "I know a lot of them do that."[38] Even Brave Bird, who would not consider an abortion herself, did not extend her views to "everyone else."[39] Some women who did not think that they would personally make the decision to abort a pregnancy or who had political reservations about Native women terminating pregnancies nonetheless believed that abortion should be available to women and that the decision had to be made by the individual.[40]

Contemporary activists and subsequent scholars have argued that the relative accessibility of sterilization versus abortion constrained Native women's options and encouraged them to "choose" more permanent measures.[41] In 1970, Congress passed, and President Richard Nixon signed, the Family Planning Services and Population Research Act, subsidizing sterilizations for Medicaid and IHS patients.[42] Nationally, there had been a decline in eugenic sterilizations during and after World War II. Anecdotally, it is clear that sterilizations still occurred in BIA (Bureau of Indian Affairs) and then IHS hospitals, but it is often difficult to discern the circumstances surrounding the operations. In the 1960s, the federal government's embrace of family planning apparently accompanied an increase in sterilization procedures, a trend that also affected African American and Latina women. On the Crow Reservation, older women privately referred to one physician as "the butcher" for his eagerness to perform such operations; women's distrust and opposition likely contributed to the physician's removal by the end of the decade.[43] Following the Family Planning Act, sterilization rates climbed dramatically. On the Navajo Nation, for example, such procedures doubled between 1972 and 1978.[44]

Many women, especially working- and middle-class white women, viewed sterilization as a liberating technology in these years, a birth control method worth fighting for in doctors' offices and courtrooms.[45] At an individual level, some Native women accepted sterilization procedures, especially the less invasive tubal ligation, with some relief in the late 1960s and early 1970s. They, too, viewed the procedure as a means of asserting a degree of reproductive control. One Native health aide in Wisconsin later recalled that before 1970, women sometimes came into his office requesting a tubal ligation, and he would have to try to talk them into having their partner get a vasectomy, a less expensive procedure.[46]

After passage of the Family Planning Act, sterilization was more accessible for these and other women. In 1972, a young woman relayed the story of an eighteen-year-old from her reservation who had had a tubal ligation after the birth of her second child. Surprised, the interviewer inquired, "And they did that without her knowing it?" The young woman was unequivocal in her refutation: "No. She wanted it done."[47] A few years later, a mother of two who had procured two abortions due to contraceptive failure went to her local IHS hospital to request a tubal ligation.[48] Christopher Doran, a student at Yale Medical School, reported that four of the thirty women he interviewed at the Gallup Indian Medical Center in New Mexico "were convinced that they had enough children and . . . wanted to have their tubes tied." One of the women was pregnant with her eighth child, another with her tenth. According to Doran, these women desired relief from "continual pregnancy" and to ensure that they would have no additional children to look after.[49] The historians Maureen Lux and Erika Dyck have documented a more public declaration of control and autonomy in Canada. Representing the local public health committee, a group of women from a small Inuit community in the eastern Arctic emphasized their personal knowledge of women's proactivity in seeking sterilization procedures: "There are those who especially ask for it."[50]

Yet the increased legitimacy of sterilization as a form of birth control ironically facilitated coercive uses of the technology, and aspects of the Yale medical student's account would have made activists who were beginning to explore the issue wary. First, Doran noted that the women did not request sterilization themselves. Their decision came only after hospital staff had presented them with the "possibility," and Doran emphasized the need for "a large measure of explanation, patience, and reassurance" on the part of the health workers. Recognizing the potential for coercion in the circumstances he described, Doran felt the need to refute the notion, although some readers likely found his assurances less than convincing. "I am not implying," Doran insisted, "that sterilization is forced on every grand-multipara who delivers at Gallup Indian Medical Center."[51] Furthermore, Doran's account underscores the extent to which women's decisions were shaped by their unreliable and inconsistent birth control options, as well as their limited options in the event of an undesired pregnancy. As other scholars have noted, it is difficult to reconcile the politics of choice that ascended in some feminist circles in these years with the colonial context that continued to shape many Native women's reproductive lives.[52] In the coming decade, Native women—as patients, professionals, and activists—grappled with this tension.

Consent and Coercion

The potential for coercion in matters of Native reproductive health did not suddenly appear in the 1970s. Decades earlier, Susie Yellowtail's experience as an employee as well as a patient within the government hospital at Crow Agency had alerted her to unethical practices, instilled a sense of urgent vigilance, and sparked a lifetime of reformist activism. As sterilization rates increased after the passage of the Family Planning Act, Native women who worked within the health care system—some of whom would have identified as activists, some of whom would not have—once again occupied the front lines in identifying and protesting unethical procedures and advancing a range of reforms to curtail abuses.

In the late 1960s, IHS began contracting with tribal governments to launch Community Health Representative (CHR) programs. Following successful pilot programs on the Northern Cheyenne and Pine Ridge Reservations, the CHR concept quickly spread to other locations.[53] As CHRs, Native women and men acted as health aides and served as liaisons among patients, local health committees, and medical providers. Women often outnumbered men in this work. In Wisconsin, for example, at least three-quarters of the state's CHRs in the late 1960s and 1970s were women.[54] CHRs did not always assume an active role in family planning programming, but they did so in some locations, such as the Crow Reservation, where Yellowtail and other women had established the precedent of active involvement in maternal and infant health services.[55] When this was the case, female CHRs, through regular and sometimes intimate exchanges with reservation women, were well positioned to remain informed regarding trends in health and health policy.

CHRs had an especially important role to play in the provision of health services for Native peoples in Wisconsin, where IHS did not operate a single service center in the late 1960s, and Native communities had no choice but to use off-reservation facilities. Early CHRs developed their own local programs, but under the leadership of Arvina Thayer, a Ho-Chunk woman who served as the state's first CHR coordinator, Wisconsin's thirteen CHRs established statewide committees to tackle priority areas including women's health.[56] Through conversations with women about their reproductive health and family planning needs, Thayer later explained, "the CHRs are the ones that found out what was going on" with sterilizations in the area. CHRs learned that sterilization procedures were far more common in some institutions than others, and they determined that institutions' protocols surrounding sterilization lacked transparency. "They were sterilizing a lot of women," Thayer recalled.[57]

CHRs alerted IHS of their concerns, and according to Thayer, "IHS came down with a rule to the doctors."[58] Based on the timing and Thayer's recollection of what the new regulations entailed, it seems likely that she was referring to guidelines HEW published in 1973. In August and then September of that year, HEW issued guidelines that established a moratorium on the sterilization of individuals under twenty-one years of age and those whom physicians deemed mentally incompetent; mandated a signed consent form that included the benefits and costs of permanent sterilization; and imposed a seventy-two-hour waiting period between formal consent and the procedure. In April 1974, HEW affirmed and strengthened these guidelines with the publication of new regulations that further required that the signed consent form specify that family planning decisions had no bearing on a woman's eligibility for benefits. In issuing these revised regulations in 1974, HEW responded to an order from a U.S. district court following the forced sterilizations of Minnie Lee and Mary Alice Relf, two African American girls who were coercively sterilized in Alabama in 1973.[59] Later investigations found that IHS employees implemented these regulations unevenly, and HEW made little effort to ensure that physicians in contract hospitals abided by the new guidelines. Ultimately, the lack of accountability surrounding medical and specifically reproductive health care led CHRs in Wisconsin and elsewhere to champion Indian-run health clinics and services.[60]

Like the CHRs in Wisconsin, Connie Pinkerton-Uri, a Choctaw and Cherokee physician, became aware of the ethically questionable circumstances surrounding sterilization through her professional experiences. In 1972, a twenty-six-year-old Native woman came into Pinkerton-Uri's Los Angeles office requesting a "womb transplant." The woman had had a hysterectomy six years earlier when she was struggling with alcoholism, but she was now sober, engaged to be married, and wanting to start a family. It was clear to Pinkerton-Uri that the woman did not understand the nature or implications of the procedure. As Pinkerton-Uri later explained in interviews, she first thought the woman's unfortunate experience was an anomaly but soon encountered similar instances and became convinced of a broader problem.[61] Pinkerton-Uri's growing awareness of sterilization abuses changed the physician's professional trajectory. She went to law school and founded Indian Women United for Social Justice to investigate the issue and provide support for women who had been sterilized coercively.[62]

Pinkerton-Uri's story has been frequently recounted, but scholars have paid less attention to what her story reveals about Native nurses' contributions to emerging sterilization-related activism. Although the anthropologist Marla Powers later highlighted tensions between Native nurses at Pine Ridge and activists who had become politicized regarding sterilization and other reproductive issues, there is some evidence that when the American Indian Nurses Association (AINA) was formally established in the early 1970s, with Susie Yellowtail as a founding member, sterilization abuse was among the group's earliest priorities.[63] By 1974, Pinkerton-Uri could proclaim, "Now, the Indian nurses . . . They do have a movement." A year earlier, Pinkerton-Uri had visited the IHS hospital in Claremore, Oklahoma, at the invitation of more than a dozen Native nurses who were protesting discriminatory labor practices and poor patient care. At Claremore, the Native physician encountered what she characterized as a "sterilization factory."[64] After reviewing the hospital's records for 1973, Pinkerton-Uri alleged that out of every four babies born in the fifty-eight-bed hospital, physicians performed one tubal ligation or hysterectomy. Pinkerton-Uri began interviewing women who had undergone the procedure; some reported having been on medication when they gave consent, others indicated that they did not understand that the procedure was irreversible, and still others implied that they had been afraid to argue with the doctor.[65] This provided Pinkerton-Uri with the evidence she needed to present her concerns to legislators.

At a rally in Los Angeles, Pinkerton-Uri cheered the "nurses' revolt against the forced sterilization of women" at Claremore.[66] Without their efforts, the physician explained, her own work would not be possible: "It was the Indian health professionals who called me in, and it's the Indian health professionals who also are feeding me information."[67] As a result, Pinkerton-Uri emphasized the need for more Native health workers inside the system acting as watchdogs. Her mission thus dovetailed with Susie Yellowtail's most urgent objective in the 1970s, that of recruiting and supporting Native nurses.

Pinkerton-Uri had likely met Yellowtail, the "grandmother of American Indian nurses," in 1973, when the American Indian Physicians Association (AIPA) held its annual meeting at Crow Fair.[68] Frustrated with the complacence of fellow Native physicians—she complained that she was the only AIPA member who supported the American Indian Movement's occupation of Wounded Knee—Pinkerton-Uri decided to give up on galvanizing Indian physicians and instead turn her energies toward the more engaged Native nurses.[69]

Pressure from Pinkerton-Uri, Native nurses, and others eventually forced the federal government's attention. Senator James Abourezk from South Dakota called for a Government Accountability Office (GAO) investigation into allegations of sterilization abuse in government hospitals. In 1976, after an investigation of IHS service areas in Albuquerque, Phoenix, Oklahoma City, and Aberdeen, South Dakota, the GAO released its report. The government's investigation relied on medical records and physician testimony, a methodology with inherent limitations because, as one scholar of post–World War II sterilizations has noted, "few sterilizations appear suspect when read through the official medical record."[70] The report stopped short of declaring that the IHS coercively sterilized Native women, but it did highlight several problems with the consent process.

Covering the period from 1973 to 1976, investigators found that HEW's 1974 regulations had had little effect. HEW failed to provide IHS with sterilization guidelines, and IHS lacked standardized consent forms, resulting in physicians' ignorance of proper protocol and variation from hospital to hospital. Some hospitals used inadequate consent forms, which did not fully explain the risks of the procedure or alternative birth control methods, and the forms did not clarify that a woman's birth control decisions had no bearing on her qualifications for government programs. IHS area offices also failed to follow HEW regulations regarding a moratorium on women under the age of twenty-one and a waiting period of seventy-two hours between consent and an operation. Staff at contract facilities violated the moratorium as well, and in almost one-third of these cases IHS authorized payment despite the failure to meet requirements.[71]

The GAO report emphasized bureaucratic missteps rather than power dynamics. In contrast, Native activists investigated the allegations by speaking with women who had been sterilized and thus focused overwhelmingly on the latter. Pinkerton-Uri and others reported a handful of incidents in which sterilization procedures appear from the patient's perspective to have been entirely forced. Native women alleged that they entered the hospital for childbirth or an unrelated surgery and did not learn that they had been sterilized until months or even years later. In one widely reported case in Montana, two young Native women claimed that they had entered a government hospital for appendectomies and received tubal ligations without their knowledge. In this especially tragic case, the women in question were not yet sixteen years old.[72] Perhaps more typically, coercion stemmed from the context of a colonial health care system and women's limited reproductive options. Some women had the false impression that the procedure was reversible. Language barriers, medical jargon, and, according to Pinkerton-Uri, physicians' deception led some women to assume that tubes that were "tied" could just as easily be untied later. A physician on the Navajo Reservation in the late 1960s remarked that "it is shocking not to find a single trained interpreter in any medical facility on the reservation."[73] This left health workers and their patients dependent on the ad hoc assistance of family members, nurses' aides, or clerks, a situation that was particularly regrettable for communication centering on intimate matters like reproduction.

Unlike private patients, who had some flexibility in selecting a provider with whom they felt comfortable, Native women were generally limited to the government services on or near their reservation or city. Women reported feeling considerable pressure to consent to an operation, and some of them were reluctant to argue with the medical staff.[74] Reliance on other federal or state services increased their susceptibility to pressure, as they feared authorities might strip them of their welfare benefits or remove their children. Mary Brave Bird alleges that physicians and social workers repeatedly asked women pointed questions: "Wouldn't it be better for you not to have more children rather than have them wind up in a faraway foster home?"[75] Even if the threat was not explicit, by the late 1960s Native children were removed from their homes and placed in white foster or adoptive homes at high enough rates to make this outcome a reasonable fear.[76]

Many Native activists also argued that the government report's quantitative findings were inadequate, in large part because the GAO restricted its investigation to four of the twelve IHS service areas. In these four service areas, investigators concluded that 3,001 American Indian women of childbearing age had been sterilized between 1973 and 1976, and about one-third of the documented sterilizations occurred in contract hospitals.[77] Pinkerton-Uri argued that if one extrapolated the government's own numbers to include all service units, it would be reasonable to estimate that physicians had sterilized at least 25 percent of Native women of childbearing age.[78] In some locations, activists suggested that the percentages climbed still higher. For example, Marie Sanchez, chief tribal judge on the Northern Cheyenne Reservation, interviewed women in her community, which had not been included in the GAO investigation. She learned that twenty-six of the fifty women she spoke with had been sterilized; many of these procedures occurred at the Crow Agency Hospital.[79] One group of activists frequently cited their estimate that 42 percent of Indian women had been sterilized.[80]

These startling percentages do not mean that all sterilizations of Native women in these years were coercive. Permanent sterilization, especially via tubal ligation, was not an inherently oppressive reproductive technology, and there is reason to believe that in assessing available options, individual women determined that this birth control method met their needs. As Native communities became aware of the scope of the issue, however, many identified a need for analyses that moved beyond the individual. When Susie Yellowtail reflected in these years on the coercive sterilizations on the Crow Reservation decades earlier, she understood the injustice on multiple levels—as deeply upsetting and sometimes traumatic for individuals, "devastating" to families, and threatening to the tribe's future.[81] Activists understood the circumstances surrounding 1970s sterilizations as similarly multilayered. In the context of a national movement for Native sovereignty and self-determination, Native women and some men advanced an analysis that underscored the centrality of reproduction to ongoing political struggles in Native America.

Political and Personal Sovereignty

In 1968, Native men and women in Minneapolis founded the American Indian Movement (AIM). AIM rejected the assimilationist pressures of preceding decades and envisioned a movement capable of unifying political struggle with cultural resurgence and spiritual rebirth.[82] AIM was characterized by its youth, but the organization also facilitated alliances between young people and elders, some of whom had spent years struggling for Native rights in different capacities. Local chapters appeared in cities from San Francisco to Cleveland, and while not welcomed on all reservations, AIM made inroads in reservation communities where tribal members had a thirst for a more militant style of Native activism. Although postwar federal policy had intended to divide urban and reservation Indians, AIM's response to these policies provided a potential avenue for coordination and shared purpose. AIM formed alliances with Six Nations activists, many of whom gathered at Loon Lake in 1977, and helped promote the five-point definition of sovereignty that came out of that meeting, which included "control of your own reproduction." In part a response to growing awareness of sterilization abuses, reproductive control encompassed a broader vision, and men and women agreed that on this issue "the women must lead."[83]

In the following decade, WARN led the public charge in the reclamation of reproductive control. Women from more than thirty Native nations gathered in Rapid City, South Dakota, for the group's founding conference in 1978, and more than 1,200 women attended a second conference in Seattle the following year.[84] The group's founding leaders had been active in AIM, and as the historian Brenda Child has demonstrated, many of these women had ample experience advocating for Native children and families.[85] WARN women emphasized that the decision to form a group for women was not akin to the separatism being championed by some white feminists at the time. Rather, as the historian Elizabeth Castle has argued, WARN allowed women to continue AIM's work at a moment when government repression had constrained the latter organization.[86]

The sex-segregated organization also facilitated work on issues that pertained to what Cook characterized as the "female side of life," foremost among them reproduction.[87] Cofounder Phyllis Young (Lakota) explained that the decision to organize separately was about restoring gender balance and "regaining our strength as women." An early promotional brochure proclaimed, "Indian women have always been in the front lines in the defense of our nations."[88] WARN was not alone in this effort. Along with the often-compatible efforts of Native health workers and reformers, other militant women's groups emerged in these years, such as the Northwest Indian Women's Council. Founded by WARN member Janet McCloud (Tulalip and Nisqually), this regional organization functioned to expand WARN's geographic reach.[89]

WARN was dedicated to ending sterilization abuse in government and contract hospitals, which members viewed as a blow to tribal sovereignty as well as to what Cook referred to as "personal sovereignty."[90] Between annual meetings and speaking tours, members studied the issue locally. In Minnesota, WARN partnered with the National Lawyers' Guild Committee on Reproductive Rights to form the Sterilization Abuse Task Force, which documented coercive sterilizations in the Twin Cities. As Connie Pinkerton-Uri had done a few years earlier, the task force advertised its contact information, encouraging women to call if they had been sterilized coercively or if they needed sterilization-related counseling.[91] These efforts enabled WARN women to identify local institutions with particularly egregious records, and it provided them with enough evidence to conclude that coercive sterilization was a serious problem in the Twin Cities—and this in a community that had been battling the removal of Native children from their homes for at least a decade.[92]

When Pat Bellanger (Ojibwe) reported these early findings at WARN's second annual meeting, however, she emphasized the challenges that she and others faced in gathering these data. *"Being sterilized is a really tender and emotional issue,"* Bellanger explained. "It's not anything where we can sit in a crowd and say how many of you have been sterilized and get any kind of information you need."[93] Women were reluctant to speak publicly about their experiences, as many felt shame and embarrassment and did not want their families and communities to know. The process of completing the questionnaire that task force members had created proved upsetting for some women, so Bellanger and others had to move slowly and dedicate significant time and energy to arranging counseling services for women who were "really ripped apart because they're no longer women in the way that they know."[94]

Activists like Pinkerton-Uri and Sanchez had hoped that Native women who had been sterilized would come forward with lawsuits as women of Mexican descent had done in Los Angeles. But only one Native woman carried a legal suit to completion, and this suit was against physicians and social service workers in western Pennsylvania. It did not involve either the BIA or IHS. In 1970, a social worker with Armstrong County Welfare Services arranged the removal of two of Norma Jean Serena's children from her home. The same year, Serena discovered that she had been sterilized without her consent when she gave birth to her fifth child. Serena initiated legal proceedings to challenge both actions, and a jury ruled in her favor in 1973 that the removal of her children had been unwarranted. Her children were returned, and she received $17,000 in damages. In 1979, however, Serena lost the case regarding her sterilization when the operating doctor contradicted the plaintiff's claims.[95] Serena's lengthy and ultimately unsuccessful legal challenge underscores the obstacles Native women faced in taking their fight to the courts. In 1977, three Northern Cheyenne women began legal proceedings but then accepted a cash settlement so that they would not have to deal with the emotional stress and publicity of a trial. The United Native Americans also threatened to file a lawsuit, but this does not seem to have made much headway.[96]

Sterilization policies and abuses became central to WARN women's indictment of the federal government, which they broadcast nationally and internationally. The group's leaders embarked on a speaking tour with the recently created Reproductive Rights National Network, an umbrella organization that linked about fifty feminist organizations.[97] Two years earlier, Sanchez, along with a handful of women who would be present at WARN's first meeting, provided testimony at the United Nations in Geneva, and many returned to the U.N. in 1981.[98] In these venues, women lambasted the federal government's domestic and international involvement in population control. Their analysis of how and why abuses occurred also dovetailed with critiques advanced by Native health workers and activists throughout the decade—and by women such as Susie Yellowtail and Annie Wauneka at the local level decades earlier. They complained that IHS lacked adequate funding and that medical staff lacked cultural sensitivity. They resented the high physician turnover rates and a health care system that relied on inexperienced doctors learning their trade on the bodies of Native peoples. As Barbara Moore, Mary Brave Bird's sister, charged, "They use Indians as guinea pigs."[99] Moore spoke publicly about her own sterilization, which occurred without her knowledge.

By mid-decade, Pinkerton-Uri publicly proclaimed that the federal government was "using the vehicle of health care as a way of genocide," and a few years later Sanchez argued that sterilization represented the "modern form" of genocide.[100] WARN women continued this charge at the end of the decade, advancing a gendered analysis of genocidal processes.[101] Like other Native activists, WARN cited the definition adopted by the United Nations Convention on the Prevention and Punishment of the Crime of Genocide in 1948.[102] The U.N. definition identifies five acts that if "committed with intent to destroy, in whole or in part, a national, ethnical, racial, or religious group, as such" constitute genocide. Scholars have documented a number of actions on the part of American settlers and soldiers, including mass killings and imposed starvation, that could be considered genocidal, but Native women pointed to the two identified acts that resonated most clearly with their own experiences and agendas. The U.N.'s fourth and fifth genocidal acts read: "Forcibly transferring children of the group to another group" and "Imposing measures intended to prevent births within the group."[103]

While the U.N. Convention placed the burden on victims of genocide to "prove" intent, many Native activists did not see the intent provision as a barrier. In interviews, WARN leaders argued that the removal of Indian children to foster care and the high sterilization rates in Native communities were part of a "planned" government effort to free up reservation land for energy development. "It's called intent to destroy," cofounder Pat Bellanger argued. "That's what genocide is, intent to destroy."[104] Lehman Brightman (Lakota and Creek) spent much of the decade studying sterilization abuses and concluded that "the sterilization campaign is nothing but an insidious scheme to get Indians' land once and for all."[105] Others approached the issue somewhat differently. Pinkerton-Uri, for example, did not think that the sterilizations she had discovered resulted from a government plan "to exterminate American Indians," yet she did not hesitate to use the label "genocide."[106] For her, as for many others, the outcomes—a sterilization rate of 25 percent or higher among women of childbearing age and the removal of as many as 25 percent of Native children in some locations from their homes—spoke for themselves.[107]

In the aftermath of the GAO report and subsequent organizing by communities of color and many feminists, HEW issued new sterilization regulations in 1978, the year of WARN's first meeting. Following a period of public comment, the regulations went into effect in February 1979. The regulations continued the moratorium on sterilizations of persons under the age of twenty-one and specified that consent must include oral and written assurance that an individual's decision was not linked to welfare or other benefits. The most notable changes were an extended waiting period—from seventy-two hours to thirty days—between consent and an operation and increased oversight in the form of regular audits.[108] Not all women's organizations were on board with the new regulations. As the historian Rebecca Kluchin has argued, "Liberal feminists' self-interest—fear of having the right to sterilization on demand removed and fear of the loss of abortion rights— led them to oppose the waiting period and age minimum in the proposed policy."[109] These feminists viewed the waiting period in particular as an infringement on a woman's reproductive "choice," and their opposition contributed to women of color's growing emphasis on "freedom" and "justice."[110]

For its part, WARN supported and promoted the new regulations, as did other Native women. Pinkerton-Uri, Sanchez, and Rayna Green (Cherokee), for example, served on the advisory board of the National Women's Health Network, an organization that dedicated tremendous energy to publicizing and promoting the new regulations.[111] The ultimate adoption of the 1979 regulations was a victory for Native women and for the many feminist organizations that lobbied for them. For individuals desiring a tubal ligation, the second hospital visit and, in some cases, the second surgical procedure could at times be an obstacle or burden; the anthropologist Marla Powers reported that some women on the Pine Ridge Reservation found the extended waiting period "annoying."[112] But most felt that the additional protections outweighed any inconvenience. In the short term, however, Native women had no reason to believe IHS would adhere to the 1979 regulations any more than practitioners had to the regulations HEW had adopted five years earlier. Activists called for continued vigilance.

A Whole Way to Be a Woman

Native women demanded that the federal government address inadequacies, abuses, and injustices within government and contract facilities, but they did not look to the federal government as the solution to the problems they had identified. When more than 1,200 Native people, mostly women, gathered for WARN's second annual meeting in 1979, they tackled a pressing question: "How will we strengthen ourselves and our families so that we may survive?" Theirs was a woman-centered vision, but the focus was on women's roles and relationships within families and communities. As one cofounder explained, "The women define the family and the family is the base of our culture and our culture, our families are under attack at every level, in every way."[113] Decolonization, as WARN women understood it, required the restoration of women's strength and the reclamation of their reproductive control.

With WARN's support, Katsi Cook launched the Women's Dance Health Program (often abbreviated as DHP in program documents) in the Twin Cities in November 1978.[114] DHP's work consisted of four primary components. First, the program promoted Native women's health education through local classes and the production and distribution of informative materials. Second, DHP prioritized the training of Native midwives, who then served as primary care providers at home deliveries, sometimes with the backup or support of an OB-GYN from Minneapolis–St. Paul New School of Family Birthing. They also sometimes acted as labor coaches for hospital births. Third, Cook and a handful of other women ran a small health clinic that provided obstetric and gynecological care to Native women. Finally, DHP supported WARN's effort to study and document sterilization abuse in the Twin Cities and to provide "counseling and advocacy" services for women who had experienced such abuse.[115]

As with much of AIM's activism, DHP emerged in an urban center—one with a long history of Native presence and the distinction of having been AIM's birthplace—and spread to reservations. The following year, a version of the program was adopted by the Oneida in Wisconsin, and Cook introduced the Women's Dance to her community after she returned to Akwesasne to give birth to her third child.[116] Its influence extended still further, as program staff and volunteers supported and coordinated with women-led community-based programs in other locations, including a well-teen clinic

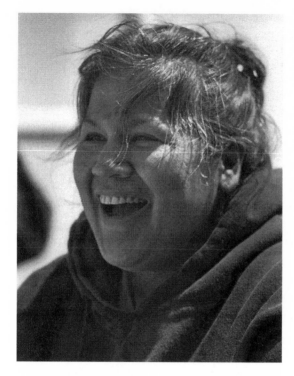

Katsi Cook attended WARN's first annual meeting in 1978 and quickly emerged as a leader in the movement to reclaim Native midwifery first in the United States and later in Canada. Photo by Millie Knapp. Reprinted with permission. Katsi Cook Papers, Sophia Smith Collection, Smith College (Northampton, Massachusetts).

on the Crow Reservation. WARN viewed the DHP as "a project aimed at the development of a new consciousness in health care for Native American women."[117] As such, it aspired to reach far beyond the localities in which the program was based.

The nature and objectives of DHP reflect Cook's response to the coercive sterilizations WARN worked to publicize and eliminate. She shared other activists' outrage, but she also challenged her peers to consider Native women's responsibility for what happened to the women in their families and communities: "Where were we when our own sisters, mothers, grandmothers, aunties, friends were under the knife, being sterilized?"[118] Drawing inspiration from self-help models advanced by feminist health activists with whom Cook had made earlier connections, she viewed DHP as a mechanism for reversing the "absolute dependency on medical systems responsible for the sterilization of over 1/3 of Native American women."[119] Not only was sterilization inextricably connected to other contemporary Native struggles, a point WARN women made frequently. For Cook, sterilization abuse was a symptom of a more fundamental problem: colonialism had diminished women's personal and social power and destabilized their understandings of the meaning of Native womanhood. "What does it mean to be a Mohawk woman? What does it mean to be a Lakotah woman? What does it mean to be a Nez Perce woman?" She explained that the answer was "a little bit different for each area but the basic underlying concepts are always the same."[120]

DHP's emphasis on women's health education in some ways mirrors the priorities of the all-female Crow Health Committee described in chapter 5. In contrast to the Crow committee's work in the 1950s, however, DHP existed outside the auspices of the federal government, and it was less concerned with promoting medical care than with restoring the ways women had historically cared for themselves and others. DHP's diagnosis of the situation—that Native women had become so reliant on professional medical authorities that they had become ignorant of their own bodies—paralleled the arguments that feminists were making through organizations such as the Boston Women's Health Book Collective, but with important nuances. Colonization was the culprit, and most answers would be found in tribal cultures. Furthermore, women's increased knowledge about their bodies, health, and sexuality was not simply about personal liberation or self-actualization. It was, many activists argued, a matter of survival. In the Twin Cities and later at Akwesasne, DHP staff and volunteers led women's health classes at Native-run survival schools as well as in women's homes, and they disseminated their curriculum and materials as widely as they were able.[121] Cook hoped to bring the curriculum together in a Women's Dance Health Book—an Indigenous take on the popular *Our Bodies, Ourselves*. Although she and a handful of others dedicated a couple of years to the project, the book did not come to fruition.[122]

The ultimate objective of this health education was to renew women's knowledge of their bodies and reproductive powers, and the curriculum approached topics such as family planning, which could sometimes be controversial, from this perspective. For example, through DHP health classes, women learned the various types of sterilization procedures, as well as their medical indications, side effects, and consequences. DHP also encouraged women to consider the topic politically: "How has sterilization become a political issue, how is it genocidal to Native people and how does it threaten the survival and sovereignty of our People?"[123] Above all, women learned their rights as patients in making these decisions. Regarding contraception, women discussed their own feelings about family planning as well as what they knew about the attitudes and practices of their grandmothers and great-grandmothers. The curriculum included detailed information on the various contraceptive methods available, instructions for use, and potential side effects, although WARN women tended to favor birth control methods that they viewed as "in keeping with our basic philosophy."[124] DHP documents specifically point to diaphragms, the rhythm method, foams, and condoms. At Akwesasne, the program partnered with a nearby feminist health center to make cervical caps available to Mohawk women. Cook explained in a funding proposal for the Akwesasne program in the early 1980s that "our women have to know that it is okay to use contraceptives, and that a support group will be available to her for the use of contraceptives which are culturally acceptable."[125]

For Cook, midwife-assisted home birth was the ultimate "expression of sovereignty" for Native women.[126] At WARN's first meeting, she called for a resurgence of Native midwifery. In the context of a meeting focused to a large degree on sterilization abuse, Cook's call parallels Susie Yellowtail's response to coercive sterilizations decades earlier. In the three years since the birth of her first child, Cook had received hands-on training at The Farm, a countercultural community in Tennessee that was emerging as a prominent location in the modern midwifery movement. She then proceeded to the University of New Mexico, where she completed a women's health specialist training program.[127] Once in the Plains in the late 1970s, she supplemented this training with the more culturally oriented education she received from her in-laws at Pine Ridge. Among other teachings, her mother-in-law, a CHR and a member of the Native American Church, introduced her to peyote as a powerful medicine to facilitate birthing. Cook incorporated the medicine into her midwifery practice when she felt it would help the mother.[128] When Cook moved to the Twin Cities, she began training Native and a few non-Native women to serve as midwives and labor coaches. Like the midwives at The Farm, these women became known as the Birthing Crew. They provided family planning services, offered prenatal care that encompassed a woman's emotions, dreams, spirituality, and personal circumstances as well as physical care, and delivered babies.[129]

Although a minority of Native women opted for or even had access to midwife-assisted childbirth in the 1970s and 1980s, Native midwifery, like the modern midwifery movement more broadly, was fueled by an intensity that surpassed its numbers. Cook had not been the only Native woman whose political activism and growing cultural consciousness had led her to seek out a new—and yet in some ways old—way of giving birth. AIM members and sympathizers on reservations in South Dakota had had similar impulses. The Lakota activist Mary Brave Bird famously gave birth during AIM's occupation of Wounded Knee in 1973. In part a response to the coercive sterilization of her sister, Brave Bird recalled, "I was determined not to go to the hospital. . . . I wanted no white doctor to touch me."[130] Two years later, another Lakota woman opted to deliver outside the hospital for similar reasons. She did not trust the government doctors, and, as the sociologist Barbara Gurr explains, her desire for a birth experience that she understood as "traditional" can be viewed as "a political assertion of identity."[131] The establishment of WARN and the founders' endorsement of Cook's message helped channel women's heretofore disparate experiences: WARN's second-annual gathering in Seattle included a midwives' meeting.[132] By the early 1980s, the Women's Dance program among the Oneida in Wisconsin and the Mohawks at Akwesasne included a midwifery component, and women in other locations displayed a similar urge to restore a sense of birthing as ceremony.[133]

Not all women were comfortable with the thought of giving birth outside a hospital or of giving birth without the supervision of a trained physician, but reclamation of control of reproduction extended beyond childbirth itself. In an era in which Native men and women were reclaiming Indianness and reincorporating cultural and spiritual knowledge and practices, women reintroduced puberty and prenatal rituals that had not disappeared but had fallen out of common practice.[134] At Crow, women called on hospital personnel to be more respectful of community members' postnatal rituals. This required, for example, that medical staff cut the umbilical cord at a length long enough for it to be taken home and beaded into a small bundle to be worn by the child to ward off illness.[135]

As it happened, IHS's introduction of nurse-midwifery in these very same years facilitated some women's quest for greater control. IHS began hiring certified nurse-midwives (CNMs) in some service units in 1969 as a cost-cutting measure and a means of mitigating continuing physician shortages. CNMs differed from many of the women who worked on Birthing Crews in Minneapolis, Akwesasne, and other locations. The latter were more likely to be lay, or direct-entry, midwives, while the former had completed academic training in nursing as well as midwifery. Most of the early CNMs were white, but a few Native women completed nurse-midwifery programs in the 1970s. Ursula Knoki-Wilson, the daughter of a Navajo midwife, graduated from the University of Utah's nurse-midwifery program in 1976 and went to work in the IHS service unit in Chinle, Arizona. Wilson recalls CNMs being welcomed into the community because women appreciated receiving care from female providers and because CNMs worked closely with Native healers to ensure women's needs were met.[136]

If Native midwifery represented the most straightforward means of re-claiming control over childbirth, Cook later emphasized that the most important outcome was for women to be "healthy enough" to exert control over their reproductive lives regardless of their birthing decisions.[137] WARN's emphasis on health—the health of women, children, families, and communities—led its work in directions that were sometimes difficult for non-Native women to understand but that made perfect sense to the women themselves, who believed that their lives could not be compartmentalized. "We can't fragment the issues as the White man would have us do," Cook insisted.[138] Nowhere was this clearer than in WARN's increasing attention to the environmental degradation of reservation land, a phenomenon that activists linked to negative reproductive health outcomes.

Marie Sanchez, the Northern Cheyenne activist who worked with AIM as well as WARN, was well positioned to illuminate connections between biological reproduction and the environment, as she worked simultaneously on both issues in the 1970s. Sanchez was among the Native activists who organized to stave off the invasion of private energy corporations that, with the federal government's assistance, opened vast swaths of reservation land to mining operations in postwar decades.[139] As the historian James Allison has demonstrated, "energy firms had gained control of hundreds of thousands of acres of Indian land" by 1973, and a second uranium mining boom a few years later accelerated this trend.[140] Economic pressures convinced some tribal leaders to favor energy development, but tribal nations were inade-quately compensated in these deals and prior to the early 1980s had little control over the process. These circumstances led Sanchez and some WARN leaders to view the coercive sterilization of Native women as a means of wiping out the Native population to meet the nation's seemingly insatiable hunger for tribal resources.

Activists identified additional intersections between environmental and reproductive politics. WARN and other Native women protested water pollution, uranium mining, and other forms of environmental degradation on reservations, all in the name of protecting their reproductive health. In 1980, WARN released a health study that revealed that uranium mining on the Pine Ridge Reservation had both long-term and short-term consequences for community health, destroying the tribal land base and exposing tribal members to low-level radiation and/or contaminated resources. Once again, the impetus for this line of inquiry came from an "insider" within the government health care system. Lorelei Decora Means (Ho-Chunk), WARN co-founder and registered nurse at the IHS hospital, spearheaded the study after she observed high rates of spontaneous abortions and birth defects in hospital patients. The resulting study alleged that in one month's time, more than one-third of pregnancies reported to IHS ended in spontaneous abortion, and more than half of children born on the reservation suffered some form of birth defect.[141] Activists discovered similar trends in other locations. Women on the Laguna Pueblo Reservation in New Mexico discovered that miscarriage rates increased after the onset of uranium mining. Native women further attributed the increase in reproductive cancers to the nuclear fuel cycle.[142]

In the coming decade, these issues would be at the forefront of many Native reproductive agendas, reflecting Cook's oft-repeated conviction that "women are the first environment."[143] Reclaiming control over reproduction was no simple matter. Native women's ability to exercise "sovereignty over their own bodies" required shoring up the political sovereignty of tribal nations to protect reservation lands and women's bodies from plunder.

THE INCREASED AVAILABILITY of the reproductive technologies of birth control, abortion, and sterilization in government and contract hospitals in the late 1960s and 1970s heightened the urgency of Native women's long-standing demands regarding competent and culturally sensitive health services. Women's attitudes toward and experiences of these technologies were shaped by individual needs, familial and community beliefs, and their political commitments—as well as their personal experiences with government health services and medical staff. By the mid-1970s, the coercive sterilization of Native women became a focal point of some women's activism in the early self-determination era, from health workers to community leaders to militant activists. In response to this and similar abuses and in the context of a broader feminist challenge to American birthing culture, women within and outside of WARN called for a reassessment of Native biological reproduction and a reincorporation of historical practices and beliefs. For some, this required a rejection of the physician or obstetrician as the foremost authority on birthing and/or a rejection of the hospital as the preferred location for childbirth.

In 1979, proponents of reproductive freedom secured a victory with HEW's adoption of regulations that established new protocols to protect women from coercion. By most accounts, coercive sterilization via tubal ligation or hysterectomy declined significantly in the aftermath of the regulations—and the public protests that produced them. Yet Native women's reproductive organizing expanded in subsequent decades. In 1990, Native women from more than eleven Northern Plains Nations descended on Pierre, South Dakota, for a three-day "collective decision-making process" in which they established an agenda for future action. The women's nineteen-plank reproductive agenda included the "right to all reproductive alternatives and the right to choose the size of our families"; the "right to give birth and be attended to in the setting most appropriate, be it home, community, clinic or hospital"; and the "right to active involvement in the development and implementation of policies concerning reproductive issues." The women further insisted that domestic violence, sexual assault, and AIDS be recognized as pressing reproductive issues.[144] This struggle for reproductive justice continues—and continues to evolve—in the twenty-first century.

Epilogue
Twenty-First-Century Stories

Many of the women who gave birth in the 1970s and 1980s are now grandmothers; some are great-grandmothers. The history recounted in this book—of the intersection of colonial and reproductive politics and of Native women's creativity, determination, and advocacy in the reproductive realm—presents no clear endpoint. In the twenty-first century, as when Native women founded the Women of All Red Nations (WARN) decades earlier, women throughout Indian Country are working to decolonize biological reproduction, an undertaking that carries subtly different meanings for diverse individuals in varying circumstances. The brief twenty-first-century stories narrated below are rooted in a much longer history; the stories presented in the preceding pages echo across the generations.

When Janine Pease's (Crow/Hidatsa) daughter gave birth to Pease's first grandchild in the 1990s, she did so under much different circumstances than Pease had two decades earlier. In the late 1970s, Pease had lived among her husband's people on the Rocky Boy Reservation, and she delivered her children in a hospital in Havre, Montana. Although she remembers her children's births as the most sacred and powerful moments of her life, the off-reservation contract hospital in which she delivered did not allow her female in-laws or her mother to join her in the delivery room. She labored and delivered in the company of the physician and nurses and missed her family's presence. Pease liked the doctor who delivered her first child, but her loneliness was made more acute by her awareness of the controversy surrounding the sterilization of Native women in these years, which heightened her desire to remain vigilant throughout her deliveries. Pease's daughter, in contrast, gave birth in the Indian Health Service (IHS) hospital at Crow Agency. Pease and her sister supported and guided her daughter throughout her pregnancy, and when the parturient woman went into labor, "absolutely everyone in the family" went to the hospital with her. The men slept in the waiting room overnight, while the women—the laboring woman's mother, aunts, grandmother, and cousins—gathered in the birthing room. For Pease, the sense that birthing should be a family affair stemmed from her dissatisfaction with aspects of her own birthing experiences.[1]

Large family gatherings like that of Pease's family for the birth of her first grandchild are not especially unusual in twenty-first-century reservation hospitals. At the Tuba City Hospital in Arizona, a facility run by the Navajo Nation and partially financed by IHS, kin from children to grandparents are often by a woman's side during labor. A non-Native nurse-midwife at Tuba City recently remarked that she has had as many as twelve family members in the delivery room: "Whoever the woman wants to be there is there." The head of midwifery concurred: "All of a sudden Mom is surrounded by women, and they're all helping her and touching her."[2] The presence of these visitors—and their general acceptance by non-Native and Native hospital staff—speaks to Native patients' long-standing insistence that birthing and healing be recognized as a social affair.

At Crow Agency, the new reservation hospital, constructed in the 1990s, was designed to facilitate visitors' presence and prominence. Pease, who served on an advisory committee during the hospital's planning and construction, recalled that the facility had "beautiful birthing rooms" with "plenty of space" and visiting areas distributed throughout the hospital, so loved ones could always be nearby. The building was well ventilated so that family members could use smudging—the burning of plants such as sage— to support positive health outcomes.[3] Since the construction of the first reservation hospital nearly a century earlier, Crows had related to the institution on their own terms and attempted with varying degrees of success to enact their vision for its use and function. The intentional design of the late twentieth-century hospital's physical space can be seen as a culmination of this multigenerational endeavor.

In the two decades since the birth of her first grandchild, Janine Pease has acted as an informal "birth coach" or "helper" for several women in her family—daughters, daughters-in-law, nieces, and also friends. She estimates that she has helped in a dozen births over the years, and her role is comparable to that of a doula. Pease encourages women throughout their pregnancies and helps them formulate a birth plan. At the hospital, Pease sometimes uses smudge and always brings sweet grass along, but mostly, she simply encourages the laboring woman and does what she can to improve her physical comfort. She also acts as a patient advocate, and women in the throes of labor are able to relax more fully knowing that Pease is monitoring the situation.[4] In Crow families, it is common for one or a few women to assume a role like Pease's, as family members appreciate their demeanor, recognize their experience and knowledge, and seek out their assistance. Although under much different circumstances, this aspect of twenty-first-century Crow birthing parallels Crow birthing in the late nineteenth-century context in which this book began.

In Pease's case, the difference between the birth of her first grandchild and the more recent deliveries she has attended is that the women she assists no longer give birth on the reservation. The obstetrics department at Crow Agency closed in 2011. The immediate cause for this reduction in services was that IHS could not find enough qualified obstetric nurses, and the hospital lacked the funds necessary to purchase up-to-date labor and delivery equipment.[5] Although many hoped the closure would be temporary, more than seven years later, Crow as well as Northern Cheyenne women continue to give birth at contract hospitals off the reservation. Hospitals and clinics on other reservations have faced similar reductions in services, a trend that has likewise plagued non-Native women living in rural areas.[6]

Native leaders protest these developments, arguing that diminishing services are an abdication of federal responsibility. At a field hearing held by Senator Max Baucus in the lobby of the Crow Hospital in 2012, Cedric Black Eagle, then chair of the Crow Nation, echoed generations of Crow leaders when he asserted that "the Crow people are entitled to get health care here. It is our right as a treaty tribe to be healed within these walls."[7] On my visits to the reservation, I have found that many Crow women are equally committed to their right to birth within the walls of their reservation hospital. As one woman explained, "I was really mad and upset when I found out that they weren't going to allow the Crow women to have their babies here. . . . I don't think we should have to go anyplace else. We have our own hospital right here."[8] This woman had been born in the Crow Agency Hospital in the 1950s and delivered her own children there in the 1970s, yet her daughters and granddaughters are now forced to leave the reservation for the same services.

In addition to federal obligations and treaty rights, Native communities can point to medical arguments in support of their demand for the full range of gynecological and obstetric services on reservations. As mounting public health research demonstrates, "Drive time affects outcomes."[9] Studies have found that women who travel more than an hour to give birth are more likely to have complicated deliveries caused by stress, and their infants have poorer health outcomes immediately following birth and throughout their first year of life. On the Crow Reservation, women living in the town of Lodge Grass, for example, should expect an hour and a half drive under good weather conditions. For other Native women, including Ojibwe women living on the Red Cliff Reservation in Wisconsin, the nearest full-service medical facility is at least two hours away. Amnesty International has argued that these circumstances directly threaten maternal health, and this is especially the case for women who suffer from other risk factors such as diabetes or high blood pressure.[10]

Such distances increase the likelihood of deliveries en route, a threat to the woman's and infant's safety. For Northern Cheyenne and other women who have not had reservation hospitals since the termination era or earlier, this is nothing new, nor has the threat of an en route delivery been out of the question for women living on dispersed reservations. At Crow, few women do not have a story to tell about a woman they know giving birth on the way to Billings in recent years. Although Janine Pease has been generally satisfied with the care her family members have received at the Billings Clinic, she acknowledges that the additional distance is "a real imposition." Pease tells the story of one young woman who delivered her child by herself in a vehicle alongside the road.[11] This problem has been especially acute for women in IHS's Great Plains Area. During a seven-month period when the Rosebud Reservation in South Dakota was without obstetric services, women delivered five babies on their way to an off-reservation hospital.[12] A Lakota woman from the Cheyenne River Reservation told the sociologist Barbara Gurr that women on her reservation give birth outside the hospital "all the time. . . . You can't get to the damn hospital!"[13] To avoid this outcome, health workers at the nearest IHS-contracted hospital prefer for women from Cheyenne River to be induced early, yet this solution brings its own problems. The American Civil Liberties Union of South Dakota contends that these inductions are often coercive in nature: women have little or no prior notice, they are not provided with adequate counseling, and they fear the consequences of their refusal.[14]

This situation is exacerbated by a shortage of physicians and especially obstetricians in IHS hospitals, but such shortages are not a new problem. IHS began employing certified nurse-midwives (CNMs) in some locations in the late 1960s as a relatively low-cost means of filling gaps in necessary health services.[15] In their first year at the IHS facility in Shiprock, New Mexico, CNMs attended 71 percent of all deliveries at the institution.[16] Although the trajectory of IHS nurse-midwifery has not proceeded linearly, nurse-midwives continue to play a large role in Native reproduction. In a master's thesis on IHS nurse-midwifery completed in the early 2000s, Gretchen Landwehr observed that "Native American women are more likely than [other ethnic groups] to deliver their infants under the care of midwives" — five times more likely than white women.[17] In some locations, CNMs coordinate with staff obstetricians and attend deliveries for which hospital staff do not anticipate complications.[18] Other IHS hospitals employ CNMs but no obstetricians. Women living on these reservations give birth at contracted hospitals off the reservation but receive their prenatal care from IHS midwives.[19]

The Native women who rely on IHS midwives for at least some portion of their reproductive health care have mixed views about these services. As noted in chapter 6, Ursula Knoki-Wilson (Navajo) is a CNM employed by IHS. For many years, Knoki-Wilson served as chief of nurse midwifery services within the Department of Obstetrics and Gynecology at the IHS facility in Chinle, Arizona. Knoki-Wilson contends that Navajos have "greatly welcomed CNMs" because of CNMs' willingness to collaborate with Native healers and because Navajo women "like being cared for by women providers."[20] But some Native women express more ambivalence about nurse-midwifery, and past and present federal policies have contributed to women's resistance. Recognizing the cost-reducing function that CNMs provide for IHS, one of the sociologist Barbara Gurr's Lakota informants resented that Pine Ridge women are stuck with midwives because they are the only practitioners IHS can afford to employ.[21] The decades of intensive propaganda touting the superiority of trained physicians and the deficiencies of Native midwives provide important context for one Crow grandmother's insistence that her great-grandchildren "be delivered by a real doctor."[22] The more recent practice of having women receive care by midwives throughout their pregnancies and then travel off the reservation to be attended by an obstetrician during delivery reinforces a perceived hierarchy of knowledge and expertise. The bottom line is that for many twenty-first-century Native women, the midwifery model is not a choice as it has been for growing numbers of American women—predominantly white women of the middle and upper classes. Rather, care by CNMs is at least in part a product of women's limited reproductive options, and this reality shapes Native women's attitudes toward this model of reproductive care.

Native women who receive health services on reservations throughout their pregnancies and/or in childbirth face the same challenges encountered by other IHS patients. The positive birthing experiences of Pease's daughter and others notwithstanding, twenty-first-century IHS hospitals are plagued by persistent underfunding and staff shortages, both of which mar patient experience. Native women and men alike complain of excessively long wait times, insensitivity on the part of hospital staff, and high employee turnover, which makes it difficult for patients to establish trusting relationships with health workers. In the most extreme cases, documented deficiencies have resulted in closures and reduction of services when the Centers for Medicare and Medicaid Services determined that it could no longer reimburse for services provided in these institutions.[23] Some of the most troubling reports pertain specifically to childbirth. In South Dakota, tribal leaders describe instances of women giving birth without medical assistance on bathroom floors.[24] Lynda Dixon, a scholar and member of the Cherokee Nation, observed one young Native woman give birth on the floor of an unnamed IHS waiting room. Dixon reported that the woman had spent four hours trying in vain to gain admittance to an examination room.[25]

Due to ongoing frustrations with IHS as well as strained historical relationships, some twenty-first-century Native women are pursuing alternative options. Zintkala Mahpiya Wi Blackowl (Lakota) gave birth to a daughter—her sixth child—in the fall of 2016. Unlike her five prior deliveries, this October birth made national headlines. Blackowl delivered her daughter in a tepee alongside the Cannonball River in North Dakota. A resident of Oregon, Blackowl and her husband and children had journeyed to North Dakota a month earlier to support the Standing Rock Sioux Nation. Water protectors gathered to protest the proposed construction of the Dakota Access Pipeline just outside the reservation through territory historically recognized as Sioux in nineteenth-century treaties. Having delivered her previous children at home with the assistance of a midwife, Blackowl had no interest in a medicalized birthing experience. In this case, she chose to deliver by herself in the family's tepee as her husband and children slept. Her sisters—one a midwife and the other a doula—were nearby, as were volunteer Native midwives who had traveled from throughout the continent to provide reproductive health services for women in the water protector camps.[26]

When Blackowl spoke of her experience to journalists, she articulated a clear link between the political struggle Native peoples waged at Standing Rock and more intimate sites of decolonization such as birthing and child-rearing. Four decades earlier, Mary Brave Bird, another Lakota woman, had also chosen to birth in a site of protest and conflict. Out of disgust with IHS and a determination to reclaim at least elements of "the Sioux way" of birthing, Brave Bird delivered her first child while she and other American Indian Movement (AIM) members occupied Wounded Knee on the Pine Ridge Reservation in South Dakota—the site of the 1890 massacre of Lakota men, women, and children, which remains the largest massacre in U.S. history.[27] Blackowl's assertion that "having babies is my act of resistance" similarly echoes Brave Bird's earlier sentiments. For Blackowl, history informed her reproductive decisions and the urgency with which she made them: "Our reproductive rights as Native women have been taken from us in so many

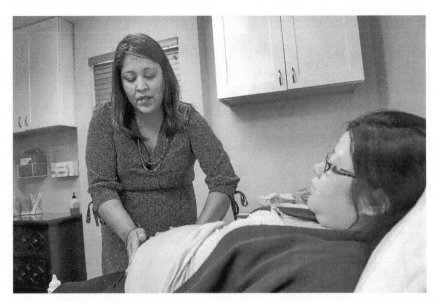

Nicolle Gonzales, founder and executive director of the Changing Woman Initiative, examines a patient. A CNM, Gonzales plans to open the first Native American birth center in the United States. Photo by Gabriela Campos. Copyright © 2018 The New Mexican, Inc. Reprinted with permission. All rights reserved.

ways." She specifically cited the history of sterilization abuses in government hospitals and federal assimilation policies aimed at the destruction of Native cultures and families.[28]

While many aspects of Blackowl's recent childbearing experience are unusual, including her desire to birth alone, she is nonetheless part of a small but growing movement of Native women who are questioning or outright challenging Western models of medicalized birthing. Nicolle Gonzales, a Navajo CNM and mother of three, delivered her first child at the age of twenty; she found the hospital setting in which she gave birth noisy, chaotic, and stressful.[29] In the following years, Gonzales pursued midwifery training and spent two years working in an IHS hospital, but she felt that Native women were treated poorly by hospital staff and providers.[30] Gonzales has increasingly felt that government bureaucracy is incompatible with many Native women's needs. She founded the Changing Woman Initiative, a Native American women's health collective of which she serves as executive director. About a year before Blackowl gave birth along the Cannonball River, Gonzales announced plans to open the first Native American birthing center in the United States.[31]

As of this writing, Changing Woman Initiative has begun offering women's health and home birth services, while the organization continues to work toward its goal of building a physical center.[32] Gonzales envisions the reproductive wellness and birth center as a space in which women can reclaim birthing as ceremony. "I'd like to see a nice building with pictures of our grandmothers, cedar welcoming you into the door, and moccasins for babies. . . . I want a place where women and families feel welcome."[33] She is also committed to providing care that is affordable to Native women, including Medicaid patients and those who are under- or uninsured.[34] Christina Castro (Jemez/Taos/Ajchamen/Chicana), an educator, writer, and mother of two, counts herself among the women invested in Gonzales's work. For Castro, a Native American birthing center is a way to "reclaim our spaces, our bodies and our voices."[35] The enthusiastic response to Gonzales's message — on social media and in the talking circles the Changing Woman Initiative organized in Pueblo communities in northern New Mexico — suggests that there is a hunger among Native women and their communities for this type of space and for the reproductive experiences Gonzales describes. Katsi Cook, the Mohawk midwife who advocated a return to Native midwifery at the first annual meeting of WARN four decades earlier, is a supporter of Gonzales's efforts. Cook has been instrumental in advancing Indigenous midwifery on the Canadian side of the border, where there is a similar, if not greater, demand for such services.[36]

For Cook, Gonzales, and many of the Native midwives who volunteered their services at Standing Rock, Indigenous midwifery is a central component of an ongoing movement for Native reproductive justice. As I have argued, WARN's political analysis and grassroots organizing should be viewed as an early articulation of Native reproductive justice. WARN's work paralleled and sometimes intersected with contemporaneous efforts by women of color. In 1994, a group of black feminists merged the terms "reproductive rights" and "social justice" to coin the label "reproductive justice."[37] Loretta Ross and other leaders in the movement have offered a three-part definition of reproductive justice: "the right to have children, not have children, and parent the children we have in safe and healthy environments."[38] In contrast to a liberal reproductive rights framework, which foregrounds the individual, reproductive justice emphasizes both individual and group rights and recognizes their intersection, an approach many Native women view as critical. Native reproductive justice proponents also stress the importance of cultural safety, arguing that Native women must be free to birth (or not) and raise their children in culturally appropriate ways. They further tend to articulate reproductive agendas through the language of sovereignty and decolonization, linking multiple forms of political struggle.

If Gonzales, Cook, and others entered the reproductive justice movement through their work as midwives, the movement's proponents also support Native women's ongoing efforts to reform and reopen hospitals and obstetric services on reservations, as well as women's rights to bring families and other elements of Indigenous birthing cultures into hospitals. As Erika Finestone and Cynthia Stirbys (Saulteaux-Cree) have emphasized, it is a matter of women having "the ability to decide how they will give birth, where they will give birth, and who will be present during the birthing process."[39] Historically, this level of autonomy has at times been denied to all or at least most American women, but it has been especially out of reach for Native women, whose reproductive autonomy has been limited by both federal "control" and "neglect."[40] Native reproductive justice further demands that the care that Native women, children, and families receive in government and government-contracted institutions be of high quality.

As the nineteen-plank platform introduced at the end of chapter 6 suggests, Native reproductive justice agendas are expansive. In most cases, such agendas include access to safe, legal, and affordable abortions. Since the late 1970s, the Hyde Amendment has limited Native women's financial access to abortion services. Over the last several years, some conservative lawmakers have attempted to double down on Hyde by making the prohibition on abortion services for federal health programs serving American Indians permanent — so far with limited success.[41] Native women on rural reservations, especially those living in conservative states, are further affected by the same trends that have limited many non-Native women's access to abortion services. Restrictive state laws, a conservative political climate, and inadequate funding have resulted in a sharp decline in the number of abortion providers operating in many regions.[42]

In 2006, Oglala Sioux President Cecelia Fire Thunder, the first female president of the Oglala Nation, responded to one such law in South Dakota by announcing plans to open a Planned Parenthood clinic on the Pine Ridge Reservation. Fire Thunder's family had relocated to California when she was a teenager, and her commitment to women's health was forged in urban centers in the 1970s. Trained as a nurse, Fire Thunder established community-based clinics in Los Angeles and San Diego before returning to Pine Ridge in 1986. The response to Fire Thunder's bold announcement two decades later underscores twenty-first-century divisions surrounding the politics of family planning and abortion services on the Pine Ridge Reservation and throughout Indian Country. Men and women alike debated Fire Thunder's proposal not through the mainstream categories of "pro-life" and "pro-choice" but rather through alternative interpretations of tradition and strategies for sovereignty. In the end, the controversy at Pine Ridge contributed to Fire Thunder's impeachment, and the Oglala Tribal Council voted to ban abortions on the reservation.[43] In the meantime, however, South Dakota's restrictive law had galvanized other Native women around the issue. Charon Asetoyer, a Comanche activist who has lived on the Yankton Sioux Reservation in South Dakota since the 1980s and worked with WARN in the group's early years, announced her bid for State Senate that year, running on a platform that supported women's reproductive rights, including the right to terminate undesirable pregnancies.[44] She did not win the election.

Despite Asetoyer's staunch support of women's reproductive freedom, she has consistently insisted that abortion politics should not subsume Native reproductive agendas, as is often the case in mainstream reproductive rights organizations.[45] For Native women, she and others argue, the "right to have children" and the right to "parent the children we have in safe and healthy environments" remain equally hard-fought. Asetoyer's work with the Native American Women's Health Education Research Center, an organization she founded in the late 1980s, has led her to conclude that some physicians are especially eager to prescribe long-acting contraceptives like Norplant and Depo-Provera for Native women, and she warns of the potential for coercion with these technologies.[46] Furthermore, in the twenty-first century, the tubal ligation rate for Native women surpasses that for white women. In 2004, 33.9 percent of Native women between the ages of eighteen and forty-four had had a tubal ligation compared with 18.7 percent of Euro-American women.[47] These statistical data do not imply that these procedures were performed coercively, but the testimony of individual women speaks to the need for continued vigilance.[48] Native children are also still removed from their homes at disproportionate rates, a situation that the Lakota People's Law Project, led in part by WARN cofounder Madonna Thunder Hawk, remains committed to documenting and challenging.[49] Throughout Indian Country, Native women are organizing in large and small ways around poverty and health disparities, rape and domestic violence, environmental justice and injustice, and police brutality and the mass incarceration of Native peoples. As Native activists have powerfully demonstrated, these issues are matters of reproductive justice.

Native women in the twenty-first century continue to adapt the work and legacy of their mothers, aunts, grandmothers, and great-grandmothers. It is perhaps fitting, then, that this book should end with the descendants of Lizzie and Susie Yellowtail. Valerie Jackson, great-granddaughter of Lizzie and granddaughter of Susie, is heartened by at least some recent trends in Native reproduction. Jackson, who resides in Arizona, counts herself among the supporters of the Changing Woman Initiative and Nicolle Gonzales's efforts to start a Native American birthing center. She believes that her grandmother would have supported this commitment to "bringing back woman-knowledge." Jackson currently receives much of her health care from the Phoenix Indian Medical Center (PIMC), and she has been pleased to learn that ongoing problems notwithstanding, Native women who have given birth at PIMC in recent years have had a number of birthing options that were unavailable to her in the 1970s, such as a water birth. Jackson is a regular speaker at workshops at PIMC, where she—like her grandmother before her—advocates for improved patient care. On the Crow Reservation, Connie Jackson, Susie Yellowtail's only living child, has been among the many Crow voices clamoring for the return of obstetric services to the reservation. A few years ago, Connie took me on a short tour of the Crow Agency Hospital, where her mother's picture rightfully hangs. As of 2018, Susie Yellowtail's descendants, including Connie, Lesley Kabotie, Jackie Yellowtail, and Tom Yellowtail, with support from other family members, honor Susie and Thomas Yellowtail's legacy through a nonprofit organization called Blue Otter, which advances a holistic approach to the revitalization of Crow families and communities. As Jackie Yellowtail, whose work centers on the needs of Crow women and children, explained, "It's our responsibility . . . to be the next bridge into the future."[50]

Notes

Abbreviations

ABMC   Ann Big Man Collection, Little Bighorn College Archives,
Crow Agency, Montana

ARCIA   Commissioner of Indian Affairs, *Annual Report* (Washington, D.C.:
Government Printing Office)

BIA   Bureau of Indian Affairs

BIA CCF   Bureau of Indian Affairs Central Classified Files, Microfilm, Record
Group 75, Labriola American Indian Center, Tempe, Arizona

BIA FNR   Bureau of Indian Affairs Field Nurses' Reports, 1931–43, Record Group
75, National Archives and Records Administration, Washington, D.C.

BIA RR   Bureau of Indian Affairs Relocation Records, Newberry Library,
Chicago, Illinois

BIA SWR   Bureau of Indian Affairs Social Workers' Reports, 1932–42, Record
Group 75, National Archives and Records Administration,
Washington, D.C.

CAGCF   Crow Agency General Correspondence Files, Record Group 75,
National Archives and Records Administration, Broomfield, Colorado

CAIOHP   Chicago American Indian Oral History Project, Newberry Library,
Chicago, Illinois

CIA   Commissioner of Indian Affairs

DD   Doris Duke American Indian Oral History Program Archives,
University of Illinois at Urbana-Champaign

EWPC   Eloise Whitebear Pease Collection, Little Bighorn College Archives,
Crow Agency, Montana

FSC   Ferdinand Shoemaker Collection, Buffalo Bill Center of the West,
Cody, Wyoming

FWVP   Fred W. Voget Papers, Mike and Maureen Mansfield Library,
University of Montana-Missoula

GAO   Elmer B. Staats, *Report to Senator James Abourezk: Investigation of
Allegations concerning Indian Health Service* (Washington, D.C.:
Government Printing Office, 1976)

HSD   Health Services Division

KCP   Katsi Cook Papers, Sophia Smith Collection, Smith College,
Northampton, Massachusetts

LBCA   Little Bighorn College Archives, Crow Agency, Montana

MHS   Montana Historical Society, Helena, Montana

MVSF	Mixed Vocational and Subject Files, 1939–1960, Billings Area Office, Record Group 75, National Archives and Records Administration, Broomfield, Colorado
NARA CO	National Archives and Records Administration, Broomfield, Colorado
NARA DC	National Archives and Records Administration, Washington, D.C.
NARA MD	National Archives and Records Administration, Baltimore, Maryland
NARG	Native American Research Group
PHS	Public Health Service
RG	Record Group
R2N2P	Reproductive Rights National Network Papers, Sophia Smith Collection, Smith College, Northampton, Massachusetts
SARL	Superintendents' Annual Reports, Microfilm, Record Group 75, Labriola American Indian Center, Tempe, Arizona
SARN	Superintendents' Annual Reports, Microfilm, Record Group 75, National Archives and Records Administration, Washington, D.C.
WARN II	WARN Annual Report 1979, Liberty Hill Foundation Records, 20th Century Organizational Files, Southern California Library for Social Studies and Research, Los Angeles, California.
WDHP	Women's Dance Health Project

Introduction

1. Lorelei Means and Janet McCloud, "Who We Are," in *Women of All Red Nations*, p. 4, KCP, Box 3, Folder 19. The epigraph for this introduction is from Tabobondung et al., "Indigenous Midwifery as an Expression of Sovereignty," 81.

2. Cook, interview by Follett.

3. Means and McCloud, "Who We Are," p. 4, KCP.

4. See Katsi Cook, WDHP Report, Apr. 1979, KCP, Box 5, Folder 7; Million, *Therapeutic Nations*, 125.

5. On reproductive justice, see Ross and Solinger, *Reproductive Justice*; and Ross et al., *Radical Reproductive Justice*.

6. See Lawrence, "The Indian Health Service"; Torpy, "Native American Women"; Carpio, "The Lost Generation: American Indian Women and Sterilization Abuse"; and Ralstin-Lewis, "The Continuing Struggle against Genocide."

7. WARN II.

8. See O'Sullivan, "Informing Red Power."

9. For a recent article on the history of Native reproduction, see Hancock, "Health and Well-Being."

10. Wolfe, "Settler Colonialism and the Elimination of the Native," 388.

11. See Murphy, *Seizing the Means of Reproduction*, 8.

12. Here I intentionally draw on and adapt Laura Briggs's language in *How All Politics Became Reproductive Politics*.

13. Brown, *Good Wives, Nasty Wenches*, 54.

14. Quoted in Green, "The Pocahontas Perplex," 699. Camilla Townsend suggests that the colonist who chose the name Rebekah for Pocahontas upon her conversion to

Christianity and marriage to Rolfe likely had in mind the biblical Rebekah's fertility and her preference for her pale son over his red twin. Townsend further emphasizes that Pocahontas's Powhatan people recognized a relationship between reproduction and political diplomacy. "In a time-honored custom, [Pocahontas] married with the enemy and bore children who owed allegiance to both sides." Townsend, *Pocahontas and the Powhatan Dilemma*, 126–27, 119.

15. See Deloria Jr., *Custer Died for Your Sins*, 3–4.

16. Green, "The Pocahontas Perplex," 702.

17. See Morgan, *Laboring Women*, ch. 1; and Brown, *Good Wives, Nasty Wenches*, 57–59.

18. Quoted in Green, "The Pocahontas Perplex," 713.

19. Report of the Joint Committee on the Conduct of War.

20. See Deer, *The Beginning and End of Rape*; Stremlau, "Rape Narratives on the Northern Paiute Frontier"; and Trafzer and Hyer, *"Exterminate Them."*

21. Trennert, *Alternative to Extinction*.

22. For a history that chronicles the lives of six Indigenous women who lived outside reservation communities in this period, see Jagodinsky, *Legal Codes and Talking Trees*.

23. The Bureau of Indian Affairs was called the Office of Indian Affairs until the 1940s. I use BIA here for consistency.

24. For two exemplary models of this work, see Cahill, *Federal Fathers and Mothers*; and Stremlau, *Sustaining the Cherokee Family*. Much of the best recent scholarship on "intimate colonialism" in the United States owes an implicit or explicit debt to the anthropologist Ann Laura Stoler. See especially Stoler, *Carnal Knowledge and Imperial Power*.

25. Cahill discusses the tension between persuasion and coercion in *Federal Fathers and Mothers*, 71–81.

26. Gurr, *Reproductive Justice*, 4, 157.

27. GAO.

28. See Untitled Report, Twin Cities Reproductive Rights Committee, 20 Mar. 1979, R2N2P, Box 6, Folder 21; and Smith, *Conquest*, 96–97.

29. Katsi Cook, "Women's Dance: A Woman's Health Book" outline, n.d., KCP, Box 6, Folder 10.

30. See Bill Donovan, "IHS Careful about Sterilizations," *Navajo Times*, 5 Dec. 1997, 2; Smith, *Conquest*, 96–97.

31. For a historical study that places the sterilization of Native American women within the context of domestic racial and gendered politics, see Kluchin, *Fit to Be Tied*. For an analysis that foregrounds global context, see Hartmann, *Reproductive Rights and Wrongs*.

32. O'Sullivan, "'We Worry about Survival,'" 178. I address some important exceptions to this scholarly trend in chapter 3.

33. Wolfe, "Settler Colonialism and the Elimination of the Native," 387.

34. Quoted in Tabobondung et al., "Indigenous Midwifery as an Expression of Sovereignty," 81.

35. Quoted in Wright, "The Woman's Lodge," 5.

36. See Cook, interview by Follett.

37. The chronology of peyote's introduction and use on reservations varied. For example, some Northern Cheyenne men and women began using peyote in the 1890s, while Crow individuals do not seem to have embraced peyotism until the 1910s. See Rzeczkowski, *Uniting the Tribes*, 146–47. The practice never took hold in some locations.

38. Yellowtail with Weatherly, "Susie Walking Bear Yellowtail."

39. Maney, interview by Cossen; and "Native Voices," pp. 132–33, 291, CAIOHP.

40. Deloria, *Indians in Unexpected Places*; O'Neill, "Rethinking Modernity and the Discourse of Development"; and McCallum, *Indigenous Women, Work, and History*. See also Barker, *Native Acts*, esp. 19–22.

41. McCallum, *Indigenous Women*, 9.

42. Katsi Cook, interview by Kim Anderson, 18 July 2001, KCP, Box 1, Folder Interviews, 1992–2001.

43. Quoted in Ross Carletta, "Chaperone Shatters Preconceptions," 44, in Hinkell, *Nurse of the Twentieth Century*.

44. Jackie Yellowtail, interview by author.

45. See Child, "Politically Purposeful Work."

46. Thomas, *Politics of the Womb*, 4.

47. Mihesuah, "Commonality of Difference," 15–16.

48. Blansett, "State of the Field" comments, 18 Oct. 2014. See also Blansett, "State of the Field" comments, 3 Nov. 2017.

49. See PHS, *Health Services for American Indians*; and HSD, *Family Planning and the American Indian*.

50. See Linderman, *Pretty-Shield*; Voget, *They Call Me Agnes*; Snell with Matthews, *Grandmother's Grandchild*; Hogan with Loeb and Plainfeather, *The Woman Who Loved Mankind*; and Yellowtail with Weatherly, "Susie Walking Bear Yellowtail."

51. I am using Crow kinship terms here, so "sisters" includes women whom Euro-Americans would call "cousins."

52. Because of the sensitive nature of some of the topics discussed in interviews, I determined that it was necessary to be sensitive to interviewees' privacy. Verbally and in writing, I informed each woman that if she chose, she could remain anonymous if I used portions of her interview in this or other publications. A few women accepted this offer, and I use pseudonyms—indicated in the first note reference—when drawing on these women's stories. Most women opted to be identified by name.

53. WARN II, 3.

Chapter 1

1. Linderman, *Pretty-Shield*, 145–48 (italics in original).

2. Barney Old Coyote Jr., Spring Crow Culture Lecture Series, 1971, p. 217, DD, Box 34.

3. In my dissertation, entitled "'The Simplest Rules of Motherhood': Settler Colonialism and the Regulation of American Indian Reproduction" (Arizona State University, 2015), I used the term "flexible mothering." I have since determined that the more

expansive "flexible childrearing" is more apt, as it encompasses the valued and necessary labor men in many Indigenous societies performed in raising, educating, and training children. My thanks to Rose Stremlau for guiding me in this direction.

4. I use Office of Indian Affairs and Indian Service interchangeably until the 1940s, when the OIA became the Bureau of Indian Affairs.

5. Medicine Crow, *From the Heart of the Crow Country*, xxi–3. More recent scholarship generally cites an earlier date for the Crow-Hidatsa split.

6. Quoted in Medicine Crow, *From the Heart of the Crow Country*, xxi.

7. McCleary, "Akbaatashee," 37–39.

8. Frederick Hoxie has characterized this period as "life in a tightening circle." Hoxie, *Parading through History*, ch. 3. On the 1825 treaty, see Kappler, *Indian Treaties*, 244–46.

9. Hoxie, *Parading through History*, ch. 3.

10. Hoxie, 175.

11. On Crow land loss, see LaGrand, *Indian Metropolis*, 20. On allotment as federal policy and local practice, see Meyer, *The White Earth Tragedy*; and Stremlau, *Sustaining the Cherokee Family*. Some reservations were never allotted, and others, such as the Northern Cheyenne Reservation, were not allotted until decades later.

12. Trennert, *Alternative to Extinction*.

13. Medicine Crow, *From the Heart of the Crow Country*, 3–4; Frey, *The World of the Crow Indians*, 28–30.

14. See Matthews, "Wherever That Singing Is Going," 113.

15. Hoxie, *Parading through History*, 133. Crows had experienced an earlier demographic crisis with the arrival of European traders in the early nineteenth century. Frank Rzeczkowski notes that Euro-American observers predicted Crows' extinction in the 1830s and 1840s, owing to either epidemics or warfare with the Blackfeet. Rzeczkowski, *Uniting the Tribes*, 32.

16. Linderman, *Pretty-Shield*, 10. Crow men made similar comments in telling their life stories. See Linderman, *Plenty-Coups*, 311; Nabokov, *Two Leggings*, 197. The philosopher Jonathan Lear considers Plenty Coups's comments at length in *Radical Hope*.

17. For the federal government's assimilation agenda, see Hoxie, *A Final Promise*.

18. Key works on Indian boarding schools include Lomawaima, *They Called It Prairie Light*; Adams, *Education for Extinction*; Child, *Boarding School Seasons*; and Gilbert, *Education beyond the Mesas*.

19. Hoxie, *Parading through History*, 105; Matthews, "Wherever That Singing Is Going," 97–99.

20. John E. Edwards to T. J. Connelly, 20 Aug. 1900, Press Copies of Letters and Directives Sent to Agency Employees, p. 345, NARA CO, RG 75, Box 2, Volume 1899; Bradley, "After the Buffalo Days," 14. See also Jacobs, *White Mother to a Dark Race*, ch. 4.

21. Quoted in Jacobs, *White Mother to a Dark Race*, 156.

22. Tobacco, interview by Lowenthal.

23. Voget, *They Call Me Agnes*, 71; Hoxie and Bernardis, "Robert Yellowtail: Crow," 58.

24. See Jacobs, *White Mother to a Dark Race*. Indeed, the health conditions at off-reservation boarding schools were often poor, and some Native children who attended them did not survive the experience. See McBride, "A Blueprint for Death."

25. Matthews, "Changing Lives."

26. Medicine Crow with Viola, *Counting Coup*, 32.

27. See Stremlau, *Sustaining the Cherokee Family*, esp. ch. 3.

28. Key works that explore the theme of gender complementarity in Native societies include Albers and Medicine, *The Hidden Half*; Tsosie, "Changing Women"; Klein and Ackerman, *Women and Power*; Mihesuah, *Indigenous American Women*.

29. Frey, *The World of the Crow Indians*, 22–25; Lowie, *The Crow Indians*, 9, 60–61. See also Foster, "Of Baggage and Bondage."

30. Old Coyote, Spring Crow Culture Lecture Series, pp. 110–11, DD.

31. Hoxie, *Parading through History*, 192.

32. Linderman, *Pretty-Shield*, 230; Crow Indian male, age eighty-eight, interview by Linton, 202–3.

33. Hogan with Loeb and Plainfeather, *The Woman Who Loved Mankind*, 124–26; Crow Indian male, age eighty-eight, interview by Linton, 202–3.

34. Lowie, *The Crow Indians*, 9.

35. See Frey, *The World of Crow Indians*, 40–58; Fred Voget, "Persistence of Crow Culture," Notecard, n.d., FWVP, Series 2, Box 7, Folder 3.

36. Lowie, *The Crow Indians*, 55. The practice of wife kidnapping—in which a member of one warrior society abducted the wife of a member of a rival society—contributed to the frequency of marriage and divorce in Crow society. See Lowie, *The Crow Indians*, 50–56.

37. Morin, interview by author.

38. Voget, *They Call Me Agnes*, 69.

39. Perdue, *Cherokee Women*, 47. Children in other matrilineal societies, such as Navajos, practiced a similar manner of reckoning female kin. See Dyk, *Left Handed*, xii.

40. Voget, *They Call Me Agnes*, 83.

41. Morin, interview by author; Voget, *They Call Me Agnes*, 66–68. Robert Yellowtail also lived with his paternal grandmother for a time during his childhood.

42. Leforge, *Memoirs of a White Crow Indian*, 165.

43. Snell with Matthews, *Grandmother's Grandchild*, 34.

44. Medicine Crow with Viola, *Counting Coup*, 28–29; and Voget, *They Call Me Agnes*, 67–69.

45. Two Crow Indians, female, ages sixty-eight and thirty-five, interview by Linton, 1–4.

46. "Crow Indians, Kay's Notes on Thrownaway Children," Notecard, 18 June 1994, FWVP, Series 2, Box 7, Folder 3.

47. McCleary, *Crow Indian Rock Art*, 146. The *iláaxe* is not an unusual concept in Native societies. Navajos have a comparable concept, for example, which the medical sociologist Stephen Kunitz translates as "soul" or "wind." See Kunitz, *Disease Change*, 123.

48. See McCleary, *Crow Indian Rock Art*, 146; and Morey and Gilliam, *Respect for Life*, 19.

49. Snell with Matthews, *Grandmother's Grandchild*, 27.

50. Voget, *They Call Me Agnes*, 36–43.

51. "Persistence of Crow Culture," Notecard, n.d., FWVP, Series 2, Box 7, Folder 3.

52. For example, Hopi women often selected a male relative to help them through deliveries. See Sekaquaptewa with Udall, *Me and Mine*, 178–80.

53. Hogan, *The Woman Who Loved Mankind*, ch. 8.

54. Voget, *They Call Me Agnes*, 83.

55. Snell with Matthews, *Grandmother's Grandchild*.

56. "Ball (f) Y-W," Notecard, 3 Aug. 1939, FWVP, Series 2, Box 7, Folder 11.

57. See Wright, "The Woman's Lodge."

58. In an autobiography published in the early 1990s, Thomas Yellowtail asserted that Crow women did seclude themselves during menstruation in "olden times." See Yellowtail with Fitzgerald, *Yellowtail*, 18. When the anthropologist Robert Lowie conducted fieldwork at Crow in the early twentieth century, he found that "opinion differs as to whether women had to dwell apart during their indisposition." Lowie, *The Crow Indians*, 45.

59. See Broker, *Night Flying Woman*, 94–95.

60. See Perdue, *Cherokee Women*, 30; Buckley, "Menstruation and the Power of Yurok Women," 47–60. For a Native feminist critique of Western discourses on Indigenous menstruation, see Baldy, "mini-k'iwh'e:n (For That Purpose—I Consider Things)."

61. Lowie, *The Crow Indians*, 44; Voget, *They Call Me Agnes*, 24. For a discussion of this type of ceremony in another community, see Baldy, *We Are Dancing for You*.

62. Moerman, *Native American Ethnobotany*, esp. 656, 765. For an analysis of the limitations of Moerman's text, see Koblitz, *Sex and Herbs and Birth Control*, 21–27.

63. Snell, interview by McCleary. For Snell's views on abortion, see Snell with Matthews, *Grandmother's Grandchild*, 136.

64. Thank you to Timothy McCleary for sharing "Akbaaúushaleelia, Colic Doctors: Infant Health and Healing in the Crow Community," the PowerPoint he has used when lecturing on this topic. Many Crow midwives were also colic specialists, a skill that they passed down to family members even as they ultimately stopped performing abortions and assisting in deliveries. Several colic doctors continue to practice on the reservation today. For more on Crow astronomy, see McCleary, *The Stars We Know*.

65. Two Crow Indians, female, ages sixty-eight and thirty-five, interview by Linton, 7.

66. Rides Horse, interview by McCleary; two Crow Indians, interview by Linton. In his 1939 master's thesis, Joseph Medicine Crow asserted that "the syphilitic woman was prevented from bearing children, through abortion." Medicine Crow, "The Effect of European Culture Contacts," 88.

67. See "Old-Dwarf Mt. Crow 7/18/39," Notecard, FWVP, Series 2, Box 7, Folder 8.

68. Holder, "Gynecic Notes," 767.

69. Morey and Gilliam, *Respect for Life*, 18.

70. Morey and Gilliam, 17.

71. Lowie, *The Crow Indians*, 34.

72. Snell with Matthews, *Grandmother's Grandchild*, 27.

73. Voget, *They Call Me Agnes*, 47.

74. Crow Indian male, age eighty-eight, interview by Linton, 71; Hogan, *The Woman Who Loved Mankind*, 234.

75. Linderman, *Pretty-Shield*, 146; Voget, *They Call Me Agnes*, 35.

76. Lowie, *The Crow Indians*, 33; Linderman, *Pretty-Shield*, 146–47.

77. Voget, *They Call Me Agnes*, 36; Lowie, *The Crow Indians*, 33. According to Lowie, one of his informants reported that some men were skilled obstetricians, but that this was a recent development. I have found no instances of Crow men delivering babies in these years, and I have spoken with multiple people on the reservation who believe that he was mistaken.

78. Snell, interview by McCleary; Lowie, *The Crow Indians*, 33; "336 Ball (f), R. Crow," Notecard, n.d., FWVP, Series 2, Box 10, Folder 21; McCleary, "*Apsáalooke Bíanne Akdia* (Crow Midwives)," 7.

79. Snell with Matthews, *Grandmother's Grandchild*, 27.

80. Many twenty-first-century Indigenous midwives continue to view water as holy. See Cavender-Wilson, "Mni Wiconi Yaktan K'a Ni Drink the Water of Life, and Live."

81. See Hoffman, "Childbirth and Abortion among the Absaroka," 9–10; Melcher, *Pregnancy, Motherhood, and Choice*, 26.

82. Hoffman, "Childbirth and Abortion among the Absaroka," 10.

83. Leavitt, *Brought to Bed*, ch. 1.

84. Voget, *They Call Me Agnes*, 36; Holder, "Gynecic Notes," 767.

85. Holder, "Gynecic Notes," 767.

86. "Yellow-woman R. Crow," Notecard, n.d., FWVP, Series 2, Box 7, Folder 13.

87. On breech births, see Cassidy, *Birth*, 119. On one Native midwife's skill in manually altering an infant's position, see Mitchell with Frisbie, *Tall Woman*, 174–75.

88. Trennert, *White Man's Medicine*, 64.

89. Bradley, "After the Buffalo Days," ch. 8.

90. Holder, "Gynecic Notes," 752, 761.

91. Holder, 752.

92. K. Tsianina Lomawaima has emphasized the extent to which federal Indian schools functioned as sites of surveillance, especially for Native girls. See Lomawaima, "Domesticity in the Federal Indian Schools."

93. Holder, "Gynecic Notes," 752–53.

94. Holder, 752–68, 44–60.

95. Engelmann, *Labor among Primitive Peoples*.

96. Jasen, "Race, Culture, and the Colonization of Childbirth"; Rich, "The Curse of Civilised Woman"; Briggs, "The Race of Hysteria."

97. Engelmann, "Pregnancy, Parturition, and Childbed," 607.

98. While generally a skeptic, Hoffman nevertheless contended that contemporary assumptions about the relative ease of childbirth applied to Crow women, largely due to Crow women's own positive reports about childbearing. Hoffman, "Childbirth and Abortion among the Absaroka," 10.

99. Holder, "Gynecic Notes," 765.

100. Holder, 762.

101. Engelmann, "Pregnancy, Parturition, and Childbed," 609.

102. See Ellinghaus, *Blood Will Tell*; and Sturm, *Blood Politics*, esp. ch. 3.

103. See Walter Q. G. Tucker to William Jones, 31 Dec. 1903, Letters to CIA, p. 415, NARA CO, RG 75, Box 6, Volume 1904.

104. See Linderman, *Pretty-Shield*, 147; Harding, "Traditional Beliefs and Behaviors," 67.

105. Engelmann, "Pregnancy, Parturition, and Childbed," 608–9.

106. For an extended discussion of how the poor health conditions on the Northern Cheyenne Reservation in the decades surrounding the turn of the century negatively affected maternal and infant health outcomes, see Campbell, "Changing Patterns of Health."

107. Snell with Matthews, *Grandmother's Grandchild*, 27.

108. See Bacon, "Pulmonary Tuberculosis as an Obstetrical Complication"; Snell with Matthews, *Grandmother's Grandchild*, 28.

109. Hoxie, *Parading through History*, 172.

110. Maureen Lux describes this cycle for a handful of Aboriginal communities in Canada during this same period. See Lux, *Medicine That Walks*, 45. See also Campbell, "Changing Patterns of Health."

111. See Hoxie, *A Final Promise*, ch. 5; Meyer, *The White Earth Tragedy*, ch. 3.

112. Bradley, "After the Buffalo Days," 51, 56; Hoxie, *Parading through History*, 239–40. Agents throughout the Northern Plains attempted to reduce the number of rations distributed on their reservations at the turn of the century, but ration issues declined especially precipitously at Crow, a trend that began before Reynolds's arrival. Frank Rzeczkowski interprets this as evidence that the Crow Reservation was more prosperous than other Montana reservations at this time. Rzeczkowski, *Uniting the Tribes*, 135–36.

113. Hoxie, *A Final Promise*, 152, 164.

114. Hoxie, *Parading through History*, 146–47.

115. Bradley, "After the Buffalo Days," 206.

116. Stremlau, *Sustaining the Cherokee Family*.

117. Bradley, "After the Buffalo Days," 130, 140; Rzeczkowski, *Uniting the Tribes*, 172; and Reynolds to William Jones, 7 Mar. 1905, Letters to CIA, p. 129, NARA CO, RG 75, Box 7, Volume Jan. 9, 1905–Oct. 2, 1905.

118. Annual Report, Crow, 1904, Letters to CIA, NARA CO, RG 75, Box 6, Volume 1904.

119. See Annual Report, Crow, 1904; Samuel Reynolds to the Farmers and Additional Farmers, 20 Sept. 1907, Letters to Agency Employees, p. 335, NARA CO, RG 75, Box 3, Volume Nov. 19 '05–Feb. 29 '08.

120. Matthews, "Changing Lives," 10.

121. Annual Report, Crow, 1904, Letters to CIA, NARA CO, RG 75, Box 6, Volume 1904.

122. Two Crow Indians, interview by Linton, 1–4.

123. Petchesky, *Abortion and Woman's Choice*, 80 (italics in original); Beisel and Kay, "Abortion, Race, and Gender."

124. Hanshew, "'You Had to Pretend It Never Happened.'"

125. Holder, "Gynecic Notes." See also Crow, *Annual Report*, 1915, SARL, FILM 3748; and Shoemaker, *American Indian Population Recovery*, 49.

126. The Native feminist scholar Sarah Deer has argued that the uncertainty, hardship, and, above all, violence that accompanied early reservation life for many Native women likely made them wary of bringing a child into the world. Deer cites the Paiute activist Sarah Winnemucca, who in her 1883 autobiography proclaimed, "My people have been so unhappy for a long time they wish now to disincrease, instead of multiply." Deer, *The Beginning and End of Rape*, 112.

127. Samuel Reynolds to William Jones, 11 July 1905, Letters to CIA, p. 341, NARA CO, RG 75, Box 7, Volume Jan. 9, 1905–Oct. 2, 1905 (emphasis in original).

128. Tucker to Jones, 31 Dec. 1903, Letters to CIA, p. 415, NARA CO, RG 75, Box 6, Volume 1904.

129. Reynolds to Jones, 11 July 1905, Letters to CIA, p. 341, NARA CO.

130. Decades later, a Crow man reported to the ethnographer Fred Voget that women no longer terminated pregnancies for fear of legal reprisal. See "Old-Dwarf Mt. Crow 7/18/39," Notecard, FWVP, Series 2, Box 7, Folder 8.

131. See Anderson, *A Recognition of Being*; Denetdale, "Chairmen, Presidents, and Princesses."

132. Perdue, *Cherokee Women*, 148.

133. Katsi Cook discusses these two positions in a 2001 interview. See Cook, interview by Kim Anderson, 18 July 2001, OFIFC Youth Sexual Health and Pregnancy Research, KCP, Box 1, Folder Interviews, 1992–2001.

134. Tucker believed abortion had declined by 1903. See Tucker to Jones, 31 Dec. 1903, Letters to CIA, NARA CO, RG 75, Box 6, Volume 1903. Crow women were also having more children in 1910 than they were in 1890, an increase that may have included more pregnancies carried to term. See Hoxie, *Parading through History*, 173.

135. Two Crow Indians, female, ages sixty-eight and thirty-five, interview by Linton, 73–74.

136. A detailed description of this meeting, including Big Medicine's quote, can be found in Hoxie, *Parading through History*, 248. Big Medicine's testimony does not mean that he opposed abortion; individual and community views regarding the termination of pregnancy remained contextual and nuanced. Evidence suggests that Big Medicine approved of abortion in at least some contexts, but I have chosen not to expand on this point to protect women's privacy.

137. Voget, *They Call Me Agnes*, 26.

138. See Leavitt, *Brought to Bed*, 38.

139. I use 1908 as Deernose's birth year because that is the year she cites in the autobiography she produced with Fred Voget. Voget, *They Call Me Agnes*, 35. More than likely, however, Deernose was born a year or two later. Her autobiography emphasizes the proximity of the hospital when describing the circumstances surrounding her birth, but government records suggest that the hospital was under construction that fall and did not begin accepting patients until November. See Samuel Reynolds to Francis Leupp, 5 Nov. 1908, Letters to CIA, p. 327, NARA CO, RG 75, Box 8, Volume May 24, 1908–Jan. 16, 1909. The historian Becky Matthews cites 1910 as the year of Deernose's birth in *Grandmother's Grandchild*, 19.

140. Medicine Crow with Viola, *Counting Coup*, 13.

Chapter 2

1. The position of agent became that of superintendent in 1908.

2. Scott reported that the system of home inspections was working well, but he was apparently blind to reservation women's subtle forms of resistance, which undermined the OIA's stated objectives regarding health and domesticity. He noted with apparent satisfaction, for example, that many of the younger women "keep 'show' rooms and in some instances will put the house in order then live in a tent to keep it so." Cheyenne and Arapaho, *Annual Report*, 1916, SARL, FILM 3748.

3. Cheyenne and Arapaho, *Annual Reports*, 1918, 1919, SARL, FILM 3748.

4. See Thomas, *Politics of the Womb*; De Barros, *Reproducing the British Caribbean*; Hunt, *A Colonial Lexicon*; Ram and Jolly, *Maternities and Modernities*; Lukere and Jolly, *Birthing in the Pacific*; Briggs, *Reproducing Empire*; and Hattori, *Colonial Dis-Ease*.

5. Thomas, *Politics of the Womb*, 4.

6. ARCIA, 1916, 5.

7. Save the Babies typically receives a few lines or a paragraph in policy and tribal histories. The best exploration of Save the Babies remains Emmerich, "'Save the Babies!'"

8. These objectives, especially those involving familial arrangements and childrearing, were not without precedent and can be viewed most clearly through the OIA field matron program, first created in 1890. See Emmerich, "'To Respect and Love'"; and Osburn, *Southern Ute Women*, esp. ch. 4.

9. On American Indian population rates, see Shoemaker, *American Indian Population Recovery*.

10. Gurr, *Reproductive Justice*, 58.

11. On medicalization as the institutional expansion of medicine and an individualized perspective on health, illness, and well-being, see Zola, "Medicine as an Institution."

12. See Dejong, "*If You Knew the Conditions*"; Putney, "Fighting the Scourge"; and Trennert, *White Man's Medicine*.

13. See Trennert, *White Man's Medicine*. On policy makers' attempt to accelerate and also temper the promised assimilation of Native peoples, see Hoxie, *A Final Promise*.

14. Putney, "Fighting the Scourge," 197.

15. See Putney, "Fighting the Scourge."

16. See Ladd-Taylor, *Mother-Work*; Lindenmeyer, "*A Right to Childhood*"; Meckel, *Save the Babies*; and Tiffin, *In Whose Best Interest?*

17. See Wertz and Wertz, *Lying-In*, 155.

18. Hoffman, *Race Traits and Tendencies*. See also Menzel, "The Political Life of Black Infant Mortality," 25, 123–52.

19. Meckel, *Save the Babies*, ch. 1. See also Molina, *Fit to Be Citizens?*

20. Meckel, *Save the Babies*, 9.

21. Circular #633, 29 Apr. 1912, Procedural Issuances of the BIA: Orders and Circulars, 1854–1915, Roll #1, NARA DC. "Save the Babies" was a relatively common refrain in the Progressive Era. See Holt and Shaw, *Save the Babies*; Meckel, *Save the Babies*.

22. On Valentine as a progressive, see Putney, "Fighting the Scourge," 104–8.

23. Quoted in ARCIA, 1912, 19.

24. In some locations, reliable data on maternal mortality did not exist until the 1930s. See Kunitz, *Disease Change*, 87.

25. Julia Lathrop quoted in Lindenmeyer, *"A Right to Childhood,"* 65.

26. Elsie Newton, Report, Crow, 21 Oct. 1914, BIA CCF, FILM 9730, Reel 8; Ferdinand Shoemaker, Medical and Sanitation Report, Jicarilla, 7 Sept. 1917, FSC, Box 1, Folder 22.

27. Emmerich, "To Respect and Love," 272. Clifford Trafzer found that employees on the Yakama Reservation began recording births in 1914, but death records were "almost nonexistent until 1924" and would not become reasonably reliable until after the 1920s. Trafzer, "Infant Mortality on the Yakama Indian Reservation," 79–81, quote on p. 92, n11.

28. Shoemaker, Report, Cheyenne River, 1 Dec. 1916, FSC, Box 1, Folder 20.

29. See Meckel, *Save the Babies*, appendix B.

30. ARCIA, 1916, 5.

31. Shaw, *A Pima Past*, 90.

32. Shoemaker, Report, Lac Courte Oreilles, 14 Nov. 1913, FSC, Box 1, Folder 11.

33. Coolidge, "Wanted," 18.

34. ARCIA, 1916, 7.

35. Sells rebooted the campaign in early 1916 with a letter to all Indian Service employees, and some sources cite 1916 as the campaign's start date. On some reservations, records do not mention the campaign or its various components until 1916.

36. Emmerich, "To Respect and Love," 275–76.

37. ARCIA, 1916, 6.

38. Crow, *Annual Report*, 1916, SARL, FILM 3748. See also Emmerich, "To Respect and Love," 274–75.

39. Shoemaker, Report, Standing Rock, 13 Nov. 1916, FSC, Box 1, Folder 20.

40. Emmerich, "To Respect and Love." See also Cahill, *Federal Fathers and Mothers*, ch. 3.

41. See Emmerich, "Right in the Midst of My Own People."

42. ARCIA, 1916, 6.

43. For attractive homemaking quote, ARCIA, 1916, 7. On field matrons' expanding involvement in OIA health initiatives, see Emmerich, "To Love and Respect," ch. 6.

44. ARCIA, 1916, 6.

45. ARCIA, 1916, 6; Woodruff, *Indian Oasis*, 123.

46. Meckel, *Save the Babies*, 6.

47. Quoted in Meckel, *Save the Babies*, 100 (italics in original).

48. Emmerich, "Save the Babies!," 397. On scientific motherhood, see Apple, *Perfect Motherhood*, ch. 2.

49. On progressive baby shows off reservations, see Meckel, *Save the Babies*, 146–51; and Lovett, *Conceiving the Future*, 136–39.

50. On the relationship between baby shows—as well as the infant welfare movement more generally—and eugenics, see Lovett, *Conceiving the Future*, ch. 6; and Meckel, *Save the Babies*, 116–18.

51. Quoted in Stidolph, "'The Hand That Rocks the Cradle,'" 67.

52. On Indian baby shows, see Emmerich, "Save the Babies!," 402–4; and Klann, "Babies in Baskets." Klann also complicates this assimilation narrative by examining Indian baby shows that doubled as tourist attractions. At the annual baby show in Yosemite National Park in California, for example, organizers welcomed markers of Indianness, such as cradleboards.

53. Circular #764, 31 July 1913; Circular #865, 20 May 1914; Circular #993, 9 June 1915; Circular #1003, 10 July 1915; Circular #1181, 9 Sept. 1916, all in BIA Orders and Circulars, NARA DC, RG 75.

54. Walter West quoted in Gurr, *Reproductive Justice*, 58.

55. See Apple, *Mothers and Medicine*, 70–71.

56. Holt, *The Care and Feeding of Children*, 35; Apple, *Mothers and Medicine*, 70–71.

57. For an example of an unusually explicit acknowledgment of this issue, see Tongue River, *Annual Report*, 1911, SARN. See also Campbell, "Changing Patterns of Health."

58. Kane and Kane, *Federal Health Care*, 5. For an example of an especially abrupt reversal at the local level, see Osburn, *Southern Ute Women*, 74–75.

59. Shoemaker, Report, Cheyenne River, 1 Dec. 1916, FSC, Box 1, Folder 20.

60. In an autobiography published shortly after leaving his position as commissioner of Indian affairs, Francis Leupp noted with both earnestness and cultural condescension that the Indian mother "loves her babies with the same fervor as if she were cultured, graceful, and white." Quoted in Emmerich, "Save the Babies!," 398.

61. See, for example, Cato Sells to C. M. Ziebach, 9 June 1916, BIA CCF, FILM 9730; and Pine Ridge, *Annual Report*, 1916, SARL, FILM 3748.

62. Emmerich addresses this tension in "To Respect and Love," ch. 7. See also Cahill, *Federal Fathers and Mothers*, esp. ch. 8.

63. ARCIA, 1911, 5.

64. Circular #764, 31 July 1913, BIA Orders and Circulars, NARA DC, RG 75. Sells's instructions specify that mothers are to receive these rations in locations "where there are rations available for issue to adult Indians." Anecdotal evidence suggests women on some reservations did not benefit from this directive. See Coolidge, "Wanted," 18–19.

65. ARCIA, 1911, 5. See Woodruff, *Indian Oasis*, 123, 209; Shoemaker, Report, Rosebud, 22 Sept. 1916, FSC, Box 1, Folder 19; Gregg, *The Indians and the Nurse*, 23–24; Osburn, *Southern Ute Women*, 76–83; Emmerich, "To Love and Respect," 277; and Hancock, "Health and Well-Being," 171.

66. On women's influence during home births, see Wertz and Wertz, *Lying-In*, 6; Litoff, *The American Midwife Debate*, 13; and Leavitt, *Brought to Bed*, 4–5.

67. See ARCIA, 1916.

68. ARCIA, 1916, 5–8.

69. Circular #1289, 30 Mar. 1917, BIA Orders and Circulars, NARA DC, RG 75; ARCIA, 1917, 18.

70. Flathead, Inspection Report, 14 July 1916, BIA CCF, FILM 9730.

71. Dejong, *"If You Knew the Conditions,"* 12; Trennert, *White Man's Medicine*, 110–11. The United States experienced a comparable explosion in hospital construction in the late nineteenth and early twentieth centuries. The nation had fewer than 200 hos-

pitals in the early 1870s; by 1909, it boasted more than 4,300. See Rosenberg, *The Care of Strangers*, 5.

72. Fort Belknap, Inspection Report, 12 July 1918, BIA CCF, FILM 9730, Reel 4.

73. Rosenberg, *The Care of Strangers*. See also Starr, *The Social Transformation of American Medicine*.

74. S. A. M. Young to Cato Sells, 16 May 1916, and Sells to Young, 17 May 1916, both BIA CCF, FILM 9730.

75. Leavitt, *Brought to Bed*, ch. 7.

76. West, *Prenatal Care*, 21.

77. Wertz and Wertz, *Lying-In*, 155.

78. ARCIA, 1917, 18. At the local level, not all employees took for granted that Indian homes were too unhygienic for childbirth. The superintendent at the Keshena Agency in Wisconsin reported in 1917 that "the practice of bringing expectant mothers into the hospital for treatment and confinement is followed in exceptional cases only. The Menominees generally have home conditions cleanly enough that it is thought better to provide for and insist upon improved sanitary conditions there, than to remove the patient to unfamiliar surroundings, away from her home and family." This somewhat unusual position seems to have been reversed in subsequent years. Keshena, *Annual Report*, 1917, SARL, FILM 3748.

79. Leavitt, *Brought to Bed*, 173–74, 182.

80. See PHS, *Health Services for American Indians*, 87.

81. Circular #1289, 30 Mar. 1917, BIA Orders and Circulars, NARA DC, RG 75.

82. Peter Paquette to Cato Sells, 24 Apr. 1916, BIA CCF, FILM 9730.

83. For favorable assessments of Native midwives in the late nineteenth century, see Hoffman, "Childbirth and Abortion among the Absaroka"; and Melcher, *Pregnancy, Motherhood, and Choice*, 26.

84. Litoff, *American Midwives*, 82.

85. The "midwife problem" became a common catchphrase in this period. See Williams, "Medical Education and the Midwife Problem in the United States."

86. Litoff, *The American Midwife Debate*, 8.

87. See Reagan, *When Abortion Was a Crime*, ch. 3.

88. See Litoff, *The American Midwife Debate*.

89. Quoted in Litoff, *American Midwives*, 29.

90. Cheyenne and Arapaho, *Annual Report*, 1919, SARL, FILM 3748.

91. ARCIA, 1916, 6.

92. See Flathead, Inspection Report, 14 Feb. 1916; Fred C. Morgan to Cato Sells, 12 May 1916; and Fred C. Morgan to Field Employees, 10 Mar. 1916, all in BIA CCF, FILM 9730.

93. Morgan to Sells, 12 May 1916, BIA CCF, FILM 9730; Guthrie, "The Health of the American Indian," 947.

94. ARCIA, 1916, 3.

95. Ferdinand Shoemaker advocated construction of hospitals on a number of reservations during his 1910s travels. See, for example, Nett Lake, Report, 11 Nov. 1913, and Lac Courte Orielles, Report, 14 Nov. 1913, both Folder 11; Yankton, Report, 3 Apr. 1914, Folder 13; Wind River, Report, 18 Sept. 1916, Folder 19, all FSC, Box 1. See

also Trafzer, "Infant Mortality on the Yakama Indian Reservation," 78. For examples of Native peoples requesting a hospital to no avail, see Fort Belknap, Inspection Report, 15 Apr. 1916, BIA CCF, FILM 9730; and Hancock, "Health and Well-Being," 172–73.

96. Trennert, *White Man's Medicine*, 110–12; Navajo, *Annual Report*, 1916, SARN.

97. Shoemaker, Report, Turtle Mountain, 10 Feb. 1917, FSC, Box 1, Folder 21.

98. On Paquette's approach to Navajo healers, see Trennert, *White Man's Medicine*, 107–8.

99. Paquette to Sells, 9 Aug. 1916, BIA CCF, FILM 9730. Public health nurses hired by the New Mexico Association on Indian Affairs (NMAIA) in the 1920s and 1930s proved especially willing to cooperate with Native midwives as well as other healers. NMAIA nurses' success resulted in an expansion of the BIA's field nursing program. See Schackel, "'The Tales Those Nurses Told!,'" 239.

100. See Thomas, *Politics of the Womb*; Hunt, *A Colonial Lexicon*; De Barros, *Reproducing the British Caribbean*; and Lukere and Jolly, *Birthing in the Pacific*.

101. Hattori, *Colonial Dis-ease*. See also DeLisle, "A History of Chamorro Nurse-Midwives."

102. See a range of primary sources surrounding this issue in Litoff, *The American Midwife Debate*.

103. See Ladd-Taylor, "'Grannies' and 'Spinsters.'"

104. Coolidge, "Wanted," 22.

105. Rude, "The Midwife Problem in the United States."

106. See Leavitt, *Brought to Bed*; Wertz and Wertz, *Lying-In*.

107. Leavitt, *Brought to Bed*, chs. 7–8.

108. Hattori, *Colonial Dis-Ease*, 201.

109. Woodruff, *Indian Oasis*, 209.

110. Osburn, *Southern Ute Women*, 83.

111. Osburn, 78, 83.

112. One of the anthropologist Robert Lowie's Crow informants explicitly addressed the loosening of gender restrictions surrounding childbirth in *The Crow Indians*, 33.

113. See, for example, Woodruff, *Indian Oasis*, 123. On Native women's varied responses to field matrons more generally, see Emmerich, "To Respect and Love," 142–46.

114. Cheyenne and Arapaho, *Annual Reports*, 1918 and 1919, SARL, FILM 3748.

115. Coolidge, "Wanted," 19–21, quote on p. 21.

116. Putney, "Fighting the Scourge," 181.

117. Crow, *Annual Reports*, 1916 and 1917, SARL, FILM 3748. Fifty-two births were recorded in 1916, and sixty-two were recorded in 1917, although it is likely that some births went unrecorded in the register. See Register of Births and Deaths, 1902–21, NARA CO, RG 75, Box 1, Vol. 2.

118. Stewart, *A Voice in Her Tribe*, 11; Young to Sells, 16 May 1916, BIA CCF, FILM 9730.

119. Navajo, *Annual Reports*, 1916, NARA DC, RG 75.

120. Paquette to Sells, 9 Aug. 1916, BIA CCF, FILM 9730. In contrast to the gains made at Fort Defiance, a later survey of 137 women living in the Tuba City area, the

western end of the reservation, suggests that no infants were born in the hospital before 1929. See Kunitz, *Disease Change*, 91.

121. Keshena, *Annual Reports*, 1916 and 1920, SARL, FILM 3748.

122. Rosebud, *Annual Report*, 1916, SARN.

123. See Rosebud, *Annual Reports*, 1916, 1917, and 1920, SARN; Trennert, *White Man's Medicine*, 112.

124. Kelm, *Colonizing Bodies*, 129. See also Lux, "We Demand 'Unconditional Surrender.'"

125. Matthews, "Changing Lives," 17–18.

126. Matthews, 18.

127. Lux, *Medicine That Walks*, 97. See also Burnett, *Taking Medicine*, 156–58.

128. Cheyenne River, *Annual Report*, 1922, SARN.

129. Flathead, Inspection Report, 5 Nov. 1926, BIA CCF, FILM 9730.

130. See Circular #1068, 4 Jan. 1916, BIA Orders and Circulars, NARA DC, RG 75.

131. Cahill, *Federal Fathers and Mothers*; and Jacobs, *White Mother to a Dark Race*.

132. See E. E. Chivers, "Among the Crow Indians," Bentley/Hubley Collection, Book 1; Kittie Deernose, "The Story of Myself," Bentley/Hubley Collection, Book 2, both Big Horn County Historical Museum, Hardin, Mont.; Matthews, "Changing Lives," 167. The OIA ultimately rescinded this order under pressure from religious organizations and the Indian Rights Association.

133. Stewart, *A Voice in Her Tribe*, 18.

134. Stewart, 19.

135. See, for example, Crow, *Annual Report*, 1917, SARL, FILM 3748; and Gertrude Sturges, Monthly Reports, Pima, July 1934, BIA FNR, Box 6.

136. The situation at Crow in these years was not necessarily "typical," but comparable patterns existed in other locations, if in some cases at a later time period. See, for example, Lux, "We Demand 'Unconditional Surrender'"; and Davies, *Healing Ways*.

137. W. S. Coleman to Cato Sells, 9 Apr. 1917; and Cato Sells to Edward Lieurance, 1 May 2017, both BIA CCF, FILM 9730.

138. Coleman to Sells, 9 Apr. 1917, BIA CCF, FILM 9730.

139. Crow, Inspection Report, 30 Oct. 1911, BIA CCF, FILM 9730.

140. Sells to Lieurance, 1 May 2017, BIA CCF, FILM 9730.

141. Coleman to Sells, 9 Apr. 1917; and Sells to Lieurance, 1 May 2017, both BIA CCF, FILM 9730; Edward Lieurance, M.D., "Autobiography" (unpublished), 14 Oct. 1937, https://www.ancestry.com/boards/localities.northam.usa.states.montana.counties .bighorn/122/mb.ashx.

142. Crow, *Annual Reports*, 1918 and 1919, SARL, FILM 3748; R. E. L. Newberne, "Report on Crow Agency Health Conditions," 22 Dec. 1920, BIA CCF, FILM 9730.

143. Crow, *Annual Report*, 1917, SARL, FILM 3748.

144. See Putney, "Fighting the Scourge," 182.

145. Osburn, *Southern Ute Women*, 75; Kunitz, *Disease Change*, 32–33.

146. ARCIA, 1918, 35.

147. Circular #1460, 14 Sept. 1918, BIA Orders and Circulars, NARA DC, RG 75.

148. See Klann, "Babies in Baskets."

149. Emmerich, "To Respect and Love," 282.

Chapter 3

1. Lindenmeyer, *"A Right to Childhood,"* 39.

2. Meriam, *The Problem of Indian Administration,* 10.

3. Meriam, 10.

4. Meriam, 88.

5. Crow, *Annual Report,* 1935, CAGCF, Box 8, Folder 051.

6. In telling Yellowtail's story, I draw on the Ho-Chunk scholar Renya Ramirez's Native feminist approach to biography. See Ramirez, "Henry Roe Cloud."

7. Connie Yellowtail Jackson, interview by author; Valerie Jackson, interview by author. For more on the sexual abuse of Indigenous children in government and religious boarding schools, see Deer, *The Beginning and End of Rape,* 69–71.

8. Connie Yellowtail Jackson, interview by author; Valerie Jackson, interview by author.

9. See Holt, *Indian Orphanages.*

10. District Replies, Statistical Data for General Superintendent's Circular No. 5, Nov. 1926, CAGCF, Box 10, Folder 052.

11. Crow, *Annual Report,* 1931, CAGCF, Box 7, Folder 051.

12. Susie Yellowtail, interviewer unknown.

13. Askins, "Bridging Cultures," 149.

14. Valerie Jackson, interview by author. See Lomawaima, *They Called It Prairie Light,* ch. 4; Lomawaima, "Domesticity in the Federal Indian Schools"; Cahill, *Federal Fathers and Mothers,* ch. 5; Haskins, *Matrons and Maids;* and Trennert, "Victorian Morality."

15. Susie Yellowtail, interviewer unknown.

16. Reverby, *Ordered to Care,* 77.

17. There is some debate about the matter, but many at Crow and a few scholars regard Susie Yellowtail as the first Native American registered nurse. For background on this debate, see Herrman, "Connecticut and the First Native American Trained Nurse"; Keller, *Empty Beds,* 98–101; and Hinkell, *Nurse of the Twentieth Century.*

18. Trennert, "Sage Memorial Hospital."

19. "Native American Students."

20. Susie Yellowtail's employment history is provided in an unsigned memorandum submitted to the Department of Health, Education, and Welfare in 1966. Yellowtail's federal employee file is held at NARA, National Personnel Records Center Annex, Valmeyer, Ill.

21. District Replies, Statistical Data for General Superintendent's Circular No. 5, Nov. 1926, CAGCF, Box 10, Folder 052.

22. See Voget, *They Call Me Agnes,* 35.

23. Crow, *Annual Report,* 1927, CAGCF, Box 16, Folder 150.

24. Voget, *They Call Me Agnes,* 119–20. On the Tobacco Society, see Lowie, *The Crow Indians,* 274–96.

25. Hogan, *The Woman Who Loved Mankind,* 234. Robert Yellowtail's first wife, Clara Spotted Horse, had died a few years earlier. Spotted Horse's mother was a respected midwife, and Clara, like Lillian, delivered her children at home. See Plenty Hoops, interview by Plainfeather.

26. Hogan, *The Woman Who Loved Mankind*, 234.

27. Melcher, "'Women's Matters.'"

28. Ethel Smith, Monthly Report, Crow Agency—Lodge Grass and Wyola District, Dec. 1933, BIA FNR, Box 1.

29. Calvin Asbury to Henrietta Crockett, 7 Apr. 1930, CAGCF, Box 50, Folder 700.

30. Josephine Yanachek, Monthly Report, Fort Peck Agency, Dec. 1934, BIA FNR, Box 6.

31. Child, *My Grandfather's Knocking Sticks*, 31–32.

32. Anna Perry, Monthly Reports, Crow Agency—Pryor District, BIA FNR, Boxes 27 and 30; Abel and Reifel, "Interactions between Public Health Nurses," 96. See also Hancock, "Healthy Vocations."

33. Crow, *Annual Report*, 1928, CAGCF, Box 7, Folder 051.

34. Morin, interview by author.

35. See Kelm, *Colonizing Bodies*, 170; and Lux, "We Demand 'Unconditional Surrender,'" 673.

36. See Mabel Morgan, Inspection Report, 14 Dec. 1931, CAGCF, Box 17, Folder 150.

37. Yellowtail with Weatherly, "Susie Walking Bear Yellowtail," ch. 4.

38. See Abel and Reifel, "Interactions between Public Health Nurses and Clients," 105.

39. Yellowtail with Weatherly, "Susie Walking Bear Yellowtail," ch. 4.

40. McCleary, "*Absáalooke Biaanne Akdia* (Crow Midwives)," 23.

41. Yellowtail with Weatherly, "Susie Walking Bear Yellowtail," ch. 4.

42. Yellowtail with Weatherly, ch. 4.

43. Cahill, *Federal Fathers and Mothers*, 113.

44. Cahill, 122–29.

45. Susie Yellowtail's application for employment as a field nurse in 1935, as well as Robert Yellowtail's endorsement and the official rejection of her application, can be found in Yellowtail's federal employment file at NARA, National Personnel Records Center Annex, Valmeyer, Ill. Robert tried again in 1937. See Robert Yellowtail to John Collier, 7 Apr. 1937, CAGCF, Box 51, Folder 706. For other nurses' experiences, see Evelyn Old Elk, interview by Pickett; and Spotted Bear, interview by McCleary.

46. Hoxie, *Parading through History*, ch. 11.

47. See Hoxie and Bernardis, "Robert Yellowtail: Crow"; and Frey, *The World of the Crow Indians*, ch. 2.

48. Weatherly, "Susie Walking Bear Yellowtail," 230.

49. Mae Takes Gun Childs, MHS interview. See also Hogan, MHS interview. On Asbury's repressive policies, see McCleary, "Akbaatashee," 44–47.

50. Interview Notes, Petzoldt 7/8/39, Field Interview Notebook, Crow, 7/8/39–7/20/39, FWVP, Series 3, Box 13, Folder 7. Many of the Yellowtails, including Robert and Susie, attended Petzoldt's church. Carson Yellowtail, Robert's brother, named his son after the missionary. On tensions between Collier and missionaries and religious organizations, see Daily, *Battle for the BIA*.

51. "Bentley (Missionary—Baptist); Crow; 7/10/39," Notecard, FWVP, Series 2, Box 11, Folder 19 (emphasis in original).

52. See Gregg, *The Indians and the Nurse*, 142–45.

53. Davies, *Healing Ways*, ch. 2.

54. On the perceived resurgence of "medicine men," see Interview Notes, Petzoldt 7/8/39, Field Interview Notebook, FWVP, Series 3, Box 13, Folder 7.

55. See Hoxie and Bernardis, "Robert Yellowtail: Crow," 67–68; Hoxie, *Parading through History*, 337–42.

56. Copies of the minutes of some 1930s Crow Tribal Council meetings are available on microfilm at Labriola American Indian Center at Arizona State University. Meeting minutes from the 1940s are available in ABMC. Euro-American and Crow observers commented on women's lack of participation in general and district councils. See Field Notes, Crow Council—Pryor 7/17/39, FWVP, Series 3, Box 9, Folder 18; and Crow Indian male, age eighty-eight, interview by Linton, 146.

57. Snell with Matthews, *Grandmother's Grandchild*, 4.

58. See Foster, "Of Baggage and Bondage," 131–32.

59. Denetdale, "Chairmen, Presidents, and Princesses"; Castle, "Black and Native American Women's Activism," 80.

60. Minutes, Crow Health Council Meeting, 9 Feb. 1935, BIA CCF, FILM 9730, Series C, Part 1, Reel 27. See also Apple, *Mothers and Medicine*, esp. ch. 5.

61. Gouveia, "'Uncle Sam's Priceless Daughters,'" 51–61. See also Bernstein, "A Mixed Record."

62. Matthews, "Wherever That Singing Is Going," 225.

63. Minnie E. Williams, "The Absaroka Indian Womens [*sic*] Federated Club," 22 Sept. 1960, ABMC, Series 2, Box 7, Folder 2.3. This copy of Williams's brief history of the women's club is incomplete.

64. Quoted in Matthews, "Wherever That Singing Is Going," 225.

65. Matthews, 261.

66. Fred Voget conducted interviews with club women in the mid-1950s. His field notes suggest that, especially outside of Crow Agency, women believed that they remained "more or less in the background" in the postwar period. See interview with Josephine Russell, Lodge Grass, 1956, FWVP, Series 2, Box 11, Folder 46.

67. J. G. Townsend to Charles Nagel, 23 Nov. 1934, CAGCF, Box 51, Folder 706.

68. Matthews, "Wherever That Singing Is Going," 226.

69. Cohen, "Stars in the Big Sky," 24.

70. Yellowtail with Weatherly, "Susie Walking Bear Yellowtail," ch. 7.

71. See John Collier to Robert Yellowtail, 8 Sept. 1934, CAGCF, Box 51, Folder 705.

72. Yellowtail with Weatherly, "Susie Walking Bear Yellowtail," ch. 7.

73. Mary McKay, Inspection Report, 26 Feb. 1936, CAGCF, Box 11, Folder 055; Charles Nagel to John Collier, 8 Aug. 1935, CAGCF, Box 10, Folder 052.

74. Report to the Committee on Indian Affairs, 1930, CAGCF, Box 18, Folder 150; Hospital Report, Aug. 1930, CAGCF, Box 53, Folder 722.2; Asbury to Crockett, 7 Apr. 1930, CAGCF, Box 50, Folder 700; Nagel to Collier, 8 Aug. 1935, CAGCF, Box 10, Folder 052.

75. Charles Rhoads to James Hyde, 8 Feb. 1933, and Hyde to Rhoads, 13 Feb. 1933, CAGCF, Box 17, Folder 150. See also Crow, *Annual Report*, 1935, CAGCF, Box 8, Folder 051.

76. Report to the Committee on Indian Affairs, 1930, CAGCF, Box 18, Folder 150; Mabel Morgan, Inspection Report, 3 Aug. 1932, CAGCF, Box 17, Folder 150; Mabel Morgan, Inspection Report, 12 Dec. 1930, CAGCF, Box 16, Folder 150; William Zimmerman to Robert Yellowtail, 16 Aug. 1934, CAGCF, Box 50, Folder 700. Woefully inadequate maternity facilities were relatively common throughout Indian Country. See Gregg, *The Indians and the Nurse*, 45, 116.

77. Yellowtail with Weatherly, "Susie Walking Bear Yellowtail," ch. 7.

78. H. J. Warner, Inspection Report, 13 Oct. 1930, CAGCF, Box 17, Folder 150. Warner's assessment of Dr. R. V. Rogers, the other physician at Crow Agency, was not much better: "His early education was evidently not much and his medical education was obtained at the old Keokuk Medical College, long since defunct." Warner allowed, however, that "in the practice of medicine [Rogers] probably is superior to Dr. Buren."

79. Crow, *Annual Report*, 1932, CAGCF, Box 7, Folder 051.

80. Yellowtail with Weatherly, "Susie Walking Bear Yellowtail," ch. 7.

81. Charles Nagel to Susie Yellowtail, 31 July 1934, CAGCF, Box 50, Folder 700.

82. Robert Yellowtail to John Collier, 8 Mar. 1938, CAGCF, Box 53, Folder Health Dr. Fullerton's Report Jan. 5, 1938.

83. Fern Rumsey to John Collier, 1 June 1935, CAGCF, Box 18, Folder 155.

84. Yellowtail with Weatherly, "Susie Walking Bear Yellowtail," ch. 7.

85. On peyotism on the Crow Reservation, see Stewart, "Peyotism in Montana." Stewart focuses primarily on male peyotists and does not mention Native women using peyote during labor.

86. Yellowtail with Weatherly, "Susie Walking Bear Yellowtail," ch. 7.

87. See Wolf, *Deliver Me from Pain*, ch. 3.

88. Vance B. Murray, Inspection Report, 11 Dec. 1933, CAGCF, Box 17, Folder 150.

89. Yellowtail with Weatherly, "Susie Walking Bear Yellowtail," ch. 4; Harding, "Traditional Beliefs and Behaviors," 65–67. See also Cook, interview by Follett.

90. Yellowtail with Weatherly, "Susie Walking Bear Yellowtail," ch. 7.

91. Yellowtail with Weatherly, ch. 7. Yellowtail's daughter Connie also discussed her mother's sterilization. Connie Yellowtail Jackson, interview by author.

92. Yellowtail with Weatherly, "Susie Walking Bear Yellowtail," ch. 4.

93. For a discussion of "Mississippi appendectomies," see Kluchin, *Fit to Be Tied*, ch. 3.

94. Charles Nagel to Robert Yellowtail, 27 Mar. 1935, CAGCF, Box 51, Folder Health and Social Relations 1935.

95. Laughlin, *Eugenical Sterilization in the United States*, 415.

96. Crow, *Annual Report*, 1935, CAGCF, Box 8, Folder 051.

97. See John Collier to R. B. Millin, 24 Apr. 1934, CAGCF, Box 17, Folder 150; Gregg, *The Indians and the Nurse*, 105.

98. Minutes, Tribal Council Meeting, 6 Feb. 1935, BIA CCF, FILM 9730, Series C, Part 1, Reel 27.

99. John Collier to Charles Nagel, 6 Nov. 1934, CAGCF, Box 51, Folder 706.

100. See Lombardo, *Three Generations, No Imbeciles*.

101. See Ladd-Taylor, *Fixing the Poor*; Kline, *Building a Better Race*, esp. ch. 4; and Gallagher, *Breeding Better Vermonters*, ch. 4.

102. O'Sullivan, "'We Worry about Survival,'" 71.

103. Gallagher, *Breeding Better Vermonters*, 7.

104. See Gonzales et al., "Eugenics as Indian Removal."

105. Stremlau, "Allotment, Jim Crow, and the State." For further discussion of Indians and eugenics in Virginia, see Coleman, *That the Blood Stay Pure*; Dorr, *Segregation's Science*; and Smith, "The Campaign for Racial Purity."

106. See Stern, *Eugenic Nation*, 52.

107. James Hyde to O. M. Spencer, 24 Aug. 1932, CAGCF, Box 50, Folder 700.

108. Hyde to Spencer, 24 Aug. 1932, CAGCF. Susan Burch has argued that resistance to assimilation made some individuals especially vulnerable to eugenic institutionalization at the Canton Indian Asylum in South Dakota, an Indian-only mental health facility operated by the federal government. Burch, "Dislocated Histories."

109. Hyde to Spencer, 24 Aug. 1932, CAGCF.

110. The sociologist Lutz Kaelber and his students at the University of Vermont have studied the eugenics program in all fifty states. Their findings with regard to Montana can be found at http://www.uvm.edu/~lkaelber/eugenics/MT/MT.html.

111. Meriam, *The Problem of Indian Administration*, 590–91. See also Lansdale, "The Place of the Social Worker."

112. My analysis stems from my review of Social Workers' Reports, Records of the Welfare Branch, NARA DC, RG 75. Because of the sensitive and personal nature of some of these records, I applied for and was granted a social science researcher exemption to view them.

113. Isabelle Robideau, Monthly Report, Consolidated Chippewa Agency, Dec. 1936, BIA SWR, Box 4. Robideau was Ojibwe. See Child, *My Grandfather's Knocking Sticks*, 177–78. Molly Ladd-Taylor was able to identify nine Native women who were sterilized in Minnesota in the 1930s. Any estimate of total numbers must be speculative because the sterilization records of the Minnesota School for the Feebleminded do not include race or tribal affiliation. See Ladd-Taylor, *Fixing the Poor*, 18.

114. Mary Kirkland, Quarterly Report, Red Lake, 31 Mar. 1940, BIA SWR, Box 6. These quotes refer to the denial of Red Lake Indians' applications for Aid to Dependent Children, which was based on the same logic.

115. Red Lake, *Annual Report*, 1937, Records of the Statistics Division, Reports and Other Records, 1933–1948, NARA DC, RG 75, Box 61.

116. See Kirkland, Annual Report, Red Lake, 1937; and Quarterly Report, Red Lake, 30 Dec. 1937, both BIA SWR, Box 6.

117. Ladd-Taylor, *Fixing the Poor*, 158. Erika Dyck similarly found that at least through the early 1940s, federal jurisdiction protected some Aboriginal men and women in Canada from eugenic sterilization. Dyck, *Facing Eugenics*, ch. 2.

118. See Sebring, "Reproductive Citizenship," 69–71.

119. See Holloway, *Sexuality, Politics, and Social Control*, 25; Lombardo, *Three Generations, No Imbeciles*, 61.

120. See Briggs, *Reproducing Empire*; and Schoen, *Choice and Coercion*.

121. "Old-Dwarf Mt. Crow 7/18/39," Notecard, FWVP, Series 2, Box 7, Folder 8.

122. WARN II. I discuss these allegations at greater length in chapter 6.

123. Yellowtail with Weatherly, "Susie Walking Bear Yellowtail," ch. 4. Susie's daughter also used "genocide" to describe the sterilizations at Crow in the years surrounding her birth. Connie Yellowtail Jackson, interview by author.

124. Wolfe, "Settler Colonialism and the Elimination of the Native."

125. Hoxie, *Parading through History*, 298–99.

126. Yellowtail with Weatherly, "Susie Walking Bear Yellowtail," ch. 4.

127. These complaints were discussed in tribal council meetings in the first months of 1935. See meeting minutes in BIA CCF, FILM 9730, Series C, Part 1, Reel 27.

128. See Torpy, "Native American Women"; and Lawrence, "The Indian Health Service."

129. Yellowtail's midwifery career is addressed in newspaper articles and biographical sketches compiled in Hinkell, *Nurse of the Twentieth Century*.

130. Yellowtail with Weatherly, "Susie Walking Bear Yellowtail," ch. 7.

131. M. Virginia Darmody, Monthly Report, Crow, Dec. 1934, BIA FNR, Box 6. Supervisor of Nurses Elinor Gregg observed that many Native Americans also favored hospitals off the reservation for other health procedures, especially surgery. Gregg, *The Indians and the Nurse*, 38.

132. Whiteman, interview by McCleary.

133. See Anna Perry, Monthly Reports, Crow, BIA FNR, Box 30.

Chapter 4

1. To protect the privacy of individuals and families, in this chapter I use pseudonyms when discussing Native people who appear in federal documents. Some notes include abbreviations rather than full names to protect anonymity. As public figures, government employees are not assigned pseudonyms.

2. This chapter draws on oral histories and social science literature pertaining to relocation and Native urbanization throughout the West, while utilizing BIA records concerning the relocation of individuals and families from Montana's seven Indian reservations. Details regarding the Browns' relocation are drawn from George Felshaw to Clyde Hobbs, 12 Sept. 1957; Thomas H. St. Clair to Clyde Hobbs, 18 Nov. 1957; George Felshaw, Home Counselor's Report, 17 Feb. 1958; Michael Keesis to Medical Officer in Charge, Crow Indian Hospital, 20 Feb. 1958; Jacob Ahtone, Memorandum, 20 Feb. 1958, all MVSF, Box 20, Folder "Assistance to Individuals (Crow, N. Cheyenne, Wind River) F. Y. 1958."

3. Rosenthal, "Native Americans and Cities." Indeed, Rosenthal's essay on the relationship between Native peoples and cities begins in pre-Columbian times.

4. Meriam, *The Problem of Indian Administration*, ch. 12; LaPier and Beck, "A 'One-Man Relocation Team.'"

5. Shaw, *A Pima Past*, 151.

6. See Shoemaker, "Urban Indians and Ethnic Choices"; and Carpio, *Indigenous Albuquerque*.

7. See Jacobs, "Diverted Mothering among American Indian Domestic Servants"; and Haskins, *Matrons and Maids*. Male boarding school graduates were also recruited to fill labor shortages in the West. See LaGrand, *Indian Metropolis*, 27.

8. See Bernstein, *American Indians and World War II*; and Townsend, *World War II and the American Indian*.

9. Fixico, interview by Zarek.

10. See Bernstein, *American Indians and World War II*, 73; Gouveia, "'Uncle Sam's Priceless Daughters,'" ch. 4; "Native Voices," pp. 38–39, CAIOHP.

11. Broker, *Night Flying Woman*, 3.

12. See Fixico, *Termination and Relocation*, ch. 1.

13. Broker, *Night Flying Woman*.

14. Fixico, *Termination and Relocation*, ch. 1.

15. Phrases like "getting out of the Indian business" were common in discussions surrounding Indian affairs during the relocation and termination era. Wilma Mankiller (Cherokee) recalled BIA employees using this language when they came to talk to her father about the program. See Mankiller with Wallis, *Mankiller*, 69.

16. Neils, *Reservation to City*, 109.

17. Urban migrants used this label themselves. Frances Gabouri, who moved to Los Angeles with her husband in 1947, described herself as "self-relocated." As she defined it, self-relocation referred to "Indians that came here completely on their own. . . . They've just simply relocated themselves here." Gabouri, interview by Brown.

18. See Miller, "Dignity and Decency," 29–30.

19. On the expansion of the relocation program, see Rosenthal, *Reimagining Indian Country*, 52. For somewhat different analyses of Dillon Myer, see Fixico, *Termination and Relocation*, ch. 4; and Drinnon, *Keeper of Concentration Camps*.

20. Quoted in Miller, "Dignity and Decency," 31. On early criticism of the relocation program, see Madigan, *The American Indian Relocation Program*, 8–9.

21. See Fixico, *The Urban Indian Experience*, 16.

22. Relocation officers in cities commented on the gap between new arrivals' expectations and reality, which they attributed to promises they had received before leaving their reservations. See, for example, C. E. Hazard to David P. Weston, 16 Aug. 1957, MVSF, Box 20, Folder Assistance to Individuals—Ft. Peck F. Y. 1957–58; Ola Beckett, Home Counselor's Report, 2 July 1957, MVSF, Box 20, Folder Assistance to Individuals—Blackfeet F.Y. 1958.

23. See LaGrand, *Indian Metropolis*, 54.

24. Deloria Jr., *Custer Died for Your Sins*, 157. Although Deloria does not mention boarding schools in this context, contemporary observers reported that the pressure facing boarding school graduates was often particularly acute. See Snyder, "The Social Environment of the Urban Indian," 220; and Officer, "The American Indian and Federal Policy," 50.

25. Mankiller with Wallis, *Mankiller*, 69.

26. Kenneth Philp and Douglas Miller place particular emphasis on migrants' motivations for and agency in moving to cities. See Philp, "Stride toward Freedom"; and Miller, "Willing Workers." While Philp is correct to emphasize that American Indians were not passive victims at the mercy of federal officials, the arguments he presents for Native agency outpace the evidence he provides, as his article incorporates few Native-produced sources. Miller's essay, in contrast, draws heavily on Native voices and perspectives.

27. Clark (pseudonym), interview by author. Minor details in Clark's personal history have been changed to protect her anonymity.

28. Knifechief, interview by Engle.

29. See Miller, "Willing Workers."

30. Rosenthal, *Reimagining Indian Country*, 51. See also Blackhawk, "I Can Carry On from Here."

31. LaGrand, *Indian Metropolis*, 75.

32. Rosenthal, *Reimagining Indian Country*, 55.

33. Clark, interview by author.

34. LaGrand, *Indian Metropolis*, 81.

35. See Blackhawk, "I Can Carry On from Here." Mary Jane Logan McCallum describes similar patterns of gendered vocational training and labor in Canada's postwar placement and relocation program. See McCallum, *Indigenous Women, Work, and History*, ch. 2.

36. James W. Boyd to Area Director, 30 Sept. 1958, MVSF, Box 18, Folder Monthly R.S. and A.V.T.S. Reports 1959.

37. Quoted in Rosenthal, *Reimagining Indian Country*, 56. See also Fixico, *Termination and Relocation*, 152–53.

38. Fixico, interview by Zarek.

39. Jacobs, "Diverted Mothering," 179.

40. See Philp, "Stride toward Freedom."

41. "Native Voices," p. 11, CAIOHP.

42. Fixico, interview by Zarek. In addition to relocating to distance themselves from spouses, some young women relocated to be free of controlling parents or grandparents. See LaGrand, *Indian Metropolis*, 89–90.

43. James W. Boyd to Area Director, 27 Feb. 1959, MVSF, Box 18, Folder Monthly R.S. and A.V.T.S. Reports 1959. See also McSwain, "The Role of Wives," 1; Snyder, "The Social Environment of the Urban Indian," 212.

44. Promotional Materials and Newspaper Clippings, n.d., BIA RR, Box 1, Folders 24–31.

45. McSwain, "The Role of Wives," 141–42. McSwain used pseudonyms in each of her nine case studies of Navajo women in Denver. I have used the pseudonyms McSwain selected throughout this chapter.

46. McSwain, "The Role of Wives," 104.

47. George Felshaw to David Weston, 9 Oct. 1957, MVSF, Box 20, Folder Assistance to Individuals — Ft Peck F.Y. 1957–1958. On maternity insurance coverage at midcentury, see Cunningham III and Cunningham Jr., *The Blues*, 14, 25, 107; and Hoffman, *Health Care for Some*, 98–99.

48. Felshaw to Weston, 9 Oct. 1957, MVSF.

49. Rosenthal, *Reimagining Indian Country*, 56.

50. George Felshaw to Clyde Hobbs, 12 Sept. 1957, MVSF, Box 20, Folder Assistance to Individuals (Crow, N. Cheyenne, Wind River) F.Y. 1958.

51. Rosenthal, *Reimagining Indian Country*, 56.

52. See Eudora Reed, Form Letter to New Arrivals, n.d., and "Summary Statement of Functions Performed by Relocation Staff of the Bureau of Indian Affairs in Assisting Indian People to Relocate," n.d., both BIA RR, Box 3, Folder 37.

53. On the history of Blue Cross and Blue Shield, see Cunningham III and Cunningham Jr., *The Blues*; and Chapin, *Ensuring America's Health*, ch. 5.

54. Thomasson, "From Sickness to Health," 233–34.

55. Hoffman, *Health Care for Some*, 94. Scholars have explored twentieth-century American health care in an attempt to understand why the United States followed a path that diverged from that of most other industrialized nations. See Hacker, *The Divided Welfare State*; Quadagno, *One Nation Uninsured*; and Gordon, *Dead on Arrival*.

56. See Adler, *Burdens of War*.

57. Chapin, *Ensuring America's Health*, ch. 5.

58. C. E. Hazard to CW, 14 Aug. 1957, MVSF, Box 20, Folder Assistance to Individuals F.Y. 1958.

59. George Felshaw, Home Counselor's Report, 8 Jan. 1958, MVSF, Box 20, Folder Assistance to Individuals F.Y. 1958.

60. George Felshaw to Clyde Hobbs, 22 Apr. 1959, MVSF, Box 20, Folder Assistance to Individuals (Crow, N. Cheyenne, Wind River) F.Y. 1959.

61. Chapin, *Ensuring America's Health*, 49; Hoffman, *Health Care for Some*, 92.

62. Rosenthal, *Reimagining Indian Country*, 70. The American Indian Council of the Bay Area (AICBA) made a similar recommendation a few years later. See Miller, "Willing Workers," 68.

63. See Madigan, *The American Indian Relocation Program*, 5; and Philp, "Stride toward Freedom," 186–87. This extension apparently did not benefit all relocatees in practice, as evidenced by the complaints presented by the AICBA in 1962.

64. Quoted in "Native Voices," p. 128, CAIOHP.

65. Hoffman, *Health Care for Some*, 90.

66. NARG, *Native American Families in the City*, 32.

67. Powell, phone conversation with author. The situation in Seattle was similar. See Sorkin, *The Urban American Indian*, 49.

68. Carpio, *Indigenous Albuquerque*, 15–17.

69. See McSwain, "The Role of Wives,"120.

70. On Native patients being turned away from Uptown hospitals, see Fixico, *The Urban Indian Experience in America*, 112.

71. Powell, phone conversation with author.

72. NARG, *Native American Families in the City*, 33. See also Fixico, *The Urban Indian Experience in America*, 111.

73. Clark, interview by author.

74. McSwain, "The Role of Wives," 65.

75. "Native Voices," p. 128, CAIOHP.

76. Miller, "Willing Workers," 55. See also Blackhawk, "I Can Carry On from Here"; Carpio, *Indigenous Albuquerque*; and O'Neill, "Rethinking Modernity."

77. McSwain, "The Role of Wives," 182–200.

78. PHS, *Health Services for American Indians*, 212–14.

79. Knifechief, interview by Engle.

80. See LaGrand, *Indian Metropolis*, 137–47; and Intertribal Friendship House, *Urban Voices*. The Los Angeles American Indian Center is an example of an urban Indian

center that emerged during the interwar period. See Rosenthal, *Reimagining Indian Country*, 111.

81. Wright, "Creating Change," 127–28. Women's service leagues were integral features of Indian life in some cities. Kent Blansett documents the existence of one such league in Brooklyn, New York, in the 1960s. See Blansett, *A Journey to Freedom*, 38.

82. Before World War II, Powell had worked among the Crow and Northern Cheyenne in Montana. Thomas and Susie Yellowtail (Crow) adopted Powell as a son.

83. See Miller, "Dignity and Decency"; LaGrand, *Indian Metropolis*, 144–45; Neog et al., *Chicago Indians*, 40; and Powell, phone conversation with author.

84. See "Native Voices," pp. 132–33, CAIOHP; Maney, interview by Cossen.

85. Danziger Jr., *Survival and Regeneration*, 115.

86. Wolf, *Deliver Me from Pain*, 110.

87. George Felshaw, Home Counselor's Report, 14 Oct. 1957, MVSF, Box 20, Folder Assistance to Individuals F. Y. 1958.

88. See Ola Beckett, Home Counselor's Report, 23 May 1958; and George Felshaw, Home Counselor's Report, 14 Feb. 1958, both MVSF, Box 20, Folder Assistance to Individuals (Crow, N. Cheyenne, Wind River) F. Y. 1958.

89. Clark, interview by author; McSwain, "The Role of Wives," 158.

90. Ray Moisa, "Relocation," 21, in Intertribal Friendship House, *Urban Voices*; Levi Beaver, Memorandum, 14 Jan. 1959, MVSF, Box 18, Folder Crow Agency Relocation Reports, F.Y. 1959.

91. Wilkinson, *Blood Struggle*, 85; Sorkin, *The Urban American Indian*, 33.

92. McSwain, "The Role of Wives," 100–104; Jackie Yellowtail, interview by author. Examples of this pattern abound. See also Red Cloud, interview by Young; and Wilkinson, *Blood Struggle*, 85.

93. Maney, interview by Cossen; "Native Voices," pp. 132–33, CAIOHP.

94. This was not entirely new to the relocation era, but this mobility became easier as the nation's transportation infrastructure improved and more Native people owned automobiles. In the interwar period, Anna Moore Shaw had returned to the Salt River Reservation for her first two deliveries, where she was attended by her mother and her husband's paternal grandmother. Phoenix's proximity to the reservation made these reproductive journeys possible. See Shaw, *A Pima Past*, 154.

95. George Felshaw, Home Counselor's Report, 24 Feb. 1958, MVSF, Box 20, Folder Assistance to Individuals — Ft. Belknap F. Y. 1959.

96. File on DR, 18 Dec. 1959, MVSF, Box 19, Folder Special Study of Returnees F. Y. 1959.

97. LaGrand, *Indian Metropolis*, 132.

98. On Navajo teachings regarding the umbilical cord, see King, *The Earth Memory Compass*, xiii, 63–64.

99. PHS, *Health Services for American Indians*, 37; Neils, *Reservation to City*, 112; DL, 18 Dec. 1959, MVSF, Box 19, Folder Special Study of Returnees F. Y. 1959.

100. NARG, *Native American Families in the City*, 32. See also Sorkin, *The Urban American Indian*, 34, 52–53.

101. James W. Boyd to Rudolph Russell, 12 Aug. 1957, MVSF, Box 20, Folder Assistance to Individuals — Ft. Peck F. Y. 1957–1958.

102. Knifechief, interview by Engle.

103. McSwain, "The Role of Wives," 64.

104. McSwain, 64–65.

105. McSwain, 131.

106. McSwain, 131, 215.

107. McSwain, 131, 215.

108. McSwain, 238.

109. Reprinted in Intertribal Friendship House, *Urban Voices*, 11.

110. Knifechief, interview by Engle.

111. Haberman, interview by Brown.

112. Ramirez, *Native Hubs*.

113. Jackie Yellowtail, interview by author.

114. File on CM, 18 Dec. 1959, MVSF, Box 19, Folder Special Study of Returnees F. Y. 1959.

115. Griffen, "Life Is Harder Here," 95–96.

116. NARG, *Native American Families in the City*, 27.

117. See Gouveia, "Uncle Sam's Priceless Daughters"; and O'Neill, "Charity or Industry?"

118. Kessler-Harris, *Out to Work*, 303.

119. Rosenthal, *Reimagining Indian Country*, 51.

120. Quoted in LaGrand, *Indian Metropolis*, 107.

121. Stanley D. Lyman to David Weston, 22 May 1957, MVSF, Box 20, Folder Assistance to Individuals — Ft. Peck F. Y. 1957–1958 (emphasis in original).

122. Jacobs, "Diverted Mothering," 183.

123. McSwain, "The Role of Wives," 49–74; Fixico, interview by Zarek.

124. Blackhawk, "I Can Carry On from Here," 22. Johnson gave birth eleven times, but two infants were stillborn.

125. Clark, interview by author.

126. McSwain, "The Role of Wives," 206.

127. McSwain, 71, 117–18, 173.

128. McSwain, 71, 200–201.

129. On fertility control and wage work, see Tempkin-Greener et al., "Surgical Fertility Regulation." On urban Indian women and family planning, see Sorkin, *The Urban American Indian*, 12–13. A 1972 survey found the trend toward lower fertility among urban Indian women to be true for Seminole women but not for Omaha women. See Liberty et al., "Rural and Urban Omaha Indian Fertility"; and Liberty et al., "Rural and Urban Seminole Indian Fertility."

130. See Lobo, "Urban Clan Mothers," 7. Many essays in this edited volume provide useful analyses of women's roles in urban Native communities.

131. See "Native Voices," pp. 85–87, CAIOHP. Julie Davis and Brenda Child have amply documented this phenomenon in Saint Paul and Minneapolis. See Davis, *Survival Schools*; and Child, *Holding Our World Together*, esp. ch. 6.

132. Knifechief and Knifechief, interview by Engle.

133. See Knifechief, interview by Engle; Broker, *Night Flying Woman*.

134. Neils, *Reservation to City*, 17.

135. On twentieth-century Indians' reconceptualization of Indigenous spaces and communities, see Rosenthal, *Reimagining Indian Country*. See also Kent Blansett's concept of "the Indian City" in *A Journey to Freedom*.

Chapter 5

1. Quoted in Askins, "Bridging Cultures," 153.
2. See Benson, "The Fight for Crow Water, Part II."
3. Quoted in Taylor, *The Bureau of Indian Affairs*, 24.
4. Arnold, *Bartering with the Bones of Their Dead*, xi. Arnold's study offers an important and relatively unique contribution to scholarly studies of termination. Unlike most tribal nations, Colvilles pursued termination, although this outcome did not come to pass.
5. PHS, *Health Services for American Indians*, 213.
6. See Kekahbah and Wood, *Life Cycle of the American Indian Family*, 31; and Rife and Dellapenna Jr., *Caring and Curing*, 39.
7. Kunitz, *Disease Change*, 91. See also PHS, *Health Services for American Indians*, 212, 214.
8. PHS, *Health Services for American Indians*, 213.
9. Spotted Bear, interview by McCleary.
10. Rides Horse, interview by McCleary.
11. Snell, interview by McCleary; Plainfeather, interview by McCleary; Dan Old Elk, interview by McCleary.
12. Connie Yellowtail Jackson, interview by author; Plainfeather, interview by McCleary; Spotted Bear, interview by McCleary; Whiteman, interview by McCleary.
13. Minnie Williams, "Health Problems on the Crow Reservation," n.d., ABMC, Series 3, Box 9, Folder 3.49.
14. Leavitt, *Brought to Bed*, 194.
15. Kunitz, *Disease Change*, 164.
16. See McCleary, "Akbaatashee," 79.
17. Calvin Asbury to Henrietta Crockett, 7 Apr. 1930, CAGCF, Box 50, Folder 700.
18. Spotted Bear, interview by McCleary.
19. McCleary, "*Apsáalooke Bíanne Akdia* (Crow Midwives)," 24.
20. See Asetoyer, interview by Follett.
21. For a discussion of medical pluralism, a concept introduced in chapter 2, see Kelm, *Colonizing Bodies*, 129.
22. McCleary, "*Apsáalooke Bíanne Akdia* (Crow Midwives)," 24.
23. Hogan with Plainfeather and Loeb, *The Woman Who Loved Mankind*, 277–78.
24. See Mabel Morgan, Inspection Report, 24 July 1946, CAGCF, Box 53, Folder 722.5.
25. Wallace, interview by author.
26. See Morgan, Inspection Report, 24 July 1946; H. W. Kassel and K. Francis Cleave, Inspection Report, 13 Feb. 1947, both CAGCF, Box 53, Folder 722.5.
27. Snell with Matthews, *Grandmother's Grandchild*, 137.
28. See Evelyn Old Elk, interview by Pickett; and Spotted Bear, interview by McCleary. I thank Tim McCleary for first bringing this trend to my attention.

29. McCallum, *Indigenous Women, Work, and History*, 196.

30. John Provinse to Crow Tribal Delegates, 2 Mar. 1948, CAGCF, Box 18, Folder 155.

31. Provinse to Crow Tribal Delegates, 2 Mar. 1948, CAGCF.

32. Matthews, "Wherever That Singing Is Going," 204; Evelyn Old Elk, interview by Pickett; Spotted Bear, interview by McCleary.

33. Davies, *Healing Ways*, 50.

34. Davies, 51; Hancock, "Health and Well-Being," 173–74.

35. Deloria Jr., "Legislation and Litigation," 87.

36. See Ulrich, *American Indian Nations from Termination to Restoration*; Peroff, *Menominee Drums*; Metcalf, *Termination's Legacy*; and Hancock, "Health and Well-Being."

37. Cordelia Big Man to Mrs. Paul Wolk, 3 Mar. 1958, Crow Indian Historical Collection, LBCA, Box 2, Folder 2.13.

38. Wilkinson, *Blood Struggle*, 58.

39. Metcalf, *Termination's Legacy*, 6.

40. Minutes, Crow Tribal Council Meeting, 30 Mar. 1944, EWPC, Box 9A.

41. Minnie Williams to Mrs. Ruth F. Kirk, 15 Feb. 1949, ABMC, Series 2, Box 7, Folder 23. Scholars have documented similar sentiments in other locations, especially in the years before Dillon S. Myer's appointment as commissioner of Indian affairs. See Humalajoki, "'What Is It to Withdraw?'"; and Philp, *Termination Revisited*.

42. Quoted in Askins, "Bridging Cultures," 153.

43. This pattern is addressed in chapter 4. See also Philp, "Stride toward Freedom."

44. Philp, *Termination Revisited*, 71–75. Zimmerman's list resembled one that John Collier had prepared three years earlier.

45. Puisto, "*This Is My Reservation*," 86–87. On Yellowtail's message of self-determination, see Hoxie, *This Indian Country*, ch. 7.

46. Puisto, "*This Is My Reservation*."

47. Puisto, 86.

48. Paul Fickinger to Gordon Macgregor, 8 Apr. 1947, CAGCF, Box 53, Folder 722.2.

49. Harry Whiteman to William Zimmerman, 3 Mar. 1947, CAGCF, Box 52, Folder 722.

50. Highwalking with Weist, *Belle Highwalking*, 27.

51. Whiteman to Zimmerman, 3 Mar. 1947, CAGCF, Box 52, Folder 722.

52. Quoted in Fixico, *Termination and Relocation*, 72.

53. Mackey, "Closing the Fort Washakie Hospital."

54. Metcalf, *Termination's Legacy*, 43; Whiteman to Zimmerman, 12 Mar. 1947, CAGCF, Box 52, Folder 722.

55. Philp, *Termination Revisited*, 154.

56. Quoted in Mackey, "Closing the Fort Washakie Hospital," 38.

57. Sidney Edelman to General Counsel Files, 15 May 1961, HEW Correspondence Relating to Indians, 1955–1969, NARA MD, RG 235, Box 2, Folder PHS—INDIAN #5 1961.

58. See Puisto, "*This Is My Reservation*," 47; Hancock, "Health and Well-Being," 173–74.

59. Public Law 568, 83rd Congress, 2d Session, HEW Correspondence Relating to Indians, 1955–1969, NARA MD, RG 235, Box 1, Folder PHS (Indian) #1 1954–1955.

60. Quoted in Dejong, *Plagues, Politics, and Policy*, 35. On tribal opposition, see Davies, *Healing Ways*, 71; and Bergman et al., "A Political History of the Indian Health Service," 578–79.

61. Davies, *Healing Ways*, 71.

62. Kunitz, *Disease Change*, 154.

63. L. C. Lippert, Report on Indian Service and Public Health Conference, 20 May 1955, CAGCF, Box 16, Folder 130.2.

64. "Health Situation on the Crow Reservation," n.d., EWPC, Box 8A, Folder Health Committee Minutes.

65. Rife and Dellapenna, *Caring and Curing*, 29; Susie Yellowtail and Eloise Pease to Edward Whiteman, 14 May 1957, EWPC, Box 8A, Folder Health Committee Minutes.

66. Report of the Health Committee, 14 July 1956, EWPC, Box 8A, Folder Health Committee Minutes.

67. Crow Health Committee Minutes, 25 Apr. and 1 May 1956, EWPC, Box 8A, Folder Health Committee Minutes.

68. Davies, *Healing Ways*, 82.

69. The first health committee on the Crow Reservation is discussed in chapter 3.

70. See Gouveia, "'Uncle Sam's Priceless Daughters.'"

71. The minutes of most tribal council meetings from this period can be found in EWPC, Box 9A.

72. Minnie Williams, "The Absaroka Indian Women's Club," 22 Sept. 1960, ABMC, Series 2, Box 7, Folder 3.51.

73. See, for example, Minutes, Crow Tribal Council, 13 Dec. 1946, EWPC, Box 9A.

74. Interview Notes, Josephine Russell, Lodge Grass, 1956, FWVP, Series 2, Box 11, Folder 46.

75. Interview Notes, Olive Venne, Crow Agency, 1956, FWVP, Series 2, Box 11, Folder 45.

76. Eloise Pease, interview by Fraser.

77. For an insightful analysis of gender, class, and Native activism, albeit in an urban context, see Howard, "Women's Class Strategies."

78. Several committee members, such as Cordelia Big Man, had worked outside the home previously, and almost all contributed in various ways to their household earnings. One woman left the committee when she obtained a position at the hospital.

79. Crow Health Committee Minutes, 2 Apr. 1957, EWPC, Box 8A, Folder Health Committee Minutes. Alma Hogan Snell later praised Cordelia Big Man, for example, for being an "industrious woman." See Snell with Matthews, *Grandmother's Grandchild*, 59.

80. Medicine Crow, interview by Lowenthal, 26–27. Years later, Susie Yellowtail told Marina Brown Weatherly, "I feel that I'm in two worlds you might say." Weatherly, "Susie Walking Bear Yellowtail," 232. Notably, Yellowtail described herself as *in* two worlds, rather than *trapped between* them. In his 1969 manifesto *Custer Died for Your Sins*, Vine Deloria Jr. complained of scholars' investment in and perpetuation of the latter trope. Deloria, *Custer Died for Your Sins*, 86. More recently, scholars have critically examined the discourse and materiality of "two worldedness" in Buss and Genetin-Pilawa, *Beyond Two Worlds*.

81. Russell, interview by LaForge.

82. Medicine Crow, interview by Lowenthal.

83. Michele Newman, "Female Activism among the Shoshone: Assimilation or Preservation?," DD, Box 39.

84. "Health Situation on the Crow Reservation," n.d., EWPC, Box 8A, Folder Health Committee Minutes.

85. "Health Situation on the Crow Reservation," n.d., EWPC.

86. Quoted in Twila Van Leer, "Room for Improvement Everywhere, Says Susie Yellowtail — Nurse, Educator," n.d., Newspaper Clipping in Susie Yellowtail Vertical File, MHS.

87. Jackie Yellowtail, interview by author.

88. Report of the Health Committee, 14 July 1956, EWPC, Box 8A, Folder Health Committee Minutes.

89. Mackey, "Closing the Fort Washakie Hospital," 38.

90. Kunitz, "The History and Politics of U.S. Health Care Policy," 1466.

91. Puisto, *This Is My Reservation.*

92. Yellowtail and Pease to Whiteman, 14 May 1957, EWPC, Box 8A, Folder Health Committee Minutes.

93. Crow Health Committee Minutes, 4 Dec. 1956, EWPC, Box 8A, Folder Health Committee Minutes.

94. Crow Health Committee Minutes, 18 Sept. 1956, EWPC, Box 8A, Folder Health Committee Minutes.

95. Dejong, *"If You Knew the Conditions,"* 4.

96. Cahill, *Federal Fathers and Mothers*, 17, 30.

97. Kappler, *Indian Treaties*, 1011; Samuel Reynolds to Francis Leupp, 21 Sept. 1904, Letters to CIA, CAGCF, Box 6.

98. Report of the Health Committee, 14 July 1956, EWPC, Box 8A, Folder Health Committee Minutes.

99. Circular, EWPC, Box 9A, Folder Crow Health Committee.

100. Yellowtail and Pease to Whiteman, 14 May 1957, EWPC, Box 8A, Folder Health Committee Minutes.

101. PHS, *Health Services for American Indians*, 210. The cited Crow rate is the average rate for 1949–53. Using the same metrics, the birth rate on the Northern Cheyenne Reservation was 242.6. The cited Montana rate is for 1950.

102. PHS, 14.

103. Wallace, interview by author; Connie Jackson, interview by author.

104. Connie Jackson, interview by author.

105. Wolf, *Deliver Me from Pain*, 120.

106. Wolf, 102, 141–42.

107. Black (pseudonym), interview by author. Minor details in Black's personal history have been changed to protect her anonymity.

108. Black, interview by author.

109. Foster (pseudonym), interview by author.

110. Crow Health Committee Minutes, 7 May 1957, EWPC, Box 8A, Folder Health Committee Minutes.

111. On intertribal tensions at the hospital, see Voget, "Note regarding Crow-Cheyenne conflict over Crow Agency hospital," n.d., FWVP, Series 2, Box 11, Folder 36.

112. Black, interview by author.

113. Report of the Health Committee, 14 July 1956, EWPC, Box 8A, Folder Health Committee Minutes.

114. See PHS, *Health Services for American Indians*, 52, 217, 234; and Audra Pambrun, "Birth to School Age Children," 32–33.

115. Rife and Dellapenna, *Caring and Curing*.

116. Crow Health Committee Minutes, 4 Dec. 1956, EWPC, Box 8A, Folder Health Committee Minutes.

117. Wolf, *Deliver Me from Pain*, 111–13.

118. PHS, *Health Services for American Indians*, 135.

119. Crow Health Committee Minutes, 4 Dec. 1956, EWPC, Box 8A, Folder Health Committee Minutes.

120. Crow Health Committee Minutes, 14 May 1957, EWPC, Box 8A, Folder Health Committee Minutes.

121. Davies, *Healing Ways*, 75. On Wauneka's career in politics and health reform, see Niethammer, *I'll Go and Do More*.

122. Report of the Health Committee, 14 July 1956, EWPC, Box 8A, Folder Health Committee Minutes.

123. Foster, interview by author.

124. Spotted Bear, interview by McCleary.

125. Two Crow Indians, female, ages sixty-eight and thirty-five, interview by Linton, 69–70; Harding, "Traditional Beliefs and Behaviors," 59.

126. Yellowtail with Weatherly, "Susie Walking Bear Yellowtail," ch. 4.

127. Jackie Yellowtail, interview by author; Connie Jackson, interview by author.

128. On the centrality of neglect in federal Indian health services, see Gurr, *Reproductive Justice*.

129. "Health Situation on the Crow Reservation," n.d.; Report of the Health Committee, 14 July 1956; Crow Health Committee Minutes, 18 Sept. 1956; Crow Health Committee Minutes, 7 May 1957, all EWPC, Box 8A, Folder Health Committee Minutes.

130. "Health Situation on the Crow Reservation," n.d.; Report of the Health Committee, 14 July 1956, both EWPC, Box 8A, Folder Health Committee Minutes.

131. WARN II, 34.

132. Big Man to Wolk, 3 Mar. 1958, Crow Indian Historical Collection, LBCA, Box 2, Folder 2.13.

133. "Health Situation on the Crow Reservation," n.d., EWPC, Box 8A, Folder Health Committee Minutes.

134. See, for example, Minutes, Crow Tribal Council, 8 Apr. 1967, ABMC, Series 1, Subseries 1, Box 1.

135. See newspaper articles and essays in Hinkell, *Nurse of the Twentieth Century*.

Chapter 6

1. Cook, interview by Follett; Silliman et al., *Undivided Rights*, 125. The title of this chapter comes from Simpson, "Birthing an Indigenous Resurgence," 29.

2. Katsi Cook to the Michener Institute, 8 Sept. 1992, KCP, Box 1, Folder "Education: Michener Institute Midwifery Program, 1992-93, 1997"; Cook, interview by Follett.

3. O'Sullivan makes a similar argument about WARN and reproductive justice in "Informing Red Power."

4. Katsi Cook, "To Take Back Our Power," in *Women of All Red Nations*, pp. 24-25, KCP, Box 3, Folder 19.

5. M. Annette Jaimes and Theresa Halsey quote WARN cofounder Lorelei DeCora Means as asserting, "Our survival, the survival of every one of us — man, woman and child — *as Indians* depends on [decolonization]." Jaimes and Halsey, "American Indian Women," 314 (italics in original).

6. On feminists' pursuit of "reproductive self-determination," see Gordon, *The Moral Property of Women*, ch. 13.

7. After attending a WARN gathering in 1980, the Cherokee scholar Rayna Green observed, "I know that my mainstream isn't that far apart from WARN's revision of the world." Green, "Diary of a Native American Feminist," 211.

8. Critchlow, *Intended Consequences*, 3.

9. On family planning in the United States, see Gordon, *The Moral Property of Women*; and Schoen, *Choice and Coercion*.

10. See HSD, *Family Planning and the American Indian*; and Doran, "Attitudes of 30 American Indian Women."

11. HSD, *Family Planning and the American Indian*, 14; Landwehr, "Nurse Midwifery within the Indian Health Service," 31.

12. Liberty et al., "Rural and Urban Omaha Indian Fertility," 70.

13. Kane and Kane, *Federal Health Care*, 71. Continued high infant mortality is also briefly acknowledged in the Omaha study. See also Liberty et al., "Rural and Urban Seminole Indian Fertility," 753.

14. HSD, *Family Planning and the American Indian*, 14.

15. Brave Bird with Erdoes, *Lakota Woman*, 78.

16. See HSD, *Family Planning and the American Indian*, 28; and Liberty et al., "Rural and Urban Omaha Indian Fertility," 64.

17. Katsi Cook, WDHP Report, Apr. 1979, KCP, Box 5, Folder 7. Cook later argued that "historically" was a better framework for assessing past practices than "traditionally," which she explained was "analytically meaningless." See Cook, interview by Kim Anderson, 18 July 2001, OFIFC Youth Sexual Health and Pregnancy Research, KCP, Box 1, Folder Interviews, 1992-2001.

18. Bergman et al., "A Political History of the Indian Health Service," 582.

19. See Harding, "Traditional Beliefs and Behaviors," 71-73; HSD, *Family Planning and the American Indian*, 27; and Doran, "Attitudes of 30 American Indian Women," 660, 662. See also Lawrence, "The Indian Health Service," 412-13.

20. See Doran, "Attitudes of 30 American Indian Women," 660–61; HSD, *Family Planning and the American Indian*, 16; Liberty et al., "Rural and Urban Omaha Indian Fertility," 65; and Liberty et al., "Rural and Urban Seminole Indian Fertility," 748–50. See also Kane and Kane, *Federal Health Care*, 71–72; Shoshone female, age twenty-one, interview by Linton, 50–51; Kay Voget Field Notes, 9 June 1968, p. 7, DD, Box 41.

21. HSD, *Family Planning and the American Indian*, 16.

22. Willis, interview by Brown.

23. HSD, *Family Planning and the American Indian*, 17.

24. HSD, 20–21. Dropout rates were similarly high in other locations. See Slocumb et al., "Complications with Use of IUD."

25. HSD, *Family Planning and the American Indian*, 20–21; and Slocumb et al., "Complications with Use of IUD," 245–47. See also Carpio, "Lost Generation: The Involuntary Sterilization," 33.

26. HSD, *Family Planning and the American Indian*, 20–22.

27. Espino, "Women Sterilized as They Give Birth," 167.

28. Foster (pseudonym), interview by author.

29. See Reagan, *When Abortion Was a Crime*.

30. Temkin-Greener et al., "Surgical Fertility Regulation," 405.

31. Petchesky, *Abortion and Woman's Choice*, 157.

32. See Asetoyer, interview by Follett, 49–50.

33. See "Close Social and Economic Ties Deleted from Health Program," *Sho-Ban News*, 27 May 1981, 6; "NIHB Requests Extension of Comment Period on IHS Abortion Regs," *Sho-Ban News*, 1 July 1981, 6; "Abortions Only for Life-Endangered," *Sho-Ban News*, 24 Feb. 1981, 1. When the changes were first published, National Indian Health Board Executive Director Jake Whitecrow expressed criticism that Indians had not been consulted regarding the new regulations, a complaint that delayed but did not prevent implementation. On *Harris*, see Petchesky, *Abortion and Woman's Choice*, 299–302.

34. Liberty et al., "Rural and Urban Omaha Indian Fertility," 65; Liberty et al., "Rural and Urban Seminole Indian Fertility," 749–50.

35. Brave Bird with Erdoes, *Ohitika Woman*, 58–59.

36. An organization that worked with WARN in Minneapolis–St. Paul characterized WARN's position on abortion as follows: "Abortion is not needed by Native American women since their extended families will care for children, but that abortion should be available for all women." Untitled Report, Twin Cities Reproductive Rights Committee, 20 Mar. 1979, R2N2P, Box 6, Folder 21. See also Shoshone female, age twenty-one, interview by Linton, 52.

37. Doran, "Attitudes of 30 American Indian Women," 660.

38. Two Crow Indians, female, ages sixty-eight and thirty-five, interview by Linton.

39. Brave Bird with Erdoes, *Ohitika Woman*, 58.

40. Valerie Jackson, interview by author. See Untitled Report, Twin Cities Reproductive Rights Committee, 20 Mar. 1979, R2N2P, Box 6, Folder 21; and WARN II.

41. See Untitled Report, Twin Cities Reproductive Rights Committee, 20 Mar. 1979, R2N2P, Box 6, Folder 21; and Smith, *Conquest*, 96–97.

42. See Petchesky, *Abortion and Woman's Choice*, 121.

43. Kay Voget Field Notes, 9 June 1968, p. 8, DD, Box 41.

44. See Davies, *Healing Ways*, 132–33.

45. See Kluchin, *Fit to Be Tied*; Schoen, *Choice and Coercion*.

46. Besaw, interview by Guglielmo, 11.

47. Shoshone female, age twenty-one, interview by Linton, 50–51.

48. Valerie Jackson, interview by author.

49. Doran, "Attitudes of 30 American Indian Women," 663.

50. Dyck and Lux, "Population Control in the 'Global North'?," 486.

51. Doran, "Attitudes of 30 American Indian Women," 663.

52. See O'Sullivan, "Informing Red Power"; and Dyck and Lux, "Population Control in the 'Global North'?"

53. Rife and Dellapenna, *Caring and Curing*, 46–49.

54. Guglielmo, "The Community Health Representative Program," 11–12.

55. HSD, *Family Planning and the American Indian*, 15. Female CHRs took part in family planning programming in Wisconsin as well. See Guglielmo, "The Community Health Representative Program," 20.

56. Guglielmo, "The Community Health Representative Program," 19–20.

57. Thayer, interview by Guglielmo, 21.

58. Thayer, 21.

59. See Lawrence, "The Indian Health Service," 405–6; Kluchin, *Fit to Be Tied*, 180–83; and GAO, 4.

60. Guglielmo, "The Community Health Representative Program," 17.

61. Gail Mark Jarvis, "The Theft of Life," in *Women of All Red Nations*, KCP, Box 3, Folder 19.

62. "Women against Sterilization," *Akwesasne Notes* 9, no. 5 (Dec. 1977): 26.

63. Powers, *Oglala Women*, 165. On Yellowtail and AINA, see Davis, "Susie Yellowtail."

64. Uri, interview by Berland.

65. "Women against Sterilization," 26; Uri, interview by Berland.

66. Quoted in Espino, "Women Sterilized as They Give Birth," 239.

67. Uri, interview by Berland.

68. American Society of Registered Nurses, "Big Heart"; Susie Yellowtail, interviewer unknown.

69. Uri, interview by Berland.

70. Kluchin, *Fit to Be Tied*, 74.

71. GAO. See also Carpio, "Lost Generation: American Indian Women and Sterilization Abuse," 48–50; and Lawrence, "The Indian Health Service," 407–9.

72. Lawrence, "The Indian Health Service," 400.

73. Kane and Kane, *Federal Health Care*, 13.

74. See Uri, interview by Berland.

75. Brave Bird with Erdoes, *Ohitika Woman*, 192.

76. See Jacobs, *A Generation Removed*; and O'Sullivan, "More Destruction to These Family Ties."

77. GAO, 4.

78. "Women against Sterilization," 26.

79. Lawrence, "The Indian Health Service," 410. WARN leaders sometimes alleged that sterilization rates on the Northern Cheyenne Reservation were as high as 80 percent, but I have not been able to trace how they came to this figure. See Pat Bellanger, Lorelei Means, and Vicki Howard, interview by Kris Melrose, *off our backs* 9, no. 5 (May 1979).

80. "Native Americans 'Warn' of Sterilization Abuse," *Reproductive Rights: Newsletter of the Philadelphia Reproductive Rights Coalition* 1, no. 2 (1981). See also "Growing Fight against Sterilization of Native Women," *Akwesasne Notes* 11, no. 1 (1979): 29.

81. Yellowtail with Weatherly, "Susie Walking Bear Yellowtail," ch. 4.

82. See Smith and Warrior, *Like a Hurricane*.

83. WARN II, 2–3.

84. *Women of All Red Nations*, KCP, Box 3, Folder 19; Million, *Therapeutic Nations*, 125.

85. See Child, *Holding Our World Together*, ch. 6.

86. Castle, "Black and Native American Women's Activism," 250. See also Katsi Cook, "Mother's Milk and First Environments Projects: Case Study Draft," p. 5, KCP, Box 4, Folder 10; and Shirley Hill Witt, "The Brave-Hearted Women," *Akwesasne Notes* 8, no. 2 (1976): 16–17.

87. Katsi Cook, "Women's Dance: A Woman's Health Book" outline, n.d., KCP, Box 6, Folder 10.

88. Young quoted in Castle, "Black and Native American Women's Activism," 252–53; "Declaration of Continuing Independence," in *Women of All Red Nations*, p. 34, KCP, Box 3, Folder 19.

89. See Jacobs, *A Generation Removed*, 107–8.

90. On coercive sterilization and tribal sovereignty, see O'Sullivan, "Informing Red Power."

91. Katsi Cook, WDHP Report, Apr. 1979, KCP, Box 5, Folder 7.

92. See Cook, interview by Follett, 68; and WARN II, 38. On child removal in the Twin Cities, see Davis, *Survival Schools*, 82–93.

93. WARN II, 38 (emphasis in original).

94. WARN II, 38. See also WDHP Report, Apr. 1979, KCP, Box 5, Folder 7.

95. On Norma Jean Serena, see Kluchin, *Fit to Be Tied*, 110–11; and Jacobs, *A Generation Removed*, 92.

96. Torpy, "Native American Women," 9; Paula Jones, "Three Million Dollar Suit against Federal Government Underway," *Akwesasne Notes* 2, no. 3 (1979): 12.

97. "Native Americans 'Warn' of Sterilization Abuse."

98. "Marie Sanchez: For the Women," *Akwesasne Notes* 2, no. 5 (1977): 14–15. Pat Bellanger was also a delegate to the 1977 United Nations conference. See "Native American Women, Forced Sterilization, and the Family: An Interview with Pat Bellanger," in Ellis, *Every Woman Has a Story*, 30–35.

99. "An Interview with Barbara Moore," *Akwesasne Notes* (Spring 1979): 11–12. The anthropologist Marla Powers was skeptical of many Lakota men and women's charges regarding physicians on the Pine Ridge Reservation: "My own opinion is that the Public Health Service doctors are no better or worse than one would expect to find off the reservation." Powers, *Oglala Women*, 220n3.

100. Uri, interview by Berland; "Marie Sanchez: For the Women," 14.

101. On gendered analyses of genocide, see Jacobs, "Bearing Witness to California Genocide." I would also argue that WARN women offered a "felt analysis" on this as well as other issues. See Million, "Felt Theory."

102. Scholars have utilized the United Nations' 1948 definition as well. See Madley, "Reexamining the American Genocide Debate"; and Madley, *An American Genocide*. See *Journal of Genocide Research* 19, no. 1 (2017) and *Western Historical Quarterly* 47, no. 4 (2016) for roundtable discussions on Madley's monograph and on genocide in U.S. history.

103. Quoted in Madley, "Reexamining the American Genocide Debate," 103.

104. Bellanger, Means, and Howard, interview.

105. Quoted in Ralstin-Lewis, "The Continuing Struggle against Genocide," 83.

106. Jarvis, "The Theft of Life," 14.

107. See "Native Americans 'Warn' of Sterilization Abuse"; Davis, *Survival Schools*, 84.

108. See Reproductive Rights Subcommittee of the Anti-Sexism Committee of the Twin Cities Chapter of the National Lawyers' Guild, "Federal Sterilization Regulations," Apr. 1979; National Women's Health Network, *Sterilization Resource Guide*, 1980, both R2N2P, Box 14, Folder 21.

109. Kluchin, *Fit to Be Tied*, 205.

110. Some radical and socialist feminist organizations supported the new regulations. See Gordon, *The Moral Property of Women*, 345–47.

111. O'Sullivan, "Informing Red Power," 975–76.

112. Powers, *Oglala Women*, 165.

113. WARN II, 1.

114. WDHP Funding Request, 1982, KCP, Box 5, Folder 7. For more on WDHP, see Silliman et al., *Undivided Rights*, 128–30.

115. Cook to the Michener Institute, 8 Sept. 1992, KCP, Box 1, Folder "Education: Michener Institute Midwifery Program"; Cook, WDHP Report, Apr. 1979, KCP, Box 5, Folder 7.

116. Cook, "Mother's Milk and First Environments Projects: Case Study Draft," p. 6, KCP, Box 4, Folder 10; Cook to the Michener Institute, 8 Sept. 1992, KCP, Box 1, Folder "Education: Michener Institute Midwifery Program."

117. Cook, WDHP Report, Apr. 1979, KCP, Box 5, Folder 7.

118. Cook, interview by Follett, 67; Cook to the Michener Institute, 8 Sept. 1992, KCP, Box 1, Folder "Education: Michener Institute Midwifery Program."

119. Cook, "Women's Dance: A Women's Health Book" outline, n.d., KCP, Box 6, Folder 10. On feminist health activists' promotion of self-help, see Kline, *Bodies of Knowledge*; Morgen, *Into Our Own Hands*; and Silliman et al., *Undivided Rights*.

120. Cook, "To Take Back Our Power," in *Women of All Red Nations*, pp. 24–25, KCP, Box 3, Folder 19; WARN II, 35.

121. On survival schools in these locations and their role as community centers and cultural hubs, see Davis, *Survival Schools*, ch. 2, 168–71; and White, *Free to Be Mohawk*.

122. Cook, "Women's Dance: A Women's Health Book" outline, n.d., KCP, Box 6, Folder 10.

123. WARN II, 42.

124. Cook, WDHP Report, Apr. 1979, KCP, Box 5, Folder 7. This, too, dovetailed with trends outside Indian Country, as a growing segment of American women pursued what they viewed as more "natural" reproductive experiences. See Kline, "Communicating a New Consciousness"; and Martucci, *Back to the Breast*.

125. Katsi Cook, "Akwesasne Community Health Project," 1982, KCP, Box 4, Folder 6A.

126. Cook, interview by Follett, 22.

127. On The Farm, see Gaskin, *Hey Beatnik!* On Cook's training in New Mexico, see Cook to the Michener Institute, 8 Sept. 1992, KCP, Box 1, Folder "Education: Michener Institute Midwifery Program."

128. Cook, interview by Follett, 71–78. See also Cook, "A Native American Response," 257. On women's peyote use during labor on the Crow Reservation, see Harding, "Traditional Beliefs and Behaviors," 64–66, 104–5.

129. Cook, WDHP Report, Apr. 1979, KCP, Box 5, Folder 7.

130. Brave Bird with Erdoes, *Lakota Woman*, 157.

131. See Gurr, *Reproductive Justice*, 94.

132. Cook, WDHP Report, Apr. 1979, KCP, Box 5, Folder 7.

133. Midwifery in Wisconsin was often stymied by a repressive political climate and the staunch opposition of local IHS personnel. See Gail Ellis to Katsi Cook, 8 May 1985, KCP, Box 1, Folder 12. Midwifery at Akwesasne is discussed in Cook, "Akwesasne Community Health Project," 1982, KCP, Box 4, Folder 6A; and "An Indian Kind of Thing," *Akwesasne Notes* 10, no. 4 (1978): 13. For an example of Native women seeking out-of-hospital birthing experiences in other locations, see Begay, "Changes in Childbirth Knowledge."

134. See McCloskey, *Living through the Generations*, 172.

135. Harding, "Traditional Beliefs and Behaviors," 23, 69, 105–6.

136. See Landwehr, "Nurse Midwifery within the Indian Health Service," 44–48. Native women's embrace of IHS CNMs has not been universal, however. I address some women's resistance to nurse-midwifery in IHS hospitals in the epilogue.

137. Cook, interview by Follett, 43.

138. Cook, "To Take Back Our Power," in *Women of All Red Nations*, p. 24, KCP, Box 3, Folder 19.

139. On Sanchez's activism on energy issues, see Allison, *Sovereignty for Survival*, ch. 4.

140. Allison, 2; Kuletz, *The Tainted Desert*, 24. See also LaDuke, *All Our Relations*, esp. chs. 4–5.

141. WDHP Funding Request, 1982, KCP, Box 5, Folder 7; Castle, "Black and Native American Women's Activism," 262.

142. Kuletz, *The Tainted Desert*, 20.

143. Katsi Cook, "Women Are the First Environment," 23 Dec. 2003, *Indian Country Today*, https://indiancountrymedianetwork.com/news/cook-women-are-the-first-environment/. See also Silliman et al., *Undivided Rights*, ch. 7; and LaDuke, *All Our Relations*, ch. 1.

144. Native American Women's Health Education Resource Center, "Reproductive Justice Agenda."

Epilogue

1. Janine Pease, interview by author.

2. Denise Grady, "Lessons at Indian Hospital about Births," *New York Times*, 6 Mar. 2010.

3. Janine Pease, interview by author. Gladys Limberhand (Cheyenne) described a similarly positive birthing experience at the Crow Agency Hospital in the mid-1990s. Limberhand, interview by author.

4. Janine Pease, interview by author.

5. Susan Olp, "Troubles Stack Up at Crow-Northern Cheyenne Hospital," *Billings Gazette*, 15 Nov. 2011, http://billingsgazette.com/news/state-and-regional/troubles -stack-up-at-crow-northern-cheyenne-hospital/article_413b2955-f1d5-5ca0-9166 -6bed377c2f96.html.

6. See Katy B. Kozhimannil and Austin Frakt, "Rural America's Disappearing Maternity Care," *Washington Post*, 8 Nov. 2017, https://www.washingtonpost.com /opinions/rural-americas-disappearing-maternity-care/2017/11/08/11a664d6-97e6 -11e7-b569-3360011663b4_story.html?utm_term=.6537004991a2; and Staci Matlock, "Rural Health Care Gaps Complicate Pregnancies for New Mexico Women," *Santa Fe New Mexican*, 30 Apr. 2016, http://www.santafenewmexican.com/news/local_news /rural-health-care-gaps-complicate-pregnancies-for-new-mexico-women/article _dab558a4-3d7f-5dab-834b-d4a782ad410f.html?mode=jqm.

7. Quoted in Susan Olp, "Baucus Promises Relief for IHS Hospital Woes," *Missoulian*, 9 Oct. 2012, http://missoulian.com/news/state-and-regional/baucus-promises -relief-for-ihs-hospital-woes/article_b6b5607e-e23f-11e1-9c7c-001a4bcf887a .html.

8. Foster (pseudonym), interview by author.

9. Kozhimannil and Frakt, "Rural America's Disappearing Maternity Care."

10. Amnesty International, *Deadly Delivery*, 61–62.

11. Janine Pease, interview by author.

12. Tanya H. Lee, "'Where You Can Legally Kill an Indian': Winnebago Treasurer on IHS Hospitals," *Indian Country Today*, 15 July 2016, https://indiancountrymedianetwork .com/news/native-news/where-you-can-legally-kill-an-indian-winnebago-treasurer -on-ihs-hospitals/.

13. Quoted in Gurr, *Reproductive Justice*, 102.

14. Gurr, 102.

15. The American College of Obstetricians and Gynecologists approved nurse-midwifery for uncomplicated maternity cases in 1971. See Cassidy, *Birth*, 44.

16. Landwehr, "Nurse Midwifery within the Indian Health Service," 40.

17. Landwehr, 1.

18. Landwehr, 34–40.

19. See Gurr, *Reproductive Justice*, 84, 92–104.

20. Landwehr, "Nurse Midwifery within the Indian Health Service," 45–48, quote on p. 48.

21. Gurr, *Reproductive Justice*, 84.

22. Foster, interview by author.

23. Lee, "Where You Can Legally Kill an Indian"; Jayme Fraser, "Indian Health Service Care Criticized as Genocidal Despite Improvement Efforts," *Billings Gazette*, 6 Sept. 2016, http://billingsgazette.com/news/state-and-regional/montana/indian-health-service-care-criticized-as-genocidal-despite-improvement-efforts/article_2d2a6c4c-9d2b-5ea5-9db0-f8277cf296b5.html.

24. Lee, "Where You Can Legally Kill an Indian."

25. Rentner et al., "Culture, Identity, and Spirituality," 50.

26. Mary Annette Pember, "Birthing the Sacred: Baby Born at Water Protector Camp Bears Hope," *Indian Country Today*, 20 Oct. 2016, https://indiancountrymedianetwork.com/culture/health-wellness/birthing-the-sacred-baby-born-at-water-protector-camp-bears-hope/.

27. Brave Bird with Erdoes, *Lakota Woman*, 159.

28. Quoted in Pember, "Birthing the Sacred."

29. Sarah van Gelder, "For Native Mothers, a Way to Give Birth That Overcomes Trauma," *Yes! Magazine*, 24 May 2017, http://www.yesmagazine.org/people-power/for-new-native-mothers-a-place-for-culture-and-comfort-20170524.

30. Prachi Gupta, "This Navajo Woman Is Planning the First Native American Birthing Center in the Country," *Cosmopolitan*, 12 Oct. 2015, https://www.cosmopolitan.com/politics/news/a47518/americas-first-native-american-birthing-center/.

31. See Miriam Zoila Pérez, "Navajo Midwives in New Mexico Plan First-Ever Native American Birthing Center," *Colorlines*, 29 Sept. 2015, https://www.colorlines.com/articles/navajo-midwives-new-mexico-plan-first-ever-native-american-birth-center.

32. Information about Changing Woman Initiative's services can be found at changingwomaninitiative.com.

33. Quoted in Pérez, "Navajo Midwives in New Mexico."

34. Cynthia Miller, "Nation's First Native Birthing Center Planned in New Mexico," *New Mexican*, 29 Apr. 2018, http://www.santafenewmexican.com/news/health_and_science/nation-s-first-native-birthing-facility-planned-in-new-mexico/article_c225ecc6-9e9f-5874-b369-1199e09ac3a7.html.

35. Quoted in Alysa Landry, "Changing Woman: Reclaiming Sovereignty over Women's Health and Rethinking Birth," *Indian Country Today*, 29 Oct. 2015, https://indiancountrymedianetwork.com/culture/health-wellness/changing-woman-reclaiming-sovereignty-over-womens-health-and-rethinking-birth/.

36. On Native midwifery in Canada, see Tabobondung et al., "Indigenous Midwifery as an Expression of Sovereignty."

37. See Ross and Solinger, *Reproductive Justice*; and Ross et al., *Radical Reproductive Justice*.

38. Quoted in Hoover et al., "Indigenous Peoples of North America," 1645.

39. Finestone and Stirbys, "Indigenous Birth in Canada," 192.

40. See Gurr, *Reproductive Justice*.

41. Michelle Chen, "Poison Pill Slipped Into Indian Health Bill," *In These Times* 32, no. 8 (2008): 8–9.

42. See Anna North, "Abortion Clinics Are Closing in Rural America. So Are Maternity Wards," *Vox*, 7 Sept. 2017, https://www.vox.com/policy-and-politics/2017/9/7

/16262182/kentucky-clinic-abortion-maternity; and Susan Scutti, "Some U.S. Women Travel Hundreds of Miles for Abortions, Analysis Finds," 4 Oct. 2017, https://www.cnn .com/2017/10/03/health/abortion-access-disparities-study/index.html.

43. See Theobald, "Settler Colonialism, Native American Motherhood, and the Politics of Terminating Pregnancies."

44. Materials related to Charon Asetoyer's Senate campaign can be found in Charon Asetoyer Papers, Box 1, Folders 17–20, and Box 2, Folders 1–3, Sophia Smith Collection, Smith College, Northampton, MA. See also Peter Rothberg, "Fighting Back in South Dakota," *The Nation*, 9 May 2006, https://www.thenation.com/article/fighting -back-south-dakota/.

45. Asetoyer, interview by Follett, 43.

46. Asetoyer, interview by Follett, 32–34, 47–49.

47. Volscho, "Sterilization, Racism, and Pan-Ethnic Disparities," 22–23.

48. See Ruth Hopkins, "Painting My Legs Red," *Indian Country Today*, 19 Apr. 2016, https://indiancountrymedianetwork.com/news/opinions/painting-my-legs-red/.

49. See Lakota People's Law Project, *The Total Title IV Solution: Sovereignty and Self-Governance in the Provision of Child and Family Services*, 8 July 2013, https://s3-us-west -1.amazonaws.com/lakota-peoples-law/uploads/LPLP-Sovereignty-and-Self -Governance.pdf.

50. Jackie Yellowtail, interview by author.

Bibliography

Manuscript Collections

Big Horn County Historical Museum, Hardin, Mont.
    Bentley/Hubley Collection
Buffalo Bill Center of the West, Cody, Wyo.
    Frederick Shoemaker Collection
Labriola American Indian Center, Tempe, Ariz.
    Records of the Bureau of Indian Affairs: Central Classified Files, 1907–1939,
        Record Group 75 (Microfilm)
    Superintendents' Annual Statistical and Narrative Reports, 1907–1938, Record
        Group 75 (Microfilm)
Little Bighorn College Archives, Crow Agency, Mont.
    Ann Big Man Collection
    Crow Indian Historical Collection
    Frederick Hoxie Collection
    Eloise Pease Whiteman Collection
Maureen and Mike Mansfield Library, Missoula, Mont.
    Fred W. Voget Papers
Montana Historical Society, Helena, Mont.
    Susie Yellowtail Vertical File
National Archives and Records Administration, Baltimore, Md.
    HEW Correspondence Relating to Indians, 1955–1969, Record Group 235
National Archives and Records Administration, Broomfield, Colo.
    Crow Agency General Correspondence Files, Record Group 75
    Mixed Vocational and Subject Files, Billings Area Office, Record Group 75
National Archives and Records Administration, Washington, D.C.
    Orders and Circulars, Record Group 75
    Reports of Field Nurses, Records of the Health Division, Record Group 75
    Social Workers' Reports, Records of the Welfare Branch, Record Group 75
    Superintendents' Annual Statistical and Narrative Reports, Record Group 75
        (Microfilm)
National Personnel Records Center Annex, Valmeyer, Ill.
    Personnel Files
Newberry Library, Chicago, Ill.
    Bureau of Indian Affairs Relocation Records
    Chicago American Indian Oral History Project, "Native Voices" Manuscript
Smith College, Northampton, Mass.
    Charon Asetoyer Papers

Katsi Cook Papers
Jennifer M. Guglielmo Papers
Reproductive Rights National Network Papers
Southern California Library for Social Studies and Research, Los Angeles, Calif.
  Liberty Hill Foundation Records, 20th Century Organizational Files
University of Illinois Archives, University of Illinois at Urbana-Champaign
  Doris Duke Field Worker Reports

Oral History Collections

American Indian Oral History Project, Part II, University of South Dakota, Vermillion
  Pease, Eloise. Interview by Willard Fraser, 10 Sept. 1968.
Chicago American Indian Oral History Project, Newberry Library, Chicago, Ill.
  Maney, Rose. Interview by Clovia Cossen, 18 Feb. 1983.
  Red Cloud, Margaret. Interview by Claire Young, 12 Feb. 1984.
Crow Expressions Oral History Project, Western Heritage Center, Billings, Mont.
  Plenty Hoops, Winona. Interview by Mardell Plainfeather, 1 June 2004.
Crow Oral History Binder, Little Bighorn College Archives, Crow Agency, Mont.
  Old Elk, Evelyn. Interview by Aldeen Pickett, n.d.
Doris Duke American Indian Oral History, University of Illinois at Urbana-Champaign
  Crow Indian male, age eighty-eight. Interview by Norma Linton, 1972.
  Medicine Crow, Joseph. Interview by Richard Lowenthal, 24 Jan. 1968.
  Old Coyote, Barney, Jr. Spring Crow Culture Lecture Series, 1971.
  Shoshone female, age twenty-one. Interview by Norma Linton, 1972.
  Tobacco, Tom. Interview by Richard Lowenthal, Summer 1967.
  Two Crow Indians, female, ages sixty-eight and thirty-five. Interview by Norma
    Linton, Nov. and Dec. 1971.
Indian Urbanization Project, Center for Oral and Public History, California State
    University, Fullerton
  Fixico, Hannah. Interview by M. J. Zarek, 14 June 1971.
  Gabouri, Frances. Interview by Georgia Brown, 5 Apr. 1971.
  Haberman, Lena. Interview by Georgia Brown, 12 May 1971.
  Knifechief, Lois, and John Knifechief. Interview by Clare Engle, 26 Oct. 1970.
  Willis, Patricia. Interview by Georgia Brown, 2 May 1971.
Jennifer M. Guglielmo Papers, Smith College, Northampton, Mass.
  Besaw, Dave. Interview by Guglielmo, 10 Mar. 1990.
  Thayer, Arvina. Interview by Guglielmo, 23 Feb. 1990.
New Deal in Montana/Fort Peck Dam Oral History, Montana Historical Society,
    Helena, Mont.
  Childs, Mae Takes Gun. Interview by Carson Walks Over Ice, 10 May 1989.
  Hogan, Effie Lillian Bullshows. Interview by Carson Walks Over Ice, 22 May 1989.
Oral History Collection, Montana Historical Society, Mont.
  Russell, Josephine Pease. Interview by Bill LaForge, 24–25 Feb. 1989.
Pacifica Radio Archives, North Hollywood, Calif.
  Uri, Connie. Interview by Jim Berland, 25 Sept. 1974.

Voices of Feminism Oral History Project, Smith College, Northampton, Mass.
Asetoyer, Charon. Interview by Joyce Follett, 1–2 Sept. 2005.
Cook, Katsi. Interview by Joyce Follett, 26–27 Oct. 2005.

Uncollected Oral Interviews

Black, Iris (pseudonym). Interview by author. Billings, Mont., 26 July 2017.
Clark, Debbie (pseudonym). Interview by author. Billings, Mont., 26 July 2017.
Foster, Annie (pseudonym). Interview by author. Hardin, Mont., 16 June 2016.
Jackson, Connie Yellowtail. Interview by author. Crow Agency, Mont., 14 Aug. 2015.
Jackson, Valerie. Interview by author. Tempe, Ariz., 26 June 2015.
Limberhand, Gladys. Interview by author. Lame Deer, Mont., 27 July 2017.
Morin, Anita. Interview by author. Fort Collins, Colo., 5 Feb. 2016.
Old Elk, Dan. Interview by Timothy McCleary. Crow Agency, Mont., 24 July 2003.
Pease, Janine. Interview by author. Hardin, Mont., 28 July 2017.
Plainfeather, Valeen. Interview by Timothy McCleary. Pryor, Mont., 22 Mar. 2018.
Powell, Peter. Phone interview by author. 22 Sept. 2017.
Rides Horse, Dora. Interview by Timothy McCleary. Crow Agency, Mont., 11 Sept. 2003.
Snell, Alma Hogan. Interview by Timothy McCleary. Fort Smith, Mont., 28 July 2003.
Spotted Bear, Dorothy. Interview by Timothy McCleary. Crow Agency, Mont., 24 Apr. 2018.
Wallace, Mary Elizabeth. Interview by author. Hardin, Mont., 22 Aug. 2015.
Whiteman, Geneva. Interview by Timothy McCleary. Crow Agency, Mont., 14 July 2017.
Yellowtail, Jackie. Interview by author. Garryowen, Mont., 21 June 2016.
Yellowtail, Susie. Interviewer unknown. In possession of Connie Yellowtail Jackson, n.d.

Newspapers

Akwesasne Notes
Billings Gazette
Indian Country Today
Missoulian
Nation
Navajo Times
New York Times
off our backs
Reproductive Rights: Newsletter of the Philadelphia Reproductive Rights Coalition
Santa Fe New Mexican
Sho-Ban News
Washington Post

Websites

American Society of Registered Nurses. "Big Heart." *Chronicle of Nursing*.
 1 Nov. 2007. http://www.asrn.org/journal-chronicle-nursing/205-big-heart.html.
Cavender-Wilson, Autumn. "Mni Wiconi Yaktan K'a Ni Drink the Water of Life, and
 Live." *Changing Woman Initiative* (blog). 6 Sept. 2016. http://www
 .changingwomaninitiative.com/blog/-mni-wiconi-yaktan-ka-ni-drink-the-water
 -of-life-and-live.
Hanshew, Annie. "'You Had to Pretend It Never Happened': Illegal Abortion in
 Montana." *Montana Women's History* (blog). Montana Historical Society, 29
 Apr. 2014. http://montanawomenshistory.org/you-had-to-pretend-it-never
 -happened-illegal-abortion-in-montana/.
Kaelber, Lutz. "Eugenics: Compulsory Sterilization in 50 American States." Accessed
 18 June 2018. https://www.uvm.edu/~lkaelber/eugenics/.
Native American Women's Health Education Resource Center. "Reproductive Justice
 Agenda." Accessed 18 June 2018. http://www.nativeshop.org/programs
 /reproductive-justice/repro-justice-agenda.html.

Government Publications

Commissioner of Indian Affairs. *Annual Reports*. Washington, D.C.: Government
 Printing Office.
Health Services Division. *Family Planning and the American Indian*. Baltimore:
 Westinghouse Learning Corporation, 1971.
Meriam, Lewis. *The Problem of Indian Administration*. Baltimore: Johns Hopkins
 University Press, 1928.
Public Health Service. *Health Services for American Indians*. Washington, D.C.:
 Government Printing Office, 1957.
Report of the Joint Committee on the Conduct of War. 2nd Session, 38th Congress.
 Washington, D.C.: Government Printing Office, 1865.
Rife, James P., and Alan J. Dellapenna, Jr. *Caring and Curing: A History of the Indian
 Health Service*. Washington, D.C.: PHS Commissioner Officers Foundation for the
 Advancement of Public Health, 2009.
Staats, Elmer B. *Report to Senator James Abourezk: Investigation of Allegations concerning
 Indian Health Service*. Washington, D.C.: Government Printing Office, 1976.

Primary Sources: Books, Articles, and Reports

Amnesty International. *Deadly Delivery: The Maternal Health Care Crisis in the U.S.A.*
 London: Amnesty International Publications, 2010.
Bacon, Charles Sumner. "Pulmonary Tuberculosis as an Obstetrical Complication."
 Journal of the American Medical Association 45 (7 Oct. 1905): 1067–70.
Brave Bird, Mary, with Richard Erdoes. *Lakota Woman*. New York: Harper Perennial,
 1991.
———. *Ohitika Woman*. New York: Grove Press, 1993.

Broker, Ignatia. *Night Flying Woman: An Ojibwe Narrative*. St. Paul: Minnesota Historical Society Press, 1983.

Cook, Katsi. "A Native American Response." In *Birth Control and Controlling Birth: Women-Centered Perspectives*, edited by Helen B. Holmes, Betty B. Hoskins, and Michael Gross, 251–58. Clifton, N.J.: Humana Press, 1980.

Coolidge, Grace. "Wanted: To Save the Babies." *American Indian Magazine: A Journal of Race Progress* 5, no. 1 (1917): 17–22.

Dyk, Walter, ed. *Left Handed, Son of Old Man Hat: A Navajo Autobiography*. Lincoln: University of Nebraska Press, 1967.

Engelmann, George. *Labor among Primitive Peoples*. St. Louis, Mo.: J. H. Chambers, 1884 (1882).

———. "Pregnancy, Parturition, and Childbed among Primitive People." *American Journal of Obstetrics and Diseases of Women and Children* 14 (1881): 602–18.

Gaskin, Stephen. *Hey Beatnik! This Is the Farm Book*. Summertown, Tenn.: Tennessee Book Publishing, 1974.

Green, Rayna. "Diary of a Native American Feminist." *Ms. Magazine*, July/Aug. 1982.

Gregg, Elinor. *The Indians and the Nurse*. Norman: University of Oklahoma Press, 1965.

Guthrie, M. C. "The Health of the American Indian." *Public Health Reports* 44, no. 16 (1929): 945–57.

Highwalking, Belle, with Katherine Weist. *Belle Highwalking: The Narrative of a Northern Cheyenne Woman*. Billings: Montana Council for Indian Education, 1979.

Hinkell, Therese, comp. *Nurse of the Twentieth Century: Susie Walking Bear Yellowtail, First Native American Registered Nurse*. Shelburne, Mass.: Therese Hinkell, 2000.

Hoffman, Frederick. *Race Traits and Tendencies of the American Negro*. New York: Macmillan, 1896.

Hoffman, Walter J. "Childbirth and Abortion among the Absoroka (or Crow) and Dakota Indians." *European Review of Native American Studies* 1, no. 1 (1888): 9–10.

Hogan, Lillian Bullshows, with Barbara Loeb and Mardell Hogan Plainfeather. *The Woman Who Loved Mankind: The Life of a Twentieth-Century Crow Elder*. Lincoln: University of Nebraska Press, 2012.

Holder, A. B. "Gynecic Notes Taken among the American Indians." *American Journal of Obstetrics and Diseases of Women and Children* 25 (1892): 752–68.

Holt, L. Emmett. *The Care and Feeding of Children: A Catechism for the Use of Mothers and Children's Nurses*. New York: D. Appleton, 1904 (1894).

Holt, L. Emmett, and Henry L. K. Shaw. *Save the Babies*. Chicago: American Medical Association, 1915.

Kane, Robert, and Rosalie Kane. *Federal Health Care (with Reservations!)*. New York: Springer, 1972.

Kappler, Charles, ed. *Indian Treaties, 1778–1883*. New York: Interland Publishing, 1972.

Lakota Law People's Project. *The Total IV Solution: Sovereignty and Self-Governance in the Provision of Child and Family Services*. 8 July 2013. https://s3-us-west-1.amazonaws.com/lakota-peoples-law/uploads/LPLP-Sovereignty-and-Self-Governance.pdf.

Lansdale, Robert. "The Place of the Social Worker in the Indian Service Program." *Hospital Social Service* 27 (1933): 96–102.

Laughlin, Harry Hamilton. *Eugenical Sterilization in the United States*. Chicago: Psychopathic Laboratory of the Municipal Court of Chicago, 1922.

Leforge, Thomas. *Memoirs of a White Crow Indian*. New York: Century, 1928.

Linderman, Frank. *Plenty-Coups: Chief of the Crows*. Lincoln: University of Nebraska Press, 2002 (1930).

———. *Pretty-Shield: Medicine Woman of the Crows*. New York: John Day, 1972 (1932).

Lowie, Robert. *The Crow Indians*. New York: Farrar & Rinehart, 1935.

Madigan, La Verne. *The American Indian Relocation Program*. New York: Association on American Indian Affairs, 1956.

Mankiller, Wilma, with Michael Wallis. *Mankiller: A Chief and Her People*. New York: St. Martin's Griffin, 1993.

Medicine Crow, Joseph, with Herman J. Viola. *Counting Coup: Becoming a Crow Chief on the Reservation and Beyond*. Washington, D.C.: National Geographic, 2006.

Mitchell, Rose, with Charlotte Frisbie. *Tall Woman: The Life Story of Rose Mitchell, a Navajo Woman*. Albuquerque: University of New Mexico Press, 2001.

Morey, Sylvester, and Olivia Gilliam, eds. *Respect for Life: The Traditional Upbringing of American Indian Children*. Garden City, N.Y.: Waldorf Press, 1974.

Nabokov, Peter. *Two Leggings: The Making of a Crow Warrior*. Lincoln: University of Nebraska Press, 1982 (1967).

Native American Research Group. *Native American Families in the City*. San Francisco: Institute for Scientific Analysis, 1975.

"Native American Students." *American Journal of Nursing* 41, no. 12 (1941): 1442–43.

Neog, Prafulla, Richard G. Woods, and Arthur M. Harkins. *Chicago Indians: The Effects of Urban Migration*. Minneapolis: University of Minnesota Press, 1970.

Rude, Anna E. "The Midwife Problem in the United States." *Journal of the American Medical Association* 81, no. 12 (1923): 987–92.

Sekaquaptewa, Helen, with Louise Udall. *Me and Mine: The Life Story of Helen Sekaquaptewa*. Tucson: University of Arizona Press, 1969.

Shaw, Anna Moore. *A Pima Past*. Tucson: University of Arizona Press, 1974.

Snell, Alma Hogan, with Becky Matthews. *Grandmother's Grandchild: My Crow Indian Life*. Lincoln: University of Nebraska Press, 2000.

Stewart, Irene, with Doris Ostrander Dawdy. *A Voice in Her Tribe: A Navajo Woman's Story*. Socorro, N.M.: Ballena Press, 1980.

Voget, Fred W. *They Call Me Agnes: A Crow Narrative Based on the Life of Agnes Yellowtail Deernose*. Norman: University of Oklahoma Press, 1995.

West, Mary Mills. *Prenatal Care*. Washington, D.C.: Government Printing Office, 1915.

Williams, J. Whitridge. "Medical Education and the Midwife Problem in the United States." *Journal of the American Medical Association* 58 (1912): 1–7.

Woodruff, Janette. *Indian Oasis*. Caldwell, Idaho: Caxton Printers, 1939.

Yellowtail, Susie, with Marina Brown Weatherly. "Susie Walking Bear Yellowtail: A Life Story." Unpublished manuscript. August 2015. Printed manuscript.

Yellowtail, Thomas, with Michael Fitzgerald. *Yellowtail: Crow Medicine Man and Sun Dance Chief*. Norman: University of Oklahoma Press, 1991.

Secondary Sources

Abel, Emily, and Nancy Reifel. "Interactions between Public Health Nurses and Clients on American Indian Reservations during the 1930s." *Social History of Medicine* 9, no. 1 (1996): 89–108.

Adams, David Wallace. *Education for Extinction: American Indians and the Boarding School Experience, 1875–1928*. Lawrence: University Press of Kansas, 1995.

Adler, Jessica. *Burdens of War: Creating the United States Veterans Health System*. Baltimore: Johns Hopkins University Press, 2017.

Albers, Patricia, and Beatrice Medicine. *The Hidden Half: Studies of Plains Indian Women*. Lanham, Md.: University Press of America, 1983.

Allison, James Robert III. *Sovereignty for Survival: American Energy Development and Indian Self-Determination*. New Haven, Conn.: Yale University Press, 2015.

Anderson, Kim. *A Recognition of Being: Reconstructing Native Womanhood*. Toronto: Sumach Press, 2000.

Apple, Rima. *Mothers and Medicine: A Social History of Infant Feeding, 1890–1950*. Madison: University of Wisconsin Press, 1987.

———. *Perfect Motherhood: Science and Childrearing in America*. New Brunswick, N.J.: Rutgers University Press, 2006.

Arnold, Laurie. *Bartering with the Bones of Their Dead: The Colville Confederated Tribes and Termination*. Seattle: University of Washington Press, 2012.

Askins, Kathryn. "Bridging Cultures: American Indian Students at the Northfield Mount Hermon School." PhD diss., University of New Hampshire, 2009.

Baldy, Cutcha Risling. "'mini-k'iwh'e:n (For That Purpose—I Consider Things): (Re)writing and (Re)righting Indigenous Menstrual Practices to Intervene on Contemporary Menstrual Discourse and the Politics of Taboo." *Cultural Studies—Critical Methodologies* 17, no. 1 (2017): 21–29.

———. *We Are Dancing for You: Native Feminisms and the Revitalization of Women's Coming-of-Age Ceremonies*. Seattle: University of Washington Press, 2018.

Barker, Joanne. *Native Acts: Law, Recognition, and Cultural Authenticity*. Durham, N.C.: Duke University Press, 2011.

Begay, R. Cruz. "Changes in Childbirth Knowledge." *American Indian Quarterly* 18, nos. 3 & 4 (2004): 550–65.

Beisel, Nicola, and Tamara Kay. "Abortion, Race, and Gender in Nineteenth-Century America." *American Sociologist Review* 69, no. 4 (2004): 498–514.

Benson, Megan. "The Fight for Crow Water, Part II: Damming the Bighorn." *Montana: The Magazine of Western History* 58, no. 1 (2008): 3–23.

Bergman, Abraham, David C. Grossman, Angela M. Erdrich, John G. Todd, and Ralph Forquera. "A Political History of the Indian Health Service." *Milbank Quarterly* 77, no. 4 (1999): 571–604.

Bernstein, Alison. *American Indians and World War II: Toward a New Era in Indian Affairs*. Norman: University of Oklahoma Press, 1991.

―――. "A Mixed Record: The Political Enfranchisement of American Indian Women during the New Deal." *Journal of the West* 23, no. 3 (1984): 13–20.

Blackhawk, Ned. "I Can Carry On from Here: The Relocation of American Indians to Los Angeles." *Wicazo Sa Review* 11, no. 2 (1995): 16–30.

Blansett, Kent. Comments, "State of the Field: American Indian History." Western History Association, Newport Beach, Calif., 18 Oct. 2014.

―――. Comments, "State of the Field: American Indian History." Western History Association, San Diego, Calif., 3 Nov. 2017.

―――. *A Journey to Freedom: Richard Oakes, Alcatraz, and the Red Power Movement.* New Haven, Conn.: Yale University Press, 2018.

Bradley, Charles Crane, Jr. "After the Buffalo Days: Documents on the Crow Indians from the 1880s to the 1920s." MA thesis, Montana State University-Bozeman, 1970.

Briggs, Laura. *How All Politics Became Reproductive Politics: From Welfare Reform to Foreclosure to Trump.* Berkeley: University of California Press, 2017.

―――. "The Race of Hysteria: 'Overcivilization' and the 'Savage' Woman in Late Nineteenth-Century Obstetrics and Gynecology." *American Quarterly* 52, no. 2 (2000): 246–73.

―――. *Reproducing Empire: Race, Sex, Science, and U.S. Imperialism in Puerto Rico.* Berkeley: University of California Press, 2002.

Brown, Kathleen. *Good Wives, Nasty Wenches, and Anxious Patriarchs: Gender, Race, and Power in Colonial Virginia.* Chapel Hill: University of North Carolina Press, 1996.

Buckley, Thomas. "Menstruation and the Power of Yurok Women: Methods in Cultural Reconstruction." *American Ethnologist* 9, no. 1 (1982): 47–60.

Burch, Susan. "'Dislocated Histories': The Canton Asylum for Insane Indians." *Women, Gender, and Families of Color* 2, no. 2 (2014): 141–62.

Burnett, Kristin. *Taking Medicine: Women's Healing Work and Colonial Contact in Southern Alberta, 1880-1930.* Vancouver: University of British Columbia Press, 2010.

Buss, James Joseph and C. Joseph Genetin-Pilawa, eds. *Beyond Two Worlds: Critical Conversations on Language and Power in Native North America.* Albany: SUNY Press, 2014.

Cahill, Cathleen. *Federal Fathers and Mothers: A Social History of the United States Indian Service, 1869-1933.* Chapel Hill: University of North Carolina Press, 2011.

Campbell, Gregory. "Changing Patterns of Health and Effective Fertility among the Northern Cheyenne of Montana, 1886-1903." *American Indian Quarterly* 15, no. 3 (1991): 339–58.

Carpio, Myla Vicenti. *Indigenous Albuquerque.* Lubbock: Texas Tech University Press, 2011.

―――. "The Lost Generation: American Indian Women and Sterilization Abuse." *Social Justice* 31, no. 4 (2004): 40–53.

―――. "Lost Generation: The Involuntary Sterilization of American Indian Women." MA thesis, Arizona State University, 1995.

Cassidy, Tina. *Birth: The Surprising History of How We Are Born*. New York: Atlantic Monthly Press, 2006.

Castle, Elizabeth. "Black and Native American Women's Activism in the Black Panther Party and the American Indian Movement." PhD diss., University of Cambridge, 2000.

Chapin, Christy Ford. *Ensuring America's Health: The Public Creation of the Corporate Health Care System*. New York: Cambridge University Press, 2015.

Child, Brenda. *Boarding School Seasons: American Indian Families, 1900-1940*. Lincoln: University of Nebraska Press, 2000.

———. *Holding Our World Together: Ojibwe Women and the Survival of Community*. New York: Viking, 2012.

———. *My Grandfather's Knocking Sticks: Ojibwe Family Life and Labor on the Reservation*. St. Paul: Minnesota Historical Society Press, 2014.

———. "Politically Purposeful Work: Ojibwe Women's Labor and Leadership in Postwar Minneapolis." In *Indigenous Women and Work: From Labor to Activism*, edited by Carol Williams, 240-53. Urbana: University of Illinois Press, 2012.

Cobb, Daniel. *Native Activism in Cold War America: The Struggle for Sovereignty*. Lawrence: University Press of Kansas, 2008.

Cohen, Betsy. "Stars in the Big Sky: A Collection of Montana's Remarkable, Forgotten Women." MA thesis, University of Montana, 1998.

Coleman, Arica. *That the Blood Stay Pure: African Americans, Native Americans, and the Predicament of Race and Identity in Virginia*. Bloomington: Indiana University Press, 2013.

Critchlow, Donald. *Intended Consequences: Birth Control, Abortion, and the Federal Government in Modern America*. New York: Oxford University Press, 1999.

Cunningham, Robert III, and Robert M. Cunningham Jr. *The Blues: A History of the Blue Cross and Blue Shield System*. DeKalb: Northern Illinois University, 1997.

Daily, David W. *Battle for the BIA: G. E. E. Lindquist and the Missionary Crusade against John Collier*. Tucson: University of Arizona Press, 2004.

Danziger, Edmund Jefferson, Jr. *Survival and Regeneration: Detroit's American Indian Community*. Detroit, Mich.: Wayne State University Press, 1991.

Davies, Wade. *Healing Ways: Navajo Health Care in the Twentieth Century*. Albuquerque: University of New Mexico Press, 2001.

Davis, Julie. *Survival Schools: The American Indian Movement and Community Education in the Twin Cities*. Minneapolis: University of Minnesota Press, 2013.

Davis, Susan. "Susie Yellowtail, 1903–1981." In *American Nursing: A Biographical Dictionary*, Vol. 2, edited by Vern L. Bullough, Lilli Sentz, and Alice P. Stein, 367-69. New York: Garland Publishing, 1992.

De Barros, Juanita. *Reproducing the British Caribbean: Sex, Gender, and Population Politics after Slavery*. Chapel Hill: University of North Carolina Press, 2014.

Deer, Sarah. *The Beginning and End of Rape: Confronting Sexual Violence in Native America*. Minneapolis: University of Minnesota Press, 2015.

Dejong, David. *"If You Knew the Conditions": A Chronicle of the Indian Medical Service and American Indian Health Care, 1908-1955*. Lanham, Md.: Lexington Books, 2008.

————. *Plagues, Politics, and Policy: A Chronicle of the Indian Health Service*. Lanham, Md.: Rowman & Littlefield Publishers, 2011.

DeLisle, Christine Taitano. "A History of Chamorro Nurse-Midwives in Guam and a 'Placental Politics' for Indigenous Feminism." *Intersections: Gender and Sexuality in Asia and the Pacific* 37 (2015). http://intersections.anu.edu.au/issue37/delisle.htm.

Deloria, Philip. *Indians in Unexpected Places*. Lawrence: University Press of Kansas, 2004.

Deloria, Vine, Jr. *Custer Died for Your Sins: An Indian Manifesto*. Norman: University of Oklahoma Press, 1988. First published 1969 by Macmillan.

————. "Legislation and Litigation concerning American Indians." *Annals of the American Academy of Political and Social Science* 436 (1978): 86–96.

Denetdale, Jennifer. "Chairmen, Presidents, and Princesses: The Navajo Nation, Gender, and the Politics of Tradition." *Wicazo Sa Review* 21, no. 1 (2006): 9–28.

Doran, Christopher. "Attitudes of 30 American Indian Women towards Birth Control." *Health Service Reports* 87, no. 7 (1972): 658–63.

Dorr, Gregory. *Segregation's Science: Eugenics and Society in Virginia*. Charlottesville: University of Virginia Press, 2008.

Drinnon, Richard. *Keeper of Concentration Camps: Dillon S. Myer and American Racism*. Berkeley: University of California Press, 1987.

Dyck, Erika. *Facing Eugenics: Reproduction, Sterilization, and the Politics of Choice*. Toronto: University of Toronto Press, 2013.

Dyck, Erika, and Maureen Lux. "Population Control in the 'Global North'? Canada's Response to Indigenous Reproductive Rights and Neo-Eugenics." *Canadian Historical Review* 97, no. 4 (2016): 481–512.

Ellinghaus, Katherine. *Blood Will Tell: Native Americans and Assimilation Policy*. Lincoln: University of Nebraska Press, 2017.

Ellis, Gayla Wadnizak, ed. *Every Woman Has a Story*. Minneapolis: Gayla Wadnizak Ellis, 1982.

Emmerich, Lisa. "Right in the Midst of My Own People: Native American Women and the Field Matron Program." *American Indian Quarterly* 15, no. 2 (1991): 201–16.

————. "'Save the Babies!': American Indian Women, Assimilation Policy, and Scientific Motherhood, 1912–1918." In *Writing the Range: Race, Class, and Culture in the Women's West*, edited by Elizabeth Jameson and Susan Armitage, 393–409. Norman: University of Oklahoma Press, 1997.

————. "'To Respect and Love and Seek the Ways of White Women': Field Matrons, the Office of Indian Affairs, and Civilization Policy, 1890–1938." PhD diss., University of Maryland, College Park, 1987.

Espino, Virginia. "Women Sterilized as They Give Birth: Population Control, Eugenics, and Social Protest in the Twentieth-Century United States." PhD diss., Arizona State University, 2007.

Finestone, Erika, and Cynthia Stirbys. "Indigenous Birth in Canada: Reconciliation and Reproductive Justice in the Settler State." In *Indigenous Experiences of Pregnancy and Childbirth*, edited by Hannah Tait Neufeld and Jaime Cidro, 176–202. Bradford, Ontario: Demeter Press, 2017.

Fixico, Donald. *Termination and Relocation: Federal Indian Policy, 1945–1960*. Albuquerque: University of New Mexico Press, 1986.

———. *The Urban Indian Experience in America*. Albuquerque: University of New Mexico Press, 2000.

Foster, Martha Harroun. "Of Baggage and Bondage: Gender and Status among Hidatsa and Crow Women." *American Indian Culture and Research Journal* 17, no. 2 (1993): 121–52.

Frey, Rodney. *The World of the Crow Indians: As Driftwood Lodges*. Norman: University of Oklahoma Press, 1987.

Gallagher, Nancy. *Breeding Better Vermonters: The Eugenics Project in the Green Mountain State*. Lebanon, N.H.: University Press of New England, 1999.

Gilbert, Matthew Sakiestewa. *Education beyond the Mesas: Hopi Students at Sherman Institute, 1902–1929*. Lincoln: University of Nebraska Press, 2010.

Gonzales, Angela, Judy Kertész, and Gabrielle Tayac. "Eugenics as Indian Removal: Sociohistorical Processes and the De(con)struction of American Indians in the Southeast." *Public Historian* 29, no. 3 (2007): 53–67.

Gordon, Colin. *Dead on Arrival: The Politics of Health Care in Twentieth-Century America*. Princeton, N.J.: Princeton University Press, 2003.

Gordon, Linda. *The Moral Property of Women: A History of Birth Control Politics in America*. Urbana: University of Illinois Press, 2002.

Gouveia, Grace Mary. "'Uncle Sam's Priceless Daughters': American Indian Women during the Great Depression, World War II, and the Postwar Era." PhD diss., Purdue University, 1994.

Green, Rayna. "The Pocahontas Perplex: The Image of Indian Women in American Culture." *Massachusetts Review* 16, no. 4 (1975): 698–714.

———. *Women in American Indian Society*. New York: Chelsea House Publishers, 1992.

Griffen, Joyce. "Life Is Harder Here: The Case of the Urban Navajo Woman." *American Indian Quarterly* 6, nos. 1/2 (1982): 90–104.

Guglielmo, Jennifer. "The Community Health Representative Program: Two Decades of American Indian Women's Health Activism." MA thesis, University of Wisconsin–Madison, 1990.

Gurr, Barbara. *Reproductive Justice: The Politics of Health Care for Native American Women*. New Brunswick, N.J.: Rutgers University Press, 2015.

Hacker, Jacob. *The Divided Welfare State: The Battle over Public and Private Social Benefits in the United States*. Cambridge: Cambridge University Press, 2002.

Hancock, Christin. "Health and Well-Being: Federal Indian Policy, Klamath Women, and Childbirth." *Oregon Historical Quarterly* 117, no. 2 (2016): 166–97.

———. "Healthy Vocations: Field Nursing and the Religious Overtones of Public Health." *Journal of Women's History* 23, no. 3 (2011): 113–37.

Harding, Rita. "Traditional Beliefs and Behaviors Affecting Childbearing Practices of Crow Indian Women." MA thesis, Montana State University-Bozeman, 1981.

Hartmann, Betsy. *Reproductive Rights and Wrongs: The Global Politics of Population Control*. Boston: South End Press, 1995.

Haskins, Victoria. *Matrons and Maids: Regulating Indian Domestic Service in Tucson, 1914-1934*. Tucson: University of Arizona Press, 2012.

Hattori, Anne Perez. *Colonial Dis-Ease: U.S. Navy Health Policies and the Chamorros of Guam, 1898-1941*. Honolulu: University of Hawaii Press, 2004.

Herrman, Eleanor. "Connecticut and the First Native American Trained Nurse: More Questions Than Answers." *Connecticut Nursing News* 73 (Feb. 2001): 7-8.

Hoffman, Beatrix. *Health Care for Some: Rights and Rationing in the United States Since 1930*. Chicago: University of Chicago Press, 2012.

Holloway, Pippa. *Sexuality, Politics, and Social Control in Virginia, 1920-1945*. Chapel Hill: University of North Carolina Press, 2006.

Holt, Marilyn Irvin. *Indian Orphanages*. Lawrence: University Press of Kansas, 2001.

Hoover, Elizabeth, Katsi Cook, Ron Plain, Kathy Sanchez, Vi Waghiyi, and Pamela Miller. "Indigenous Peoples of North America: Environmental Exposures and Reproductive Justice." *Environmental Health Perspectives* 120, no. 12 (2012): 1645-49.

Howard, Heather. "Women's Class Strategies as Activism in Native Community Building in Toronto, 1950-75." In *Keeping the Campfires Going: Native Women's Activism in Urban Communities*, edited by Susan Krouse and Heather Howard, 134-53. Lincoln: University of Nebraska Press, 2009.

Hoxie, Frederick. *A Final Promise: The Campaign to Assimilate the Indians, 1880-1920*. Lincoln: University of Nebraska Press, 1984.

———. *Parading through History: The Making of the Crow Nation in America, 1805-1935*. Cambridge: Cambridge University Press, 1995.

———. *This Indian Country: American Indian Activists and the Place They Made*. New York: Penguin Books, 2012.

Hoxie, Frederick, and Tim Bernardis. "Robert Yellowtail: Crow." In *The New Warriors: Native American Leaders Since 1900*, edited by R. David Edmunds, 55-78. Lincoln: University of Nebraska Press, 2001.

Humalajoki, Reetta. "'What Is It to Withdraw?': Klamath and Navajo Tribal Councils' Tactics in Negotiating Termination Policy, 1949-1964." *Western Historical Quarterly* 48, no. 4 (2017): 415-38.

Hunt, Nancy Rose. *A Colonial Lexicon of Birth Ritual, Medicalization, and Mobility in the Congo*. Durham, N.C.: Duke University Press, 1999.

Intertribal Friendship House. *Urban Voices: The Bay Area American Indian Community*. Edited by Susan Lobo. Tucson: University of Arizona Press, 2002.

Jacobs, Margaret. "Bearing Witness to California Genocide." *Journal of Genocide Research* 19, no. 1 (2017): 143-49.

———. "Diverted Mothering among American Indian Domestic Servants." In *Indigenous Women and Work: From Labor to Activism*, edited by Carol Williams, 179-92. Urbana: University of Illinois Press, 2012.

———. *A Generation Removed: The Fostering and Adoption of Indigenous Children in the Postwar World*. Lincoln: University of Nebraska Press, 2014.

———. *White Mother to a Dark Race: Settler Colonialism, Maternalism, and the Removal of Indigenous Children in the American West and Australia, 1880-1940*. Lincoln: University of Nebraska Press, 2009.

Jagodinsky, Katrina. *Legal Codes and Talking Trees: Indigenous Women's Sovereignty in the Sonoran and Puget Sound Borderlands, 1854–1946.* New Haven, Conn.: Yale University Press, 2016.

Jaimes, M. Annette, and Theresa Halsey. "American Indian Women: At the Center of Resistance in Indigenous Resistance in North America." In *The State of Native America: Genocide, Colonization, and Resistance*, edited by M. Annette James, 311–44. Boston: South End Press, 1992.

Jasen, Patricia. "Race, Culture, and the Colonization of Childbirth in Northern Canada." *Social History of Medicine* 10, no. 3 (1997): 383–400.

Kekahbah, Janice, and Rosemary Wood, eds. *Life Cycle of the American Indian Family.* Norman, Okla.: American Indian/Alaska Native Nurses Association, 1980.

Keller, Jean. *Empty Beds: Indian Student Health at Sherman Institute, 1902–1922.* East Lansing: Michigan State University Press, 2002.

Kelm, Mary-Ellen. *Colonizing Bodies: Aboriginal Health and Healing in British Columbia, 1900–1950.* Vancouver: University of British Columbia Press, 1998.

Kessler-Harris, Alice. *Out to Work: A History of Wage-Earning Women in the United States.* New York: Oxford University Press, 1982.

King, Farina. *The Earth Memory Compass: Diné Landscapes and Education in the Twentieth Century.* Lawrence: University Press of Kansas, 2018.

Klann, Mary. "Babies in Baskets: Motherhood, Tourism, and American Indian Identity in Indian Baby Shows, 1916–1949." *Journal of Women's History* 29, no. 2 (2017): 38–61.

Klein, Laura, and Lillian Ackerman, eds. *Women and Power in Native North America.* Norman: University of Oklahoma Press, 1995.

Kline, Wendy. *Bodies of Knowledge: Sexuality, Reproduction, and Women's Health in the Second Wave.* Chicago: University of Chicago Press, 2010.

———. *Building a Better Race: Gender, Sexuality, and Eugenics from the Turn of the Century to the Baby Boom.* Berkeley: University of California Press, 2001.

———. "Communicating a New Consciousness: Countercultural Print and the Home Birth Movement of the 1970s." *Bulletin of the History of Medicine* 89, no. 3 (2015): 527–56.

Kluchin, Rebecca. *Fit to Be Tied: Sterilization and Reproductive Rights in America, 1950–1980.* New Brunswick, N.J.: Rutgers University Press, 2009.

Koblitz, Ann Hibner. *Sex and Herbs and Birth Control: Women and Fertility Regulation through the Ages.* Seattle: Kovalesvskaia Fund, 2014.

Kuletz, Valerie. *The Tainted Desert: Environmental Ruin in the American West.* New York: Routledge, 1998.

Kunitz, Stephen. *Disease Change and the Role of Medicine: The Navajo Experience.* Berkeley: University of California Press, 1983.

———. "The History and Politics of U.S. Health Care Policy for Native Americans and Alaska Natives." *American Journal of Public Health* 86, no. 10 (1996): 1464–73.

Ladd-Taylor, Molly. *Fixing the Poor: Eugenic Sterilization and Child Welfare in the Twentieth Century.* Baltimore: Johns Hopkins University Press, 2017.

———. "'Grannies' and 'Spinsters': Midwife Education under the Sheppard-Towner Act." *Journal of Social History* 22, no. 2 (1988): 255–75.

———. *Mother-Work: Women, Child Welfare, and the State, 1890-1930*. Urbana: University of Illinois Press, 1994.

LaDuke, Winona. *All Our Relations: Native Struggles for Land and Life*. Chicago: Haymarket Books, 1999.

LaGrand, James. *Indian Metropolis: Native Americans in Chicago, 1945-1975*. Urbana: University of Illinois Press, 2002.

Landwehr, Gretchen. "Nurse Midwifery within the Indian Health Service." MA thesis, Yale University, 2002.

LaPier, Rosalyn, and David Beck. "A 'One-Man Relocation Team': Scott Henry Peters and American Indian Urban Migration in the 1930s." *Western Historical Quarterly* 45, no. 1 (2014): 17-36.

Lawrence, Jane. "The Indian Health Service and the Sterilization of Native American Women." *American Indian Quarterly* 24, no. 3 (2000): 400-419.

Lear, Jonathan. *Radical Hope: Ethics in the Face of Cultural Devastation*. Cambridge, Mass.: Harvard University Press, 2006.

Leavitt, Judith Walzer. *Brought to Bed: Childbearing in America, 1750 to 1950*. New York: Oxford University Press, 1986.

Liberty, Margot, David V. Hughey, and Richard Scaglion. "Rural and Urban Omaha Indian Fertility." *Human Biology* 48, no. 1 (1976): 59-71.

———. "Rural and Urban Seminole Indian Fertility." *Human Biology* 48, no. 4 (1976): 741-55.

Lindenmeyer, Kriste. *"A Right to Childhood": The U.S. Children's Bureau and Child Welfare, 1912-46*. Urbana: University of Illinois Press, 1997.

Litoff, Judy Barrett. *The American Midwife Debate: A Sourcebook on Its Modern Origins*. New York: Greenwood Press, 1986.

———. *American Midwives, 1860 to the Present*. Westport, Conn.: Greenwood Press, 1978.

Lobo, Susan. "Urban Clan Mothers: Key Households in Cities." In *Keeping the Campfires Going: Native Women's Activism in Urban Communities*, edited by Susan Krouse and Heather Howard, 1-21. Lincoln: University of Nebraska Press, 2009.

Lomawaima, K. Tsianina. "Domesticity in the Federal Indian Schools: The Power of Authority over Body and Mind." *American Ethnologist* 20, no. 2 (1993): 227-40.

———. *They Called It Prairie Light: The Story of Chilocco Indian School*. Lincoln: University of Nebraska Press, 1994.

Lombardo, Paul. *Three Generations, No Imbeciles: Eugenics, the Supreme Court, and Buck v. Bell*. Baltimore: Johns Hopkins Press, 2008.

Lovett, Laura L. *Conceiving the Future: Pronatalism, Reproduction, and the Family in the United States, 1890-1938*. Chapel Hill: University of North Carolina Press, 2007.

Lukere, Vicki, and Margaret Jolly, eds. *Birthing in the Pacific: Beyond Tradition and Modernity?* Honolulu: University of Hawaii Press, 2002.

Lux, Maureen. *Medicine That Walks: Disease, Medicine, and Canadian Plains Native People, 1880-1940*. Toronto: University of Toronto Press, 2001.

———. "We Demand 'Unconditional Surrender': Making and Unmaking the Blackfoot Hospital." *Social History of Medicine* 25, no. 3 (2012): 665-84.

Mackey, Mike. "Closing the Fort Washakie Hospital: A Case Study in Federal Termination Policy." *Wyoming History Journal* 67, no. 2 (1995): 36–42.

Madley, Benjamin. *An American Genocide: The United States and the California Indian Catastrophe, 1846–1873*. New Haven, Conn.: Yale University Press, 2016.

———. "Reexamining the American Genocide Debate: Meaning, Historiography, and New Methods." *American Historical Review* 120, no. 1 (2015): 98–139.

Martucci, Jessica. *Back to the Breast: Natural Motherhood and Breastfeeding in America*. Chicago: University of Chicago Press, 2015.

Matthews, Becky. "Changing Lives: Baptist Women, Benevolence, and Community on the Crow Reservation, 1904–60." *Montana: The Magazine of Western History* 61, no. 2 (2011): 3–29.

———. "Wherever That Singing Is Going: The Interaction of Crow and Euro-American Women, 1880–1945." PhD diss., Auburn University, 2002.

McBride, Preston. "A Blueprint for Death in U.S. Off-Reservation Boarding Schools: Rethinking Institutional Mortalities at Carlisle Indian Industrial School, 1879–1918." MA thesis, Dartmouth, 2013.

McCallum, Mary Jane Logan. *Indigenous Women, Work, and History, 1940–1980*. Winnipeg: University of Manitoba Press, 2014.

McCleary, Katherine Nova. "*Apsáalooke Bíaanne Akdia* (Crow Midwives): Empowering *Bia* ("Women") and Resisting United States Health Care, 1907–1947." Senior essay, Yale University, 2018.

McCleary, Timothy. "Akbaatashee: The Oilers Pentecostalism among the Crow Indians." MA thesis, University of Montana, 1993.

———. *Crow Indian Rock Art: Indigenous Perspectives and Interpretations*. Walnut Creek, Calif.: Left Coast Press, 2016.

———. *The Stars We Know: Crow Astronomy and Lifeways*. Long Grove, Ill.: Waveland Press, 1996.

McCloskey, Joanne. *Living through the Generations: Continuity and Change in Navajo Women's Lives*. Tucson: University of Arizona Press, 2007.

McSwain, Romola Mae. "The Role of Wives in the Urban Adjustment of Navajo Migrant Families to Denver, Colorado." MA thesis, University of Hawaii, 1965.

Meckel, Richard. *Save the Babies: American Public Health Reform and the Prevention of Infant Mortality, 1850–1925*. Baltimore: Johns Hopkins University Press, 1990.

Medicine Crow, Joseph. "The Effect of European Culture Contacts upon the Economic, Social and Religious Life of the Crow Indians." MA thesis, University of Southern California, 1939.

———. *From the Heart of Crow Country*. New York: Orion Books, 1992.

Melcher, Mary. *Pregnancy, Motherhood, and Choice in Twentieth-Century Arizona*. Tucson: University of Arizona Press, 2012.

———. "'Women's Matters': Birth Control, Prenatal Care, and Childbirth in Rural Montana, 1910–1940." *Montana: The Magazine of Western History* 41, no. 3 (1991): 47–56.

Menzel, Annie. "The Political Life of Black Infant Mortality." PhD diss., University of Washington, 2014.

Metcalf, Warren. *Termination's Legacy: The Discarded Indians of Utah*. Lincoln: University of Nebraska Press, 2002.

Meyer, Melissa L. *The White Earth Tragedy: Ethnicity and Dispossession at a Minnesota Anishinaabe Reservation, 1889-1920*. Lincoln: University of Nebraska Press, 1994.

Mihesuah, Devon. "Commonality of Difference: American Indian Women and History." *American Indian Quarterly* 20, no. 1 (1996): 15-27.

———. *Indigenous American Women: Decolonization, Empowerment, Activism*. Lincoln: University of Nebraska Press, 2003.

Miller, Douglas. "Dignity and Decency: Father Peter Powell and American Indian Relocation to Chicago." In *Native Americans and the Legacy of Harry S. Truman*, edited by Brian Hosmer, 25-46. Kirksville, Mo.: Truman State University Press, 2010.

———. "Willing Workers: Urban Relocation and American Indian Initiative, 1940s-1960s." *Ethnohistory* 60, no. 1 (2013): 51-76.

Million, Dian. "Felt Theory: An Indigenous Feminist Approach to Affect and History." *Wicazo Sa Review* 24, no. 2 (2009): 53-76.

———. *Therapeutic Nations: Healing in an Age of Indigenous Human Rights*. Tucson: University of Arizona Press, 2013.

Moerman, Daniel. *Native American Ethnobotany*. Portland, Ore.: Timber Press, 1998.

Molina, Natalia. *Fit to Be Citizens? Public Health and Race in Los Angeles, 1879-1939*. Berkeley: University of California Press, 2006.

Morgan, Jennifer L. *Laboring Women: Reproduction and Gender in New World Slavery*. Philadelphia: University of Pennsylvania Press, 2004.

Morgen, Sandra. *Into Our Own Hands: The Women's Health Movement in the United States, 1969-1990*. New Brunswick, N.J.: Rutgers University Press, 2002.

Murphy, Michelle. *Seizing the Means of Reproduction: Entanglements of Feminism, Health, and Technoscience*. Durham, N.C.: Duke University Press, 2012.

Neils, Elaine M. *Reservation to City: Indian Migration and Federal Relocation*. Chicago: Department of Geography, University of Chicago, Research Paper No. 131, 1971.

Niethammer, Carolyn. *I'll Go and Do More: Annie Dodge Wauneka, Navajo Leader and Activist*. Lincoln: University of Nebraska Press, 2001.

Officer, James. "The American Indian and Federal Policy." In *The American Indian in Urban Society*, edited by Jack Waddell and O. Michael Watson, 8-65. Boston: Little, Brown, 1971.

O'Neill, Colleen. "Charity or Industry? American Indian Women and Work Relief in the New Deal Era." In *Indigenous Women and Work: From Labor to Activism*, edited by Carol Williams, 193-209. Urbana: University of Illinois Press, 2012.

———. "Rethinking Modernity and the Discourse of Development in American Indian History, an Introduction." In *Native Pathways: American Indian Culture and Economic Development in the Twentieth Century*, edited by Brian Hosmer and Colleen O'Neill, 1-20. Boulder: University Press of Colorado, 2004.

Osburn, Katherine M. B. *Southern Ute Women: Autonomy and Assimilation on the Reservation, 1887-1934*. Albuquerque: University of New Mexico Press, 1998.

O'Sullivan, Meg Devlin. "Informing Red Power and Transforming the Second Wave: Native American Women and the Struggle against Coerced Sterilization in the 1970s." *Women's History Review* 25, no. 6 (2016): 965–82.

———. "More Destruction to These Family Ties: Native American Women, Child Welfare, and the Solution of Sovereignty." *Journal of Family History* 41, no. 1 (2016): 19–38.

———. "'We Worry about Survival': American Indian Women, Sovereignty, and the Right to Bear and Raise Children in the 1970s." PhD diss., University of North Carolina at Chapel Hill, 2007.

Pambrun, Audra. "Birth to School Age Children." In *Life Cycles of the American Indian Family*, edited by Janice Kekahbah and Rosemary Wood, 27–40. Norman, OK: American Indian/Alaska Native Nurses Association, 1980.

Perdue, Theda. *Cherokee Women: Gender and Culture Change, 1700-1835*. Lincoln: University of Nebraska Press, 1998.

Peroff, Nicholas. *Menominee Drums: Tribal Termination and Restoration, 1954-1974*. Norman: University of Oklahoma Press, 1982.

Petchesky, Rosalind Pollack. *Abortion and Woman's Choice: The State, Sexuality, and Reproductive Freedom*. Boston: Northeastern University Press, 1990 (1984).

Philp, Kenneth. "Stride toward Freedom: The Relocation of Indians to Cities, 1952-1960." *Western Historical Quarterly* 16, no. 2 (1985): 175–90.

———. *Termination Revisited: American Indians on the Trail to Self-Determination, 1933-1953*. Lincoln: University of Nebraska Press, 1999.

Powers, Marla. *Oglala Women: Myth, Ritual, and Reality*. Chicago: University of Chicago Press, 1986.

Puisto, Jaakko. *"This Is My Reservation, I Belong Here": The Salish Kootenai Indian Struggle against Termination*. Pablo, Mont.: Salish Kootenai College Press, 2016.

Putney, Diane. "Fighting the Scourge: American Indian Mobility and Federal Indian Policy, 1897-1928." PhD diss., Marquette University, 1980.

Quadagno, Jill. *One Nation Uninsured: Why the U.S. Has No National Health Insurance*. Oxford: Oxford University Press, 2005.

Ralstin-Lewis, D. Marie. "The Continuing Struggle against Genocide: Indigenous Women's Reproductive Rights." *Wicazo Sa Review* 20, no. 1 (2005): 71–95.

Ram, Kalpana, and Margaret Jolly, eds. *Maternities and Modernities: Colonial and Postcolonial Experiences in Asia and the Pacific*. Cambridge: Cambridge University Press, 1998.

Ramirez, Renya. "Henry Roe Cloud: A Granddaughter's Native Feminist Biographical Account." *Wicazo Sa Review* 24, no. 2 (2009): 77–103.

———. *Native Hubs: Culture, Community, and Belonging in Silicon Valley and Beyond*. Durham, N.C.: Duke University Press, 2007.

Reagan, Leslie. *When Abortion Was a Crime: Women, Medicine, and Law in the United States, 1867-1973*. Berkeley: University of California Press, 1997.

Rentner, Terry L., Dinah A. Tetteh, and Lynda Dixon. "Culture, Identity, and Spirituality in American Indians and Native People of Alaska Pregnancy Campaigns." In *Indigenous Experiences of Pregnancy and Birth*, edited by Hannah Tait Neufeld and Jaime Cidro, 50–69. Bradford, Ontario: Demeter Press, 2017.

Reverby, Susan. *Ordered to Care: The Dilemma of American Nursing, 1850–1945*. Cambridge: Cambridge University Press, 1987.

Rich, Miriam. "The Curse of Civilised Woman: Race, Gender, and the Pain of Childbirth in Nineteenth-Century American Medicine." *Gender and History* 28, no. 1 (2016): 57–76.

Rosenberg, Charles. *The Care of Strangers: The Rise of America's Hospital System*. New York: Basic Books, 1987.

Rosenthal, Nicholas. "Native Americans and Cities." In *Oxford Research Encyclopedia of American History*, 1–18. Oxford: Oxford University Press, online pub. Mar. 2015.

———. *Reimagining Indian Country: Native American Migration and Identity in Twentieth-Century Los Angeles*. Chapel Hill: University of North Carolina Press, 2012.

Ross, Loretta, Lynn Roberts, Erika Derkas, Whitney Peoples, and Pamela Bridgewater Toure. *Radical Reproductive Justice: Foundations, Theory, Practice, Critique*. New York: Feminist Press, 2017.

Ross, Loretta, and Rickie Solinger. *Reproductive Justice: An Introduction*. Berkeley: University of California Press, 2017.

Rzeczkowski, Frank. *Uniting the Tribes: The Rise and Fall of Pan-Indian Community on the Crow Reservation*. Lawrence: University Press of Kansas, 2012.

Schackel, Sandra K. "'The Tales Those Nurses Told!': Public Health Nurses among the Pueblo and Navajo Indians." *New Mexico Historical Review* 65 (Apr. 1990): 225–49.

Schoen, Johanna. *Choice and Coercion: Birth Control, Sterilization, and Abortion in Public Health and Welfare*. Chapel Hill: University of North Carolina Press, 2005.

Sebring, Serena. "Reproductive Citizenship: Women of Color and Coercive Sterilization in North Carolina, 1950–1980." PhD diss., Duke University, 2012.

Shoemaker, Nancy. *American Indian Population Recovery in the Twentieth Century*. Albuquerque: University of New Mexico Press, 1999.

———. "Urban Indians and Ethnic Choices: American Indian Organizations in Minneapolis, 1920–1950." *Western Historical Quarterly* 19, no. 4 (1988): 431–77.

Silliman, Jael, Marlene Gerber Fried, Elena Gutiérrez, and Loretta Ross. *Undivided Rights: Women of Color Organize for Reproductive Justice*. Cambridge, Mass.: South End Press, 2004.

Simpson, Leanne. "Birthing an Indigenous Resurgence: Decolonizing Our Pregnancy and Birthing Ceremonies." In *"Until Our Hearts Are on the Ground": Aboriginal Mothering, Oppression, Resistance and Rebirth*, edited by D. Memee Lavell-Harvard and Jeannette Corbiere Lavell, 25–33. Toronto: Demeter Press, 2006.

Slocumb, John C., Stephen J. Kunitz, and Charles L. Odoroff. "Complications with Use of IUD and Oral Contraceptives among Navajo Women." *Public Health Reports* 94, no. 3 (1979): 243–47.

Smith, Andrea. *Conquest: Sexual Violence and American Indian Genocide*. Cambridge, Mass.: South End Press, 2005.

Smith, J. Douglas. "The Campaign for Racial Purity and the Erosion of Paternalism in Virginia, 1922–1930: 'Nominally White, Biologically Mixed, and Legally Negro.'" *Journal of Southern History* 68, no. 1 (2002): 65–106.

Smith, Paul Chaat, and Robert Warrior. *Like a Hurricane: The Indian Movement from Alcatraz to Wounded Knee*. New York: New Press, 1996.

Snyder, Peter. "The Social Environment of the Urban Indian." In *The American Indian in Urban Society*, edited by Jack O. Waddell and O. Michael Watson, 206–43. Boston: Little, Brown, 1971.

Sorkin, Alan. *The Urban American Indian*. Lexington, Mass.: Lexington Books, 1978.

Starr, Paul. *The Social Transformation of American Medicine*. New York: Basic Books, 1982.

Stern, Alexandra. *Eugenic Nation: Faults and Frontiers of Better Breeding in Modern America*. Berkeley: University of California Press, 2005.

Stewart, Omer. "Peyotism in Montana." *Montana: The Magazine of Western History* 33, no. 2 (1983): 2–15.

Stidolph, Julie. "'The Hand That Rocks the Cradle': Shoshone and Arapaho Women in the Wind River Region and Assimilation Policy, 1880–1932." MA thesis, University of Wyoming, 2008.

Stoler, Ann Laura. *Carnal Knowledge and Imperial Power: Race and the Intimate in Colonial Rule*. Berkeley: University of California Press, 2002.

Stremlau, Rose. "Allotment, Jim Crow, and the State: Reconceptualizing the Privatization of Land, the Segregation of Bodies, and the Politicization of Sexuality in the Native South." *Native South* 10 (2017): 60–75.

———. "Rape Narratives on the Northern Paiute Frontier: Sarah Winnemucca, Sexual Sovereignty, and Economic Autonomy, 1844–1891." In *Portraits of Women in the American West*, edited by Dee Garceau-Hagen, 37–60. New York: Routledge, 2005.

———. *Sustaining the Cherokee Family: Kinship and the Allotment of an Indigenous Nation*. Chapel Hill: University of North Carolina Press, 2011.

Sturm, Circe. *Blood Politics: Race, Culture, and Identity in the Cherokee Nation of Oklahoma*. Berkeley: University of California Press, 2002.

Tabobondung, Rebeka, Sara Wolfe, Janet Smylie, Laura Senese, and Genevieve Blais. "Indigenous Midwifery as an Expression of Sovereignty." In *Mothers of the Nations: Indigenous Mothering as Global Resistance, Reclaiming and Recovery*, edited by D. Memee Lavell-Harvard and Kim Anderson, 71–87. Bradford, Ontario: Demeter Press, 2014.

Taylor, Theodore W. *The Bureau of Indian Affairs: Public Policies toward Indian Citizens*. Boulder, Colo.: Westview Press, 1984.

Temkin-Greener, Helena, Stephen J. Kunitz, David Broudy, Marlene Haffner. "Surgical Fertility Regulation among Women on the Navajo Indian Reservation." *American Journal of Public Health* 71, no. 4 (1981): 403–7.

Theobald, Brianna. "Settler Colonialism, Native American Motherhood, and the Politics of Terminating Pregnancies." In *Transcending Borders: Abortion in the Past and Present*, edited by Shannon Stettner, Katrina Ackerman, Kristin Burnett, and Travis Hay, 221–37. London: Palgrave-Macmillan, 2017.

Thomas, Lynn. *Politics of the Womb: Women, Reproduction, and the State in Kenya*. Berkeley: University of California Press, 2003.

Thomasson, Melissa. "From Sickness to Health: The Twentieth-Century Development of U.S. Health Insurance." *Explorations in Economic History* 39, no. 3 (2002): 233–53.

Tiffin, Susan. *In Whose Best Interest? Child Welfare Reform in the Progressive Era*. Westport, Conn.: Greenwood Press, 1982.

Torpy, Sally. "Native American Women and Coerced Sterilization: On the Trail of Tears in the 1970s." *American Indian Culture and Research Journal* 24, no. 2 (2000): 1–22.

Townsend, Camilla. *Pocahontas and the Powhatan Dilemma*. New York: Hill and Wang, 2004.

Townsend, Kenneth William. *World War II and the American Indian*. Albuquerque: University of New Mexico Press, 2000.

Trafzer, Clifford. "Infant Mortality on the Yakama Indian Reservation, 1914–1964." In *Medicine Ways: Disease, Health, and Survival among Native Americans*, edited by Clifford Trafzer and Diane Weiner, 76–94. Walnut Creek, Calif.: AltaMira Press, 2001.

Trafzer, Clifford, and Joel R. Hyer, eds. *"Exterminate Them": Written Accounts of the Murder, Rape, and Slavery of Native Americans during the California Gold Rush, 1848–1868*. East Lansing: Michigan State University Press, 1999.

Trennert, Robert. *Alternative to Extinction: Federal Indian Policy and the Beginnings of the Reservation System, 1846–51*. Philadelphia: Temple University Press, 1975.

———. "Sage Memorial Hospital and the Nation's First All-Indian School of Nursing." *Journal of Arizona History* 44, no. 4 (2003): 353–74.

———. "Victorian Morality and the Supervision of Indian Women Working in Phoenix, 1906–1930." *Journal of Social History* 22, no. 1 (1988): 113–28.

———. *White Man's Medicine: Government Doctors and the Navajo, 1863–1955*. Albuquerque: University of New Mexico Press, 1998.

Tsosie, Rebecca. "Changing Women: The Crosscurrents of American Feminine Identity." In *Unequal Sisters: A Multicultural Reader in U.S. Women's History*, edited by Vicki Ruiz and Ellen Carol DuBois, 508–30. New York: Routledge, 1994.

Ulrich, Roberta. *American Indian Nations from Termination to Restoration, 1953–2006*. Lincoln: University of Nebraska Press, 2010.

Volscho, Thomas. "Sterilization, Racism, and Pan-Ethnic Disparities of the Past Decade: The Continued Encroachment on Reproductive Rights." *Wicazo Sa Review* 25, no. 1 (2010): 17–31.

Weatherly, Marina Brown. "Susie Walking Bear Yellowtail: A Life Story." *North Dakota Quarterly* 67 (2000): 229–41.

Wertz, Richard W., and Dorothy C. Wertz. *Lying-In: A History of Childbirth in America*. New York: Free Press, 1977.

White, Louellyn. *Free to Be Mohawk: Indigenous Education at the Akwesasne Freedom School*. Norman: University of Oklahoma Press, 2015.

Wilkinson, Charles. *Blood Struggle: The Rise of Modern Indian Nations*. New York: Norton, 2005.

Wolf, Jacqueline. *Deliver Me from Pain: Anesthesia and Birth in America*. Baltimore: Johns Hopkins University Press, 2009.

Wolfe, Patrick. "Settler Colonialism and the Elimination of the Native." *Journal of Genocide Research* 8, no. 4 (2006): 387–409.

Wright, Mary C. "Creating Change, Reclaiming Indian Space in Post-World War II Seattle: The American Indian Women's Service League and the Seattle Indian Center, 1958–1978." In *Keeping the Campfires Going: Native Women's Activism in Urban Communities*, edited by Susan A. Krouse and Heather A. Howard, 125–45. Lincoln: University of Nebraska Press, 2009.

———. "The Woman's Lodge: Constructing Gender on the Nineteenth-Century Pacific Northwest Plateau." *Frontiers* 24, no. 1 (2003): 1–18.

Zola, Irving. "Medicine as an Institution of Social Control." In *The Sociology of Health and Illness—Critical Perspectives*, edited by Peter Conrad and Rochelle Kern, 379–70. New York: St. Martin's Press, 1986.

Index

Abenakis, 91
abortion: decline in, 41, 95, 194n134;
  federal policies surrounding, 16;
  and government threats of punitive
  measures, 40, 194n130; herbs used
  for, 30; illegality of, 39, 40; individual and community views
  regarding, 58, 153, 194n136; Native
  men on, 40–41; Native women on,
  152–53, 171, 218n33; obstacles in
  procuring, 8, 181–82; physicians'
  antiabortion campaign, 39, 58; U.S.
  Supreme Court on, 152; WARN on,
  218n36; women's reasons for ending
  pregnancy, 30–31, 39, 191n66,
  194n126
Abourezk, James, 158
adoption: for parents grieving loss of
  child, 27–28, 38–39; for sickly
  children, 28; temporary and long-
  term adoption procedures, 26, 38–39
African American communities, infant
  mortality rates in, 47
African American women: and reproductive justice, 180; sterilization of,
  89, 153, 156
akbaawasée (baby doctors), 125
Akwesasne, New York, 165, 167–69
Alan Guttmacher Institute, 152
Albuquerque, New Mexico, Native
  peoples' migration to, 101
Allison, James, 170
allotment: and Crow Reservation,
  38–39, 41, 126; Crow women's interest
  in, 40; land questions related to
  morality, 37–39; and men as heads-
  of-household, 38; and privatization of
  Indian land, 20, 37

American Association for the Study and
  Prevention of Infant Mortality, 47
American Civil Liberties Union of South
  Dakota, 176
American College of Obstetricians and
  Gynecologists, 223n15
American Indian Center of Chicago, 112
American Indian Council of the Bay
  Area (AICBA), 209nn62–63
American Indian Movement (AIM), 1,
  149, 158, 160–61, 165, 168, 178
American Indian Nurses Association
  (AINA), 157
American Indian Physicians Association
  (AIPA), 158
American Indian Women's Service
  League (Seattle), 112–13
*American Journal of Obstetrics and
  Diseases of Women and Children*, 34
Amnesty International, 175–76
Anderson, Joy (Assiniboine) (pseud-
  onym), 116
Arapahoes, 132–33, 138
Arapaho women, 44–45, 59
Arapooish (Crow chief), 19
Arnold, Laurie, 212n4
Asbury, Calvin, 73, 82
Asetoyer, Charon (Comanche), 182
assimilation. *See* cultural assimilation
Assiniboine women, 78
Australia, 3

baakáatawaxiia ("throwaway"
  ceremony), 28
Bacone Indian School, Oklahoma, 23, 74
Baptists, as missionaries, 24, 66, 82
Battle of the Little Bighorn, 18
Baucus, Max, 175

federal relocation program, 99–100, 102–10, 112, 114, 116, 119, 121, 123, 209nn62, 63; field nursing program of, 199n99; gendered familial model promoted by, 107, 118–19; and "getting out of the Indian business" language, 207n15; hospitals closed by, 131–32; Native employees steered away from home reservations, 80; as obstacle to Native progress, 129; and politics of blame, 6–7; promotional material on urban life, 102, 105; records of Crow Reservation, 15; and reduction of program responsibilities, 133, 146; reproduction-related policies and practices of, 6, 7, 16, 99–100; on reservation employment for Native peoples, 127–28; and termination policies, 130; and "well-baby" care, 143. *See also* Office of Indian Affairs (OIA)

Buren, Charles, 87, 204n78
Burke, Charles, 70
Burns, Elsie (Navajo) (pseudonym), 111–12, 117, 120–21

Cahill, Cathleen, 80, 139
Campbell, Maria (Metís), 4, 9–10
Canada: Aboriginal communities of, 193n110, 205n117; Indian hospitals of, 127; Indigenous women's birthing experiences in, 66; Inuit women on sterilization, 154; nationwide health program in, 108; relocation program of, 208n35; as settler-colonial society, 3
Canton Indian Asylum, South Dakota, 205n108
Carlisle Indian School, Pennsylvania, 23, 68, 85
Carpenter, James (Crow), 90
Carpio, Myla Vicenti, 110
Carson, Mary (Crow) (pseudonym), 109
Castle, Elizabeth, 161
Castro, Christina (Jemez/Taos/Ajchamen/Chicana), 180

Catholics, 24, 73
Centers for Disease Control, 152
Centers for Medicare and Medicaid Services, 177–78
Chamorro peoples, 62
Changing Woman Initiative, 179–80, 183
Chapin, Christy Ford, 109
Cherokee Council, 40–41
Cherokee men, 40–41
Cherokees, 26
Cheyenne, 20, 142
Cheyenne and Arapaho Agency, Oklahoma, 44, 63
Cheyenne River Reservation, South Dakota, 48, 66, 176
Cheyenne women: reproductive experiences of, 45, 141–42; resistance to hospital childbirth, 59; and Save the Babies campaign, 44
Chicago, Illinois: and federal relocation program, 104, 109–13, 115; Indian centers in, 112–13; Ruth Maney in, 11–12, 115
Child, Brenda (Ojibwe), 78–79, 161
childbirth: as stage in broader reproductive process, 11. *See also* hospital childbirth; pregnancy and childbirth
child mortality, 27, 41. *See also* infant mortality
Childs, Mae Takes Gun (Crow), 82
Christianity, 22, 24, 41
civilization: and evolutionary theory, 34–35, 42; and gender roles, 38, 51; and infant feeding practices, 52–53; and role of field matrons, 50
Claremore, Oklahoma, 157
Clark, Debbie (Cheyenne) (pseudonym), 103–4, 110–12, 114, 120, 208n27
Cold War, 129
Coleman, W. S., 68–69
colic, Crow midwives as colic specialists, 125, 191n64
Collier, John, 16, 75, 80–83, 90–91, 100, 129

colonialism: and Crow reproductive practices, 33–36, 39–41; cultural processes disrupted by, 9–10; economic pressures caused by, 75; and eugenics, 72; and flexibility of colonial power, 3–4; flexible child-rearing mitigating effects of, 26–27; forms of, 3, 6; and health conditions on reservations, 46; and imposition of patriarchal relationships, 83; and infant mortality, 27, 51; intimate colonialism, 178, 187n24; and meanings attached to Native women's bodies, 5, 34, 39; of medical institutions, 13; and midwives' training, 61; and patriarchal and biological line of inheritance of land, 38; and reservation hospitals, 124; and Save the Babies campaign, 44; settler colonialism, 3–5, 14; and sterilization abuses, 96, 159

Colvilles, 212n4

commonality of difference, 14

Community Health Representative (CHR) programs, 155–56, 168, 219n55

Conference on the Care of Dependent Children (1909), 46–47

Congregationalists, as missionaries, 24

Consolidated Chippewa Agency, Minnesota, 94, 95

Consolidated Salish and Kootenai Tribes, 131, 139

contraception. *See* birth control

contract hospitals: Indian Health Service's use of, 8, 175, 177; regulations of, 173; sterilization abuses in, 96, 147, 161

Cook, Katsi (Mohawk): on assessing past practices, 150, 194n133, 217n17; on birth control methods, 169; on environmental issues, 171; and midwifery, 148, 168, 170, 180–81; on sovereignty, 147, 161, 168; on sterilization abuse, 8, 166, 168; on termination policies, 145; and WARN,

1, 161, 169; Women's Dance Health Program, 165–69, 222n124

Coolidge, Grace, 62, 64

Crabbe, Theodore, 127

cradleboards, 51, 197n52

Critchlow, Donald, 148

Crow Agency: annual agricultural fair, 42; boarding school of, 22–23, 73; and Crow Tribal Council, 83; A. B. Holder as physician of, 33–36, 39–40; and Indian self-sufficiency, 37; Lodge Grass district, 24, 78, 135, 175; physicians of, 31, 33, 66, 79, 82–83, 86–87, 204n78; Pryor district, 33, 73, 77–78, 97, 125–26, 144; Reno district, 126; and reproductive autonomy of Crow women, 31; Samuel G. Reynolds as agent, 36–41, 44, 193n112; W. W. Scott as superintendent, 44, 195n1; Walter Q. G. Tucker as physician, 39–40; Wyola district, 86, 97, 138, 141

Crow Agency Hospital: construction of, 64, 66; construction of new hospital, 174; Crow hospital matron of, 68; Crows' negotiations with, 68–69, 134, 137–39, 141, 169, 173, 183, 200n136; Crows' use of, 75, 128; Crow women's involuntary sterilization at, 72, 86, 93, 96, 153; Crow women's resistance to hospital childbirth at, 78; Crow women's use of, 79–80, 98, 141; head nurse of, 68–69; inadequacies of, 79, 86–87, 134, 175; mistreatment of Crows at, 80; obstetric practices at, 141–42, 146, 175; proposed closure of, 131–33, 137, 140, 146; and sterilization abuses, 72, 96–97, 160; Susie Yellowtail as nurse in, 72, 75, 79–80, 86, 92, 127, 128, 155, 201n20, 202n45; Susie Yellowtail's birthing experiences in, 72

Crow birthing culture: and bonds between patrilineal and matrilineal kin, 28–29; and gender restrictions,

199n112; A. B. Holder's research on, 34–36; key features of, 18, 174–75; parameters of, 15, 19; and reservation system, 18, 29–33, 35–36, 39, 194n126; role of female kin in, 28, 31, 68, 77, 87–88. *See also* Crow reproductive practices

Crow children: boarding school for, 22; charges of maternal neglect, 28, 143–45; and flexible childrearing, 19, 26–27, 38, 41–42, 53–54, 73, 93, 145, 188–89n3; name selection, 28; and "rightful homes" policy, 38; "throwaway" ceremony for sickly children, 28

Crow cosmology, 30

Crow Fair, 81, 158

Crow families and households: marriage and divorce of Crows, 25–26, 38, 190n36; Samuel G. Reynolds's approach to, 37, 38–39

Crow Health Committee, 134–46, 167

Crow health council, 84–85, 134–35

Crow Indian Women's Club: on Crow Agency Hospital, 87; Crow Agency Women's Club, 129, 135, 146; founding of, 85–86; Lodge Grass Women's Club, 135; on treaty rights, 139; Fred Voget on, 203n66

Crow men: celebration of men's achievements, 25; and Crow Tribal Council, 83, 97; government's threats of punitive measures, 40; institutionalization of, 93–94; on life during reservation era, 189n16; men who dressed and lived as women, 25; opposition to cession of additional land, 41; Samuel G. Reynolds's linking of reproductive and land politics, 39–41; role of father's clan and kin, 25

Crow Nation: divisions among tribal leaders, 41; land cession of 1904, 37, 140; loss of homeland during allotment era, 20, 37; separation from Hidatsa, 19

Crow reproductive practices: autonomy in, 16, 30–31; and colonial scrutiny, 33–36, 39–41; federal intervention in, 15–16, 37, 42; and flexible childrearing, 19, 26–27, 29, 38, 41–42, 53–54, 73, 93, 145, 188–89n3; land politics linked to, 39–41; and Save the Babies campaign, 51–52; as sex-segregated process, 29; as social, cultural, and spiritual process, 19; and wealth measured in relatives, 28; Robert Yellowtail on, 84. *See also* Crow birthing culture

Crow Reservation, Montana: and allotment era, 38–39, 41, 126; assimilation pressures of, 16, 22; birth rates of, 36, 140, 194n134, 215n101; bureaucratic districts of, 20; and congregation of Crows in camps, 37; and Crow women's activism, 72, 85; cultural lifeways on, 81–83, 85; and demographic decline, 21–22, 189n15; and eugenic language and logic, 92, 153; government rations of, 36–37, 193n112; headquarters along Little Bighorn River, 18, 20; health services of, 122; and hospital childbirth, 64, 199n117; and infant mortality, 48; land cessions of, 20, 37, 140; missionaries living on, 24, 82; obstetrics and gynecology on, 85–91; reservation hospitals on, 42–43, 194n139; and reservation politics in 1930s, 80–85; and restrictions on mobility, 21–22, 30, 49; "rightful homes" policy, 38; and settlement groups of band and kin networks, 20; study of reproduction on, 13–15; and termination policies, 130, 131; towns of, 126; transportation available on, 126; white ranchers and farmers leasing reservation land, 37; and white settlers' demand for land, 41

Crows: clan and kinship networks of, 25–29, 41–42; demographic decline

Crows (*continued*)

of, 21, 189n15; formal relationship with federal government, 20; horses acquired by, 19; migration from northeastern North America, 19; mobility of, 21–22, 30, 49, 126; and practice of wife kidnapping, 190n36; reductions in Crow land, 20, 37; relationships with Euro-American fur traders, 20, 189n15; resistance to allotment, 37; treaties with United States, 20, 123; wealth measured in relatives, 28

Crow Tribal Council: and complaints regarding hospital staff and policies, 83–84, 96–97, 206n127; and Crow women's hospital childbirth experiences, 83–84; Crow women's participation in, 83, 135, 138–39, 203n56; and termination policies, 129, 131, 133

Crow women: activism of, 72, 85, 128, 135; and allotment issues, 40; and appeals to tribal council, 83–84; breastfeeding habits of, 84; female kin's role in childrearing, 26, 29, 52, 54; female kin's role in pregnancies, 31, 68, 77, 142, 144; gender roles of, 24, 29, 93; government obstetric services rejected by, 40; government physicians' surveillance of women's bodies and pregnancies, 40–41; grandmothers assuming responsibility for child care, 26, 29, 38, 54; grandmothers' role in birth, 28; as healers, 29, 30, 42, 125; and hospital childbirth, 79, 83–84, 89, 96, 98, 124–27, 141, 145–46; and matrilineal clan system, 25–26; memoirs of, 15; and menarche, 29–30; as midwives, 29; midwives valued by, 125; participation in Crow Tribal Council, 83, 135, 138–39, 203n56; pregnancy and childbirth in early reservation years, 29–33, 35–36, 192n98; resistance to

hospital childbirth, 78–79; resources controlled by, 25; sexual and reproductive autonomy of, 16, 30–31; sterilization of, 72, 86, 89–90, 93, 95–96, 98; value of women's role, 25, 41; as warriors, 25

cultural assimilation: and American Indian Movement, 160; and baby shows, 51, 197n52; biological reproduction as marker of, 7, 42; and boarding schools, 22, 83; John Collier on, 80–81; competing pressures regarding, 16, 22, 42; and eugenic campaigns, 8, 93, 205n108; federal government's assimilationist agenda, 19, 22, 24, 80–81, 99, 179; as form of violence, 6; and gender roles, 24, 93; gradual approaches to, 37; and health conditions on reservations, 46; and health insurance, 108; and A. B. Holder, 35; and hospital childbirth, 57, 61, 66, 110, 126; and Native healers, 57, 59–61; Native peoples' erasure through, 92; of Native women, 126; pessimism regarding, 9; and rejection of Native spiritual systems, 24; and reservation hospitals, 108; resistance to, 136; and Samuel G. Reynolds, 37; and Save the Babies campaign, 44, 51; and termination policies, 129, 145; and World War II, 101

cultural lifeways: on Crow Reservation, 81–83, 85; Native women's role in reproduction of, 4, 10; repression or suppression of, 6, 49

Custer, George Armstrong, 18

Dakota Access Pipeline, 178
Dallas, Texas, 108
Danziger, Edmund Jefferson, Jr., 113
Davies, Wade, 82, 128
Deer, Sarah, 194n126
Deernose, Agnes (Crow), 26, 29, 42, 77, 194n139

Deloria, Philip, 12

Deloria, Vine, Jr., 103, 128, 207n24, 214n80

Denetdale, Jennifer, 83

Denison, Inez Running Bear (Rosebud Sioux), 109–11, 113

Denver, Colorado, 105–6, 111, 114, 117, 120

Department of Health, Education, and Welfare (HEW): failure to provide oversight at contract hospitals, 8; and family planning services of Indian Health Service, 148, 156, 158; sterilization regulations of, 164, 171

Department of Health and Human Services (DHHS), 152

Department of the Interior, Office of Indian Affairs in, 20

Depression, 75, 91, 98

Detroit, Michigan, 113

Dixon, Lynda (Cherokee), 178

domestic imperialism, 24, 50, 51

Doran, Christopher, 154–55

Dyck, Erika, 154, 205n117

Edwards, Lowell, 144

Eisenhower, Dwight, 133

elimination campaigns, 9, 16, 96, 152

Emmerich, Lisa, 51

Emmons, Glenn, 132–33

Engelmann, George, 34–35, 36

environmental degradation, 3, 170–71

Espino, Virginia, 151

eugenic campaigns, 8–9, 72, 90–96, 98, 153, 205n108, 205n110

European colonies, and midwifery, 61

evolutionary theory, discourse of, 34–35, 42

extractive colonialism, 3

Family Planning Services and Population Research Act (1970), 153–55

The Farm, 168

federal government: abortion policies of, 16; Crows' formal relationship with, 20; efforts to "get out of Indian business," 102, 122, 207n15; intervention in biological reproduction, 7; intervention in Crow reproductive practices, 15–16, 37, 42; Native peoples' relationship with, 3, 6; privatization of Indian land, 20; promotion of hospital childbirth, 11, 44, 45–46, 62, 70, 75; relocation program to urban centers, 16, 98, 99, 101–11, 113, 121, 207n24; on reservation hospitals, 11, 44–45, 55–68, 70; restructuring efforts in Native families and households, 7, 45, 195n8. *See also* reservation system; *and specific government departments*

Felshaw, George, 99, 106

field matrons: childbirth supervised by, 56, 63; field nurses replacing, 70; home visits of, 44, 51, 58, 195n2; and hospital childbirth, 55, 69, 126; on infant feeding practices, 53; on infant mortality, 48–49; and maternalism, 49–52, 54; Native women's trust in, 66; and prenatal care, 54–55; and Save the Babies campaign, 49, 50–52, 54; training of, 54

field nurses: attendance at home births, 87–88; and Crow women's health initiatives, 85; education of Native women, 70; and eugenics campaigns, 93; hospital childbirth advocated by, 78; on "illegitimate" pregnancies, 78–79; Susie Yellowtail's application for work as, 80, 202n45

field relocation officers (FROs), 99, 107, 109, 112, 119–20

Finestone, Erika, 181

Fire Thunder, Cecelia (Oglala Sioux), 181–82

Fixico, Hannah (Lakota), 101, 104, 120

Flagstaff, Arizona, 119

Flathead Reservation, Montana, 56, 67, 130–31, 139

flexible childrearing: and Crow repro-
ductive practices, 19, 26–27, 29, 38,
41–42, 53–54, 73, 93, 145, 188–89n3;
and family planning services, 152–53,
218n36; government employees on,
54, 73, 93; and Native women's
migration to urban centers, 119, 120
Fond du Lac Indian Hospital, Cloquet,
Minnesota, 75, 79
Fort Belknap Reservation, Montana, 69,
90, 115
Fort Defiance, Arizona, 60, 64
Fort Defiance School and Agency,
Arizona, 60
Fort Laramie Treaty (1851), 20
Fort Laramie Treaty (1868), 20, 140
Fort Peck Reservation, Montana, 78
Fort Washakie Hospital, Wyoming, 132,
138
Franklin County Memorial Hospital,
Greenfield, Massachusetts, 74
fur trade, 20, 189n15

Gabouri, Frances, 207n17
Gallup Indian Medical Center, New
Mexico, 153–55
gender roles: and BIA's expectations
regarding work, 103; "civilized"
gender roles, 38, 51; complementarity
of, 25; of Crow women, 24, 29, 93;
and cultural assimilation, 24, 93;
federal Indian policy destabilizing,
40; and federal relocation program,
103, 104, 107, 119–20; and imposition
of patriarchal relationships, 40; in
Native families, 24, 25–29; of Native
men, 24, 38, 103, 105, 107, 120; and
nuclear family model, 38, 107,
118–19, 121; and politics, 39, 98;
Samuel G. Reynolds's approach to, 37,
38; and role of field matrons, 44,
50–51; and tribal health committees,
134; and tribal political structure,
83–84, 135; and vocational training,
103–4, 208n35

General Allotment Act of 1887, 20, 37
General Federation of Women's Clubs,
135
germs and germ transmission, 57
Glenn, John (Crow), 134
Goes Ahead (Crow), 18
Goes Ahead, Helen (Crow), 32
Gonzales, Nicolle (Navajo), 179–81,
183
Government Accountability Office
(GAO) investigation, 158–59, 164
government employees: and antiabortion campaign, 39; and John Collier's
policies, 82–83; condescending
attitudes of, 79, 109; on Crow health
council, 84; Crow women's pregnancies scrutinized by, 19, 40–41, 104;
eugenic language and logic used by,
92; expectations of, 22; fascination
with Native reproduction, 19; on
flexible childrearing, 54, 73, 93;
hospital childbirth promoted by, 56,
62, 78–79, 126; on hospital construction, 60, 198n95; institutionalization
of Crow men and women, 93–94;
interventions in pregnancy and
childbirth, 19, 40–42, 45, 61; on land
ownership and politics as concern of
men, 40; and land questions related
to morality, 37–39; and maternal
education, 51; on Native healers, 59,
82; on Native women as field matrons,
50; opposition to seclusion during
menstruation, 29; physicians and
hospitals advocated by, 7; promotion
of federal relocation program, 102,
207n22
government hospitals. See reservation
hospitals
Great Britain: colonies of, 61; nationwide health program in, 108
Great Plains Area (IHS), 176
Green, Rayna (Cherokee), 5, 164, 217n7
Gregg, Elinor, 206n131
Griffen, Joyce, 119

Linderman, Frank B., 15
Lippert, L. C., 131
Little Bighorn College Library, 15
Lomawaima, K. Tsianina, 192n92
Lone Wolf v. Hitchcock (1903), 37
Los Angeles, California, Native men and women migrating to, 99, 103–4, 112, 114–15, 117–18, 121
Los Angeles Indian Center, 109, 209–10n80
Lowie, Robert, 191n58, 192n77, 199n112
Lumbee women, 95
Lux, Maureen, 66, 154, 193n110

McCallum, Mary Jane Logan, 12, 127, 208n35
McCleary, Katherine Nova (Little Shell Chippewa-Cree), 80
McCleary, Timothy, 28, 191n64
McCloud, Janet (Tulalip and Nisqually), 161
McSwain, Romola Mae, 117, 121, 208n45
malnutrition: effect on infant mortality, 49; and government rations, 36, 55; and reservation system, 6, 21, 33
Maney, Rose (Ho-Chunk), 11–12, 115
Manifest Destiny, 5
Mankiller, Wilma (Cherokee), 103, 207n15
maternal health, 6–7, 71
maternal mortality, 32, 47–48, 196n24
matrilineal clan system, 25–26, 28–29
Matthews, Becky, 85, 194n139
Mattson, Margaret (Navajo) (pseudonym), 111, 117, 120
Means, Lorelei Decora (Ho-Chunk), 170–71, 217n5
Medicaid, 110, 153, 180
medical pluralism, 65, 126, 174
Medicine Crow, Joseph (Crow), 19, 24, 26, 136, 191n66
medicine men. *See* Native healers
Melany, Fazly A., 143–45
menarche, 29–30, 34

Menominees, 198n78
Menominee women, 65
Meriam, Lewis, 71–72, 100
Meriam Report, 71–72, 94, 100
Mexican American women, 151, 162
midwives and midwifery: abortion associated with, 58; adaptation and expansion of practices over time, 10–11, 42, 60–61, 98, 199n99; attendance preceding birth, 31; and breech births, 33; certified nurse midwives, 169, 176–77, 179, 222n136, 223n15; coexistence with hospital childbirth, 72, 77, 78, 97–98, 126–27, 174; as colic specialists, 125, 191n64; community's faith in, 29; decline in use of, 125, 126, 141; Euro-American observers' recognition of skills of, 32, 58; federal government's disparagement of, 71–72; as immigrants, 58–59; and Indian Health Service, 169, 176–77, 222n133, 222n136; influence on hospital childbirth, 65, 70; knowledge of women's health, 30, 33; legal threats to, 126; licensing of, 61, 62; limitations of, 32–33; modern midwifery movement, 147, 165, 168, 169, 174; as patient advocates, 11; payment of, 31; peyote used by, 11, 88–89; as political act of resistance for women, 13, 44; replacement of, 7, 43, 58; and reservation births, 33, 43, 59, 72; and ritual use of umbilical cord, 80; social commentators against, 58–59, 61–62, 198n85; spiritual component of, 59; techniques of, 32; "tradition" as historical process, 12; training of, 60–61, 165, 168–69, 179; on water as holy, 192n80; Robert Yellowtail on, 72, 77; Susie Yellowtail as midwife, 97–98, 125, 141, 206n129; Susie Yellowtail's use of, 88. *See also* pregnancy and childbirth
Mihesuah, Devon, 14
Miller, Douglas K., 111, 207n26

Minneapolis, Minnesota, 101, 160, 169
Minneapolis–St. Paul (Twin Cities), Minnesota, 14–15, 101, 121, 161–62, 165, 167–68
Minneapolis–St. Paul New School of Family Birthing, 165
Minnesota: sterilization of Native women in, 94–95, 205n113; WARN's Native midwifery training in, 14–15, 165, 168–69
Minnesota School for the Feeble-minded, Faribault, 94–95, 205n113
missionaries: as agents of domestic imperialism, 24, 51; and boarding schools, 74; on Crow Reservation, 24, 82; day schools of, 38; expectations of, 22; and government's assimilation campaign, 24; and hospital child-birth, 66, 126; Native women's trust in, 66; opposition to political and cultural consciousness on reserva-tions, 82; opposition to seclusion during menstruation, 29; on physi-cians and hospitals, 7; and "rightful homes" policy, 38; training of Indigenous birth attendants, 61
Mitchell, Rose (Tall Woman) (Navajo), 22
Modoc women, 35
Mohawk, John (Seneca), 147
Mohawk women, 168–69
Montana: abortion criminalized in, 39, 40; compulsory eugenic sterilization law of, 93; Indian birth rate in, 140; non-Native women's use of midwifery in, 78
Montana Inter-Tribal Policy Board, 130–31
Montana State Mental Hospital, Warm Springs, 69, 93
Montana State Training School, Boulder, 93
Moore, Barbara (Lakota), 163
Moore, Molly (Pima), 49
morality: Crow Agency Hospital used as jail for women, 87; and family

planning services, 148–49; field nurses on "illegitimate" pregnancies, 78–79; government employees' relating land questions to, 37–39; perceived sexual immorality of Native communities, 67; and physicians' antiabortion campaign, 39, 58; and pronatalism, 44; and punishment of Crow families and households, 38; Samuel G. Reynolds on, 38
Morin, Anita (Crow), 79
Mountain Crow, 19
Myer, Dillon S., 102, 131–32, 213n41

Nagel, Charles Edward, 84, 88–92, 96
National Center for Health Statistics, 48
National Lawyers' Guild Committee on Reproductive Rights, 161
National Women's Health Network, 164
Native American Church, 168
Native American Research Group, 119
Native American Women's Health Education Research Center, 182
Native children: and coercive methods for enforcing attendance at boarding schools, 22–24, 67, 200n132; compul-sory school attendance, 62; dangers of toddlerhood and early childhood, 48; federal policies on childrearing, 45, 195n8; and federal relocation program, 104–6, 118–21; and health conditions at boarding schools, 190n24; removal to white foster and adoptive homes, 3, 159, 162–64, 182. *See also* infant mortality
Native families and households: allotment as means of reform of, 37–38; and federal government's assimilationist agenda, 19, 22, 24; federal government's restructuring efforts, 7, 45, 195n8; and federal relocation program, 99–105, 113, 117–18; and flexible childrearing, 19, 26–27, 29, 38, 41–42, 53–54, 73, 93, 119, 120, 188–89n3; and gender roles,

24–29; nuclear family unit imposed on, 24, 38, 54, 113, 118–19, 121; separation of Native children at boarding schools, 22–24

Native feminist scholars, 40, 201n6. *See also specific scholars*

Native healers: certified nurse-midwives working with, 169, 177; Crow women as healers, 29–30, 42, 125; cultural assimilation allegedly hindered by, 57, 59–60, 61; and eradication of Native health ways, 45, 60, 82; health outcomes attributed to, 46; and medical pluralism, 65, 126, 174; and pregnancy and childbirth, 54, 113; public health nurses' cooperation with, 199n99; spiritual component of work, 59

Native men: on abortions, 40–41; emasculation of, 4; and eugenic campaigns, 9; and family planning services, 149–50; and federal relocation program, 107; and flexible childrearing, 189n3; gender roles of, 24, 38, 103, 105, 107, 120; as head of household, 24, 38, 103, 105, 107, 119, 120; migration to urban centers, 99–101, 103, 105, 107, 110, 113, 119–21, 206n7; and partner's child-bearing decisions, 117–18, 149–50

Native nurses: and sterilization-related activism, 157–58; as watchdogs and patient advocates, 13, 127–28

Native peoples: bureaucratic erasure of, 92; and colonial imposition of patriarchal relationships, 83; cultural identity of, 73, 80, 91, 116, 121, 129, 145, 169; diseases affecting, 46; displacement of Native peoples residing in West, 5; and eugenic sterilization, 91–96; family and kinship of, 4, 7, 10, 24; federal government's relationship with, 3, 6; health ways of, 45; physicians' relationship to, 33, 65, 67, 71–72;

population decline in, 45; population growth in, 9; reservation hospitals' relationship to, 65, 67–68, 79, 110–11; treaty rights of, 13, 139–40, 175, 178; in urban centers, 100, 206n3

Native women: on abortions, 152–53, 171, 218n33; activism of, 72, 85, 121, 168; agency of, 10–13, 95; birth stories of, 9–10; and commonality of difference, 14; Crow kinship terms, 15, 188n51; and eugenic campaigns, 9, 72; Euro-American "knowledge" of, 34; and federal family planning services, 148–55, 218n24; as field matrons, 50; gender roles of, 24; guidance from female kin, 8, 11, 51–52, 54, 67, 69; and home visits, 44, 51, 54, 59, 195n2; and hospital childbirth, 11–12, 16, 45–46; and infant feeding practices, 52–53; and infant mortality, 49, 51, 70; migration to urban centers, 16, 99–105, 208n42; and motherhood, 13, 15, 50–51, 54, 58, 67, 197n60; on Native men's interference on reproductive matters, 41; negotiations with hospital staff, 69; physicians' evaluation of, 54; and private physicians off reservation, 8, 86, 95, 98, 206n131; reproductive histories of, 10; reproductive-related activism of, 12–13; resistance to home inspections, 195n2; resistance to hospital childbirth, 59, 60, 62–65, 67–69, 75, 77, 78, 199–200n120; role in families and communities, 10, 59; role in reproduction of cultural lifeways, 4, 10; and tribal politics, 83; younger women choosing hospital childbirth, 66–67

Native women's bodies: colonial meanings attached to, 5, 34, 39; eliminatory logic expressed through assaults on, 9; federal and state power over, 94; and federal relocation program, 107; Barbara Gurr on

Ojibwe women: and infant mortality, 49; medical facilities for, 175; sterilization of, 94, 95

Old Coyote, Barney, Jr. (Crow), 18

Omaha women, surveys of, 149, 152, 217n13

O'Neill, Colleen, 12

Osburn, Katherine M. B., 63

Other Medicine, Alice (Crow), 85, 127

Paiute women, 63

Paquette, Peter, 60–61, 64

patrilineal descent, 4, 28–29, 38

Pease, Eloise Whitebear (Crow), 134, 135

Pease, Janine (Crow/Hidatsa), 173–77

Penn, Cornelia (Lakota), 104

Perdue, Theda, 26, 40–41

Petchesky, Rosalind, 39

Petzoldt, William, 82, 202n50

peyote: chronology of introduction and use of, 188n37; Crow men's use of, 204n85; midwives' use of, 11, 88–89

Philp, Kenneth, 130, 207n26

Phoenix, Arizona, Native peoples' migration to, 100–101, 210n94

Phoenix Indian Medical Center (PIMC), 183

Phoenix Indian School, 101

physicians: antiabortion campaign of, 39, 58; attendance at home births, 87–88, 124; boarding school teachers advocating, 7, 67; of Crow Agency, 31, 33, 66, 79, 82–83, 86–87, 204n78; and Crow health council, 84; and Crow Tribal Council, 83; evaluation of Native mothers, 54; on midwives, 58, 60–62, 126; Native peoples' relationship to, 33, 65, 67, 71–72; Native women's resistance to, 63; Native women's use of, 63, 65–66; private physicians off reservation, 8, 86, 95, 98, 110, 206n131; role in women's reproductive lives, 11; shortage of, 176; and sterilization abuses, 89–90,

153; supervision of pregnancy and childbirth, 55–56, 63; surveillance of women's bodies and pregnancies, 40–41; unreliability of, 79–80, 86–87, 204n78; Robert Yellowtail on, 72, 88

Pine-fire (Crow), 18

Pine Ridge Reservation, South Dakota, 155, 157, 164, 168, 170, 177–78, 181–82, 220n99

Pinkerton-Uri, Connie (Choctaw and Cherokee), 156–59, 161–64

Planned Parenthood, 181

Pocahontas, 5, 186–87n14

Popenoe, Paul, 92

poverty, 6, 47, 50, 95, 102

Powell, Peter John, 110, 113, 210n82

Powers, Marla, 157, 164, 220n99

pregnancy and childbirth: and birthing locations, 31–32, 63, 125–26, 171; birthing positions, 18, 32, 35; and breech births, 33; continuity in approach to, 42; dangers of childbirth, 32–33; and delivery of placenta, 18, 33; difficulty of, 35–36, 192n98; in early reservation years, 29–33; and federal relocation program, 99–100; female kin's role in, 31, 51–52, 77, 115, 118, 142, 144, 173–74; government employees' interventions in, 19, 40–42, 45, 61; "illegitimate" pregnancies, 78–79, 93–94; medicalization of, 16, 45, 54–62, 64, 65, 69, 71–72, 75; and medical pluralism, 65; men's role in, 32–33, 192n77; and need for land, 41; older women's role in, 18, 29–30, 33, 35–36, 59, 61, 63–64, 67, 78, 84, 127; physician supervision of, 55–56, 63; and postpartum care, 31; and Public Health Service, 143; romanticization of, 42; as sex-segregated process, 29, 63, 77, 199n112; and umbilical cord, 80, 116, 169; and women's role as life givers, 32, 41, 96, 97. See also hospital childbirth; midwives and midwifery

Presbyterians, 74–75

Pretty Shield (Crow): birth of first child, 18, 19, 31; and birth of Helen Goes Ahead's child, 32; and boarding school attendance, 22; collaboration with Frank Linderman, 15; and dislocation to reservation, 21–22; as grandmother, 29, 127; herbs used by, 30; as midwife, 31, 125

Price, Hiram, 33

Progressive era: federal Indian policy during, 45; and midwives, 58; movement for infant and maternal health, 44; and pronatalism in Indian Country, 46–55, 60, 70, 143; and "Save the Babies" as refrain, 195n21

pronatalism: in Indian Country, 46–55, 60, 70, 143, 196n35; and Save the Babies campaign, 44–45, 47–55, 143, 195n2, 196n35

public health officials, 47, 50, 57

Public Health Service (PHS): and Crow Health Committee, 138, 140, 143–45; Division of Indian Health, 133; maternal and infant welfare efforts of, 143–45; and maternity-related debt of Native women, 99; Native peoples' use of, 107, 121, 139–41; and reservation sanitation, 143. *See also* Indian Health Service (IHS)

puerperal fever, 32

Puisto, Jaakko, 131

Putney, Diane T., 46, 64

Pyramid Lake Reservation, Nevada, 63

Ramirez, Renya (Ho-Chunk), 118, 201n6

Red Cliff Reservation, Wisconsin, 175

Red Lake Indians, 94, 205n114

Red Lake Reservation, Minnesota, 78, 94–95

Red Power movement, 3

Reese, Mary (Navajo) (pseudonym), 114

Relf, Mary Alice, 156

Relf, Minnie Lee, 156

relocation: in Canada, 208n35; in Chicago, 104, 109–13, 115; field relocation officers, 99, 107, 109, 112, 119–20; and gender roles, 103–4, 107, 119–20; government employees' promotion of, 102, 207n22; and Native children, 104–6, 118–21; and Native families and households, 99–105, 113, 117–18; Native self-relocation, 102, 111, 130, 207n17; and pregnancy and childbirth, 99–100; and reservation system, 102–3; vocational training for, 102–5

reproduction: disruption of traditional/modern dichotomy, 10–11; government intervention in Native reproduction, 42; histories of, 3–4, 10, 15; implementation of reproduction-related policies, 14; justice in, 172; questions of scale, 13; and sovereignty, 147, 161, 169; view of Indigenous reproduction as marker of difference, 5. *See also* biological reproduction

reproductive autonomy: of Crow women, 16, 30–31; and eugenics, 91–96; Native women's attempts to regain control of reproduction, 16–17, 180–81

reproductive health services, from private physicians, 8, 86, 95, 98, 110, 206n131

reproductive justice: in twenty-first century, 4, 17, 180–81; WARN articulating early vision of, 1, 4, 180

reproductive labor, forms of, 4

reproductive politics, 4, 6, 9, 13, 186n12

Reproductive Rights National Network, 163

reservation hospitals: building of, 7, 56, 60, 63, 65, 198n95; and colonialism, 124; on Crow Reservation, 42–43, 194n139; and cultural assimilation, 108; federal government's vision of, 11, 44–45, 55–68, 70; inadequacy of staff and facilities in, 65, 67, 78–79, 110, 128, 134, 204n76; Native peoples' relationship to, 65, 67–68, 79, 110–11; Native women as nurses in, 75; Native women returning from urban centers for childbirth, 117; Native women's access to, 78; sterilizations in, 89–90, 95, 147, 161; terminationist priorities threatening, 16, 124, 128, 131–34, 137–40, 146, 176

reservation system: as alternative to extinction, 21; and biological reproduction, 6–7, 42; and birth rates, 36; and Crow birthing culture, 18, 29–33, 35–36, 39, 194n126; cultural and political resurgence on, 9; and disease and illness rates, 21, 33, 36, 46, 49; economic underdevelopment of, 6, 100–101, 122; and eugenics, 9, 72; and federal management of Native life, 15, 20; and federal paternalism, 78, 101, 104, 129, 130; and federal relocation program, 102–3; government employees' interventions in Indigenous pregnancy and childbirth, 19, 40–42, 45, 61; and government-managed health care, 108; and government rations, 36–37, 55, 193n112, 197n64; health conditions of, 46, 57, 71, 132; and home inspections, 44, 195n2; and infant mortality, 45–49; and introduction of medicalized pregnancy and childbirth, 16; and medical pluralism, 65, 126; and morbidity and mortality rate, 36, 42, 45, 54; and Native treaty rights, 13, 139–40, 175, 178; and Native women's reproductive experiences shaped by colonial policies, 6; and Native women's reproductive health services, 8; and punishment methods, 38, 40; and Save the Babies campaign, 44–45, 47–55, 195n2, 196n35; scrutiny and surveillance of Native women's

reproductive bodies and lives, 6–7, 40, 42, 45; and tribal enrollment, 116. *See also* Bureau of Indian Affairs (BIA); field matrons; field nurses; government employees; Office of Indian Affairs (OIA); *and specific reservations*

resistance: Crows' resistance to allotment, 37; Crow women's resistance to government's imposition of gender roles, 24; Crow women's resistance to hospital childbirth, 78–79; to cultural assimilation, 136; midwifery as political act of resistance, 13, 44; Native peoples' turning government positions into politicized sites of, 80; Native resistance to termination policies, 16, 130–33, 135, 139, 146, 212n4; Native women's resistance to home inspections, 195n2; Native women's resistance to hospital childbirth, 59–60, 62–65, 67–69, 75, 77, 78, 199–200n120

Reverby, Susan, 74

Reynolds, Samuel G., 36–41, 44, 73, 81, 193n112

River Crow, 19

Riverside, California, boarding school in, 23

Rocky Boy Reservation, Montana, 173

Roe v. Wade (1973), 152

Rogers, R. V., 204n78

Rolfe, John, 5, 187n14

Roosevelt, Franklin, 80

Rosebud Reservation, South Dakota, 40, 65, 104, 176

Rosenberg, Charles, 56

Rosenthal, Nicholas, 100, 103, 107, 119, 206n3

Ross, Loretta, 180

Roundface, Matilda (Crow), 97–98, 125, 126

Rumsey, Fern, 88

Russell, Josephine (Crow), 134–36

Rzeczkowski, Frank, 189n15, 193n112

and eugenic logic, 9, 72, 90–96, 98,
153; as genocide, 206n123; history of,
10; and James Hyde, 92–93; involun-
tary sterilizations, 9, 89–90; scholar-
ship on, 8; and terminationist
priorities of postwar policies, 16;
WARN's protests against, 1, 3, 8, 16,
147, 161–63, 165–66, 168, 170, 220n79
Sterilization Abuse Task Force, 161
Stewart, Irene (Navajo), 67
Stewart, Kate (Crow), 85, 204n85
Stirbys, Cynthia (Saulteaux-Cree), 181
Stoler, Ann Laura, 187n24
Stremlau, Rose, 37, 92, 189n3
Sun Dance, 81, 132, 136

Taft, William Howard, 48, 56
Takes the Gun, Mary (Crow), 26, 29, 31,
84, 88, 127
termination policies: and health
services, 124, 128, 131–34, 137–40,
146, 176; Native resistance to, 16,
130–33, 135, 139, 146, 212n4;
priorities of, 16, 122–24, 130, 145–46;
and self-determination, 146; termination of tribes, 129, 131, 137; timeline
for, 130
Thayer, Arvina (Ho-Chunk), 156
Thomas, Lynn M., 13, 44
Thomasson, Melissa, 108
Thunder Hawk, Madonna, 182
Tobacco, Tom (Crow), 22
Tobacco Society, 77
tourism, and baby shows, 197n52
Townsend, Camilla, 186–87n14
trachoma, 46, 71
Trafzer, Clifford, 196n27
Trennert, Robert, 33
tribal enrollment, 116
truant officers, tribal policemen as,
22–23
Tsosie, May (Navajo) (pseudonym), 117,
120
Tuba City, Arizona, 125, 199–200n120
Tuba City Hospital, Arizona, 174

tuberculosis, 36, 46, 60, 71, 87
Tucker, Walter Q. G., 39–41, 194n134
Turns Back Plenty, Lucy (Crow),
65–66
Turtle Mountain Reservation, North
Dakota, 60
Twin Cities (Minneapolis–St. Paul),
Minnesota, 14–15, 101, 121, 161–62,
165, 167–68

Umpqua women, 35
Unitarians, as missionaries, 24
United Nations, 163
United Nations Convention on Indig-
enous Rights in Geneva, Switzerland, 1
United Nations Convention on the
Prevention and Punishment of the
Crime of Genocide, 163, 221n102
United Native Americans, 162
United States: Crows' treaties with, 20,
123; hospital construction in, 56, 60,
197–98n71; as settler-colonial society,
3; trends in rural to urban migration,
101. See also federal government
U.S. Army, 5–6
U.S. Children's Bureau, 47–48, 51, 57,
71
U.S. Congress: on abortion, 152, 181;
appropriations for Indian affairs, 71,
128, 132; on assimilation of Native
peoples, 123; and family planning
services, 153; on federal relocation
program, 102; funding for Indian
health services, 56, 163; reservation
land policies of, 37; and termination
policies, 129
U.S. Navy, 61
U.S. Supreme Court, 37, 91, 152
urban centers: boarding school graduates migrating to, 101, 104, 207n24;
federal relocation program, 16,
98–99, 101–11, 113, 121, 207n24;
health insurance market in, 16, 100,
106–10, 116–17, 122, 209n55,
209nn62–63, 209n67; health services

urban centers (*continued*)
in, 105, 110–13, 116–18, 121–22; Indian centers in, 109, 112–13, 121, 209–10n80; and infant mortality rates, 47; and midwives, 59; and motivations of Native migrants, 103–4, 122, 130, 207n26, 208n42; Native cultural and political resurgence in, 9; Native men migrating to, 99–101, 103, 105, 107, 110, 113, 119–21, 206n7; and Native motherhood, 118–21; Native mothers migrating to, 104–6; and Native return migration, 114–17, 122; Native self-relocation to, 102, 111, 130, 207n17; Native women giving birth in, 12, 16, 99–100, 105, 110, 112; Native women migrating to, 16, 99–105, 113, 121; Native women's birth control options in, 120–21, 211n129; and Native women's child-care needs, 104, 107, 114, 119–20; Native women's employment in, 104, 107, 119–20, 121; Native women's options for reproductive care in, 8, 105–12, 117–18, 121–22; and Native women's pregnancies, 99–100, 107, 116; and Native women's service leagues, 112–13, 210n81; Native women's ties to female kin in, 113–14, 119, 120; and Native women's ties to reservations and reservation-based kin, 16, 100, 115–19, 121; and progressivism, 46; unmarried Native mothers migrating to, 104, 107; and urban leisure culture, 104

Valentine, Robert G., 47–48, 50–51, 54
venereal disease, 34, 95, 96, 191n66
Venne, Olive (Crow), 135
Vermont, 91
veterans' health service, 108
Virginia, 91–92
vocational training: and boarding schools, 23, 74; for federal relocation program, 102–5; and gender roles,

103–4, 208n35; nurses' aid training, 61, 74, 128
Voget, Fred W., 29, 194n130, 194n139, 203n66

Warner, H. J., 204n78
War Relocation Authority, 102
Watkins, Arthur, 129, 133
Wauneka, Annie (Navajo), 134, 144, 163
Weatherly, Marina Brown, 86
West, Mary Mills, 57
West, Walter G., 56
Whistling Water clan, 73
Whitecrow, Jake, 218n33
White Horse, Jane (Crow), 73
Whiteman, Edward Posey (Crow), 134
Whiteman, Geneva (Crow), 97
Whiteman, Harry (Crow), 129
Wilkinson, Charles, 129
Williams, Minnie (Crow), 85, 125, 129–30, 135, 213n41
Wind River Reservation, Wyoming, 62, 64, 132, 136–37
Winnebago Reservation, Nebraska, 115
Winnemucca, Sarah (Paiute), 194n126
Wisconsin, 155–56, 165, 219n55, 222n133
Wolf, Jacqueline, 141
Wolfe, Patrick, 3, 9, 96
Women Accepted for Voluntary Emergency Service, 101
Women of All Red Nations (WARN): on abortion, 218n36; and anticolonial coalitions, 4; and Charon Asetoyer, 182; on birth control methods, 168; and environmental degradation, 170–71; establishment of, 147–48, 161, 169, 173; and gendered analysis of genocidal processes, 163, 221n101; health emphasized by, 170; legacy of, 3; Native midwifery training sponsored by, 14–15, 165, 168–69; and Native women's reproductive-related activism, 12–13, 147–48, 161, 165, 171; and reproductive justice, 1, 4, 180; on self-determination, 3, 16, 147;

on sterilization abuses, 1, 3, 8, 16, 147, 161–63, 165–66, 168, 170, 220n79; and woman-centered vision, 165–66; on women's dependence on medical systems, 8

Women's Dance Health Program (DHP), 165–69, 222n124

Woodruff, Janette, 63

Work, Hubert, 71

World Health Organization, 4

World War I, 69–70

World War II, 70, 98, 101, 128

Yakama Reservation, 196n27

Yankton Sioux Reservation, South Dakota, 182

Yellowtail, Amy (Crow), 26, 42–43

Yellowtail, Bruce (Crow), 86–87, 123

Yellowtail, Carson (Crow), 202n50

Yellowtail, Clara Spotted Horse (Crow), 201n25

Yellowtail, Elizabeth (Lizzie) (Crow), 26, 31, 42, 88, 183

Yellowtail, Jackie (Crow), 12–13, 138, 183

Yellowtail, Margaret Pickett (Crow), 79

Yellowtail, Robert (Crow): attendance at boarding school, 23, 74; and Baptists, 202n50; campaign to remove James Hyde, 81; on Crow women as health workers, 127; and cultural assimilation, 73; daughter's explanation of flexible childrearing, 26; and female kin, 26; living with paternal grandmother in childhood, 190n41; on midwifery, 72, 77, 84; paternal grandmother's avoidance of boarding school education for, 22–23; promotion of hospital childbirth, 84, 87, 90; on self-determination, 130; as superintendent of reservation, 72, 81–84, 90, 92, 96–97, 139; on termination policies, 130; Susie Yellowtail's field nurse application endorsed by, 80, 202n45

Yellowtail, Susie Walking Bear (Crow): advocacy for pregnant and childbearing women, 12–13, 86, 88–90, 96, 98, 135, 144–46, 155, 157–58, 183; and Baptists, 202n50; at boarding schools, 73–74; children's urban migration and return, 114–15, 119, 123; and cultural assimilation, 73; family background of, 73; health-related roles of, 124, 134–36, 138, 140–41, 144–46; on Indians' lack of militancy, 12; on land claims, 123; legacy of, 183; marriage of, 79, 85–86, 88, 145; as midwife, 97–98, 125, 141, 206n129; as nurse, 72, 74–75, 79–80, 85, 89, 92, 128, 146, 155, 201n17, 201n20, 202n45; as nursing student, 74; and Peter Powell, 210n82; pregnancies and births of, 86–88, 127; and proposed dam construction, 123, 129; re-embracement of Crow lifeways, 81–82; reformist agenda of, 13; reproductive trajectory of, 11; on self-determination, 130; on sterilization abuses, 160, 163, 168; sterilization of, 89, 95–97, 204n91; and termination policies, 124; two worldedness of, 136, 214n80; on unreliability of physicians, 79–80

Yellowtail, Thomas (Crow): attendance at Bacone Indian School, Oklahoma, 23; on Crow women's seclusion during menstruation, 191n58; legacy of, 183; and Peter Powell, 210n82; Susie Yellowtail's marriage to, 79, 85–86, 88, 145

Yellowtail, Virjama (Crow), 86

Yosemite National Park, California, 197n52

Young, Phyllis (Lakota), 161

Young, S. A. M., 56, 64

Zimmerman, William, 130–31